WM 220
10/14

D1579353

Clinical Manual of Neuropsychiatry

Clinical Manual of Neuropsychiatry

Edited by

Stuart C. Yudofsky, M.D.
Robert E. Hales, M.D., M.B.A.

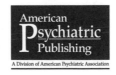

American Psychiatric Publishing
A Division of American Psychiatric Association

Washington, DC
London, England

Note: The authors have worked to ensure that all information in this book is accurate at the time of publication and consistent with general psychiatric and medical standards, and that information concerning drug dosages, schedules, and routes of administration is accurate at the time of publication and consistent with standards set by the U.S. Food and Drug Administration and the general medical community. As medical research and practice continue to advance, however, therapeutic standards may change. Moreover, specific situations may require a specific therapeutic response not included in this book. For these reasons and because human and mechanical errors sometimes occur, we recommend that readers follow the advice of physicians directly involved in their care or the care of a member of their family.

Books published by American Psychiatric Publishing (APP) represent the findings, conclusions, and views of the individual authors and do not necessarily represent the policies and opinions of APP or the American Psychiatric Association.

If you would like to buy between 25 and 99 copies of this or any other American Psychiatric Publishing title, you are eligible for a 20% discount; please contact Customer Service at appi@psych.org or 800-368-5777. If you wish to buy 100 or more copies of the same title, please e-mail us at bulksales@psych.org for a price quote.

Copyright © 2012 American Psychiatric Association
ALL RIGHTS RESERVED

Manufactured in Canada on acid-free paper
15   14   13   12   11   5   4   3   2   1
First Edition

Typeset in Adobe's Garamond and Formata

American Psychiatric Publishing,
a Division of American Psychiatric Association
1000 Wilson Boulevard
Arlington, VA 22209-3901
www.appi.org

Library of Congress Cataloging-in-Publication Data
Clinical manual of neuropsychiatry / edited by Stuart C. Yudofsky, Robert E. Hales.
— 1st ed.
      p. ; cm.
   Includes bibliographical references and index.
   ISBN 978-1-58562-429-4 (pbk. : alk. paper)
   I. Yudofsky, Stuart C. II. Hales, Robert E. III. American Psychiatric Association.
   [DNLM: 1. Mental Disorders—physiopathology. 2. Nervous System Diseases.
WM 140]
   LC classification not assigned
   616.89—dc23
                                                                  2011032144

British Library Cataloguing in Publication Data
A CIP record is available from the British Library.

Contents

8 HIV-1 Infection of the Central Nervous System **265**

Brian Giunta, M.D., Ph.D., Jun Tan, M.D., Ph.D., and Francisco Fernandez, M.D.

9 Dementias Associated With Motor Dysfunction **287**

Alan J. Lerner, M.D., and David Riley, M.D.

10 Alzheimer's Disease and Other Dementing Illnesses. .311

*Liana G. Apostolova, M.D., M.S., and
Jeffrey L. Cummings, M.D.*

11 Psychopharmacological Treatments for Patients With Neuropsychiatric Disorders. .339

*Paul E. Holtzheimer III, M.D.,
Mark Snowden, M.D., M.P.H., and
Peter P. Roy-Byrne, M.D.*

List of Tables and Figures

Contributors

Liana G. Apostolova, M.D., M.S.
Associate Professor in Neurology, Mary S. Easton Center for Alzheimer's Disease Research, David Geffen School of Medicine, University of California at Los Angeles, Los Angeles, California

Frank Y. Chen, M.D.
Houston Adult Psychiatry, Houston, Texas

Jeffrey L. Cummings, M.D.
Augustus S. Rose Professor of Neurology; Professor of Psychiatry and Biobehavioral Neurosciences; Director, Mary S. Easton Center for Alzheimer's Disease Research; Director, Deane F. Johnson Center for Neurotherapeutics, David Geffen School of Medicine, University of California at Los Angeles, Los Angeles, California; Director, Lou Ruvo Center for Brain Health, Cleveland Clinic, Las Vegas, Nevada

Francisco Fernandez, M.D.
Professor and Chair, Department of Psychiatry and Neurosciences; Director, Institute for Research in Psychiatry, University of South Florida, Tampa, Florida

Ronald E. Fisher, M.D., Ph.D.
Assistant Professor, Departments of Radiology and Neuroscience, Baylor College of Medicine; Director of Nuclear Medicine, The Methodist Hospital, Houston, Texas

Michael D. Franzen, Ph.D.
Associate Professor of Psychiatry, Drexel University College of Medicine, Allegheny General Hospital, Pittsburgh, Pennsylvania

Brian Giunta, M.D., Ph.D.
Assistant Professor and Director, Neuroimmunology Laboratory, Department of Psychiatry and Neurosciences, University of South Florida, Tampa, Florida

Kenneth L. Goetz, M.D.
Geriatric Psychiatrist, Pittsburgh, Pennsylvania

Robert E. Hales, M.D., M.B.A.
Joe P. Tupin Professor and Chair, Department of Psychiatry and Behavioral Sciences, University of California–Davis School of Medicine, Sacramento, California; Medical Director, Sacramento County Mental Health Services; Editor-in-Chief, American Psychiatric Publishing, Inc.

Paul E. Holtzheimer III, M.D.
Assistant Professor of Psychiatry, Emory University School of Medicine, Atlanta, Georgia

Diane B. Howieson, Ph.D.
Associate Professor of Neurology and Psychiatry, Oregon Health and Science University, Portland, Oregon

Robin A. Hurley, M.D., F.A.N.P.A.
Professor, Departments of Psychiatry and Radiology, Wake Forest University School of Medicine, Winston-Salem, North Carolina; Clinical Associate Professor, Department of Psychiatry, Baylor College of Medicine, Houston, Texas; Associate Chief of Staff for Research and Education, W. G. "Bill" Hefner VA Medical Center, Salisbury, North Carolina; Associate Director, Education, Mid-Atlantic Mental Illness Research, Education and Clinical Center, Salisbury, North Carolina

H. Florence Kim, M.D., M.S.
Houston Adult Psychiatry, Houston, Texas

Alan J. Lerner, M.D.
Professor of Neurology, Case Western Reserve University School of Medicine; Director, Memory and Cognition Center, Neurological Institute, University Hospitals Case Medical Center, Cleveland, Ohio

Muriel D. Lezak, Ph.D.
Professor Emerita, Neurology, Oregon Health and Science University, Portland, Oregon

Mark R. Lovell, Ph.D.
Professor and Chief, Division of Sports Medicine, Department of Orthopaedic Surgery, University of Pittsburgh School of Medicine; Director, Sports Medicine Concussion Program, UPMC Center for Sports Medicine, Pittsburgh, Pennsylvania

David J. Meagher, M.D., M.R.C.Psych.
Consultant Psychiatrist and Director of Clinical Research, Department of Psychiatry, Midwestern Regional Hospital, Dooradoyle, Limerick, Ireland

Trevor R.P. Price, M.D.
Private practice of psychiatry, Bryn Mawr, Pennsylvania

David Riley, M.D.
Professor of Neurology, Case Western Reserve University; Director, Movement Disorders Center, Neurological Institute, University Hospitals Case Medical Center, Cleveland, Ohio

Robert G. Robinson, M.D.
Paul W. Penningroth Chair, Professor and Head, Department of Psychiatry, University of Iowa College of Medicine, Iowa City, Iowa

Peter P. Roy-Byrne, M.D.
Professor and Vice-Chair, Department of Psychiatry and Behavioral Sciences, University of Washington; Director, Harborview Center for Healthcare Improvement for Addictions, Mental Illness and Medically Vulnerable Populations; and Chief of Psychiatry, Harborview Medical Center, Seattle, Washington

Jonathan M. Silver, M.D.
Clinical Professor of Psychiatry, New York University School of Medicine, New York, New York

Mark Snowden, M.D., M.P.H.
Associate Professor, Department of Psychiatry and Behavioral Sciences, University of Washington, Seattle, Washington

Sergio E. Starkstein, M.D., Ph.D.
Professor of Psychiatry and Clinical Neurosciences, University of Western Australia, Fremantle, Australia

Katherine H. Taber, Ph.D., F.A.N.P.A.
Research Professor, Division of Biomedical Sciences, Virginia College of Osteopathic Medicine, Blacksburg, Virginia; Adjunct Associate Professor, Department of Physical Medicine and Rehabilitation, Baylor College of Medicine, Houston, Texas; Assistant Director, Education, Mid-Atlantic Mental Illness Research, Education and Clinical Center, Salisbury, North Carolina; Research Scientist, W. G. "Bill" Hefner VA Medical Center, Salisbury, North Carolina

Jun Tan, M.D., Ph.D.
Robert A. Silver Chair in Developmental Neurobiology and Professor, and Director, Developmental Neurobiology Laboratory, Silver Child Development Center, Department of Psychiatry and Neurosciences, University of South Florida, Tampa, Florida

Paula T. Trzepacz, M.D.
Senior Medical Fellow, Neurosciences Research, Lilly Research Laboratories; Clinical Professor of Psychiatry, Indiana University School of Medicine, Indianapolis, Indiana

Gary J. Tucker, M.D. (deceased)
Department of Psychiatry and Behavioral Sciences, University of Washington, Seattle, Washington

Stuart C. Yudofsky, M.D.
D. C. and Irene Ellwood Professor and Chairman, Menninger Department of Psychiatry and Behavioral Sciences, and Drs. Beth K. and Stuart C. Yudofsky Presidential Chair of Neuropsychiatry, Baylor College of Medicine; Chairman, Department of Psychiatry, The Methodist Hospital, Houston, Texas

Disclosure of Competing Interests

The following contributors to this book have indicated a financial interest in or other affiliation with a commercial supporter, a manufacturer of a commercial product, a provider of a commercial service, a nongovernmental organization, and/or a government agency, as listed below:

Jeffrey L. Cummings, M.D.—*Consultant (pharmaceutical companies):* Abbott, Acadia, Acerra, ADAMAS, Anavex, Astellas, Avanir, Baxter, Bristol-Myers Squibb, Eisai, Elan, EnVivo, Forest, Genentech, GlaxoSmithKline, Janssen, Lilly, Lundbeck, Medivation, Medtronics, Merck, Merz, Neurokos, Novartis, Pfizer, Prana, QR Pharma, Sonexa, Takeda, Toyama; *Consultant (assessment companies):* Bayer, Avid, GE, MedAvante, Neurotrax, UBC; *Stock:* ADAMAS, MedAvante, Neurokos, Neurotrax, Prana, QR Pharma, Sonexa; *Speaker/Lecturer:* Eisai, Forest, Janssen, Lundbeck, Novartis, Pfizer; *Assessment instrument copyright owner:* Neuropsychiatry Inventory; Expert witness/legal consultation: Expert witness consultation regarding olanzapine and ropinerol.

Paul E. Holtzheimer III, M.D.—*Consultant fees from:* St. Jude Medical Neuromodulation.

Alan J. Lerner, M.D.—*Research grants:* Allon, Baxter, Ceregene, Forest, Pfizer/Medivation; *Book royalties:* Elsevier, Springer

David Riley, M.D.—*Research support:* Cleveland Medical Devices; *Honararia for presentations and consulting:* Allergan, Ipsen, Lundbeck, Merz, Teva. Dr. Riley has no equity ownership in these or other health care businesses, or in health care–oriented mutual funds. He may possibly have some health care stocks as a component of multi-industry mutual funds held in retirement accounts. Dr. Riley has no other relationships with commercial interests in the health care field.

Robert G. Robinson, M.D.—*Consultant:* Avanir Pharmaceuticals.

Peter P. Roy-Byrne, M.D.—*Editor-in-Chief: Journal Watch Psychiatry* (Massachusetts Medical Society; *Depression and Anxiety* (Wiley-Liss), and *UpToDate Psychiatry* (UpToDate).

The following contributors to this book indicated that they have no competing interests or affiliations to declare:

Liana G. Apostolova, M.D., M.S.
Francisco Fernandez, M.D.
Ronald E. Fisher, M.D., Ph.D.
Michael D. Franzen, Ph.D.
Brian Giunta, M.D., Ph.D.
Kenneth L. Goetz, M.D.
Robert E. Hales, M.D., M.B.A.
Diane B. Howieson, Ph.D.
Robin A. Hurley, M.D., F.A.N.P.A.
H. Florence Kim, M.D., M.S.
Muriel D. Lezak, Ph.D.
Trevor R.P. Price, M.D.
Jonathan M. Silver, M.D.
Mark Snowden, M.D., M.P.H.
Katherine H. Taber, Ph.D., F.A.N.P.A.
Jun Tan, M.D., Ph.D.
Paula T. Trzepacz, M.D.
Stuart C. Yudofsky, M.D.

1

The Neuropsychological Evaluation

Diane B. Howieson, Ph.D.

Muriel D. Lezak, Ph.D.

Neuropsychologists assess brain function by making inferences from an individual's cognitive, sensorimotor, emotional, and social behaviors. Neuropsychological measures are useful diagnostic indicators of brain dysfunction for many conditions and will remain the major diagnostic modality for some conditions (Farah and Feinberg 2000; Lezak et al. 2011; Mesulam 2000). However, methods for determining brain structure and function have become increasingly accurate in recent decades (see, e.g., Kamitani and Tong 2005). Advances in quantitative and functional neuroimaging have enriched understanding of pathological disturbances of the brain (Damasio and Damasio 2003; Levin et al. 1996; Stern and Silbersweig 2001). Precisely placed, reversible "lesions" can be produced to study how the remainder of the brain functions without a designated cortical area (Deouell et al. 2003; Grafman and

Wassermann 1999). These developments have allowed a shift in the focus of neuropsychological assessment from the diagnosis of possible brain damage to a better understanding of specific brain-behavior relationships and the psychosocial consequences of brain damage.

Indications for a Neuropsychological Evaluation

Patients referred to a neuropsychologist for assessment typically fall into one of three groups. The first and probably largest group consists of patients with known brain disorders, such as stroke or Parkinson's disease. A neuropsychological evaluation can be useful in defining the nature and severity of the associated behavioral and emotional problems. The assessment provides information about patients' cognition, personality characteristics, social behavior, emotional status, and adaptation to their conditions. Patients' potential for independent living and productive activity can be inferred from these data. Information about their behavioral strengths and weaknesses provides a foundation for treatment planning, vocational training, competency determination, and counseling for both patients and their families (Bennett and Raymond 2003; Diller 2000; Kalechstein et al. 2003; Sloan and Ponsford 1995).

The second group of patients is composed of persons with a known risk factor for brain disorder in whom a change in behavior might be the result of such a disorder. In these cases, a neuropsychological evaluation might be used both to provide evidence of brain dysfunction and to describe the nature and severity of problems.

In the third group, brain disease or dysfunction may be suspected when a person's behavior changes without an identifiable cause (i.e., the patient has no known risk factors for brain disorder) and other diagnoses have been excluded. The most common application of the neuropsychological evaluation in older adults without obvious risk factors for brain disease—other than age—is for early detection of progressive dementia, such as Alzheimer's disease (Knopman and Selnes 2003; Kramer et al. 2003). Neuropsychological assessment is useful in evaluating whether problems noted by the family or the individual are age related, are attributable to other factors such as depression, or are suggestive of early dementia.

Neuropsychological signs and symptoms that are possible indicators of a pathological brain disorder are presented in Table 1–1. Confidence in diagnoses

Table 1–1. Neuropsychological signs and symptoms that may indicate a pathological brain process

Functional class	Symptoms and signs
Speech and language	Dysarthria Dysfluency Marked change in amount of speech output Paraphasias Word-finding problems
Academic skills	Alterations in reading, writing, calculating, and number abilities Frequent letter or number reversals
Thinking	Perseveration of speech Simplified or confused mental tracking, reasoning, and concept formation
Motor	Weakness or clumsiness, particularly if lateralized Impaired fine motor coordination (e.g., changes in handwriting) Apraxias Perseveration of action components
Memory[a]	Impaired recent memory for verbal or visuospatial material or both Disorientation
Perception	Diplopia or visual field alterations Inattention (usually left-sided) Somatosensory alterations (particularly if lateralized) Inability to recognize familiar stimuli (agnosia)
Visuospatial abilities	Diminished ability to perform manual skills (e.g., mechanical repairs and sewing) Spatial disorientation Left-right disorientation Impaired spatial judgment (e.g., angulation of distances)
Emotions[b]	Diminished emotional control with temper outburst and antisocial behavior Diminished empathy or interest in interpersonal relationships Affective changes Irritability without evident precipitating factors Personality change

Table 1–1.   Neuropsychological signs and symptoms that may indicate a pathological brain process *(continued)*

Functional class	Symptoms and signs
Comportment[b]	Altered appetites and appetitive activities
	Altered grooming habits (excessive fastidiousness or carelessness)
	Hyperactivity or hypoactivity
	Social inappropriateness

[a]Many emotionally disturbed persons complain of memory deficits, which most typically reflect the person's self-preoccupation, distractibility, or anxiety rather than a dysfunctional brain. Thus, memory complaints in themselves do not necessarily warrant neuropsychological evaluation.

[b]Some of these changes are most likely to be neuropsychologically relevant in the absence of depression, although they can also be mistaken for depression.

Source.   Reprinted from Howieson DB, Lezak MD: "The Neuropsychological Evaluation," in *Essentials of Neuropsychiatry and Behavioral Neurosciences,* 2nd Edition. Edited by Yudofsky SC, Hales RE. Washington, DC, American Psychiatric Publishing, 2010, pp. 29–54. Used with permission. Copyright © 2010 American Psychiatric Association.

based on neuropsychological evidence will be greater when risk factors for brain dysfunction exist or the patient shows signs and symptoms of brain dysfunction than when the neuropsychological diagnoses rely solely on exclusion of other diagnoses.

One of the greatest challenges for a neuropsychologist is to determine whether patients with psychiatric illness show evidence of an underlying neurological disorder. Many psychiatric patients without neurological disease suffer from cognitive disruptions and behavioral or emotional aberrations. Cognitive impairment is highly prevalent in patients with schizophrenia (Heinrichs and Zakzanis 1998; Hill et al. 2001), particularly impairment in attention, processing speed, memory, problem solving, cognitive flexibility, and abilities for organization and planning (Goldman et al. 1996). Obsessive-compulsive disorders are often accompanied by mild cognitive impairment. For patients with these disorders, areas of difficulty may include nonverbal memory, use of strategies, visuospatial skills, and selected executive functions (Deckersbach et al. 2000; Greisberg and McKay 2003; Savage et al. 2000). Both schizophrenia and obsessive-compulsive behavior have been linked to dysfunction of frontal-subcortical circuits (Abbruzzese et al. 1995; Chamberlain et al. 2005), and temporal lobe structures have also been implicated (Adler et al. 2000; Post 2000).

Compared with control subjects, depressed patients often underperform on measures of speed of processing, mental flexibility, and executive function (Veiel 1997; Weiland-Fiedler et al. 2004). Memory impairment occurs less consistently (Basso and Bornstein 1999; Boone et al. 1995), and memory performance may be intact even when memory complaints are present (Dalgleish and Cox 2000; Kalska et al. 1999). Although a number of psychological explanations have been proposed to explain cognitive deficits in mood disorders, such as self-focused rumination associated with dysphoria (Hertel 1998), underlying structural and functional abnormalities have been reported in the neural pathways that modulate mood (Ali et al. 2000; Strakowski et al. 1999).

The Assessment Process

Interview and observation provide the data of neuropsychological evaluations. The interview is the basic component of the evaluation (Lezak et al. 2011; Luria 1980; Sbordone 2000). Its main purposes are to elicit the patient's and family's complaints, understand the circumstances in which these problems occur, and evaluate the patient's attitude toward these problems.

The presenting problems and the patient's attitude toward them may also provide important diagnostic information. Patients with certain neuropsychological conditions lack awareness of their problems or belittle their significance (Markova and Berrios 2000; Prigatano and Schacter 1991). Many patients with right hemisphere stroke, Alzheimer's disease, or frontal lobe damage are unaware of or unable to appreciate the problems resulting from their brain injury. In the extreme form of right hemisphere stroke, some patients with hemiplegia are unable to comprehend that the left side of their body is part of them, let alone that they cannot use it.

The interview provides an opportunity to observe the patient's appearance, attention, speech, thought content, and motor abilities, and to evaluate his or her affect, appropriateness of behavior, orientation, insight, and judgment. The interview can provide information about the patient's premorbid intellectual ability and personality, occupational and school background, social situation, and ability to use leisure time.

The tests used by neuropsychologists are simply standardized observational tools that in many instances have the added advantage of providing normative data to aid in interpreting the observations. A variety of assessment approaches are available, but they all have in common the goals of determining whether the patient shows evidence of brain dysfunction, identifying the nature of problems detected, and determining which functions have been preserved and, thus, what the patient's cognitive strengths are.

Cognitive performance is only one aspect of an assessment. A full evaluation of the individual assesses emotional and social characteristics as well. Many patients with brain injuries experience changes in personality, mood, or ability to control emotional states (Gainotti 2003; Heilman et al. 2003; Ochoa et al. 2003), as well as problems with social relationships (Dikmen et al. 1996; Lezak 1988a). Depression is a common and sometimes serious complication of brain disease. Unusually high incidences of depression occur with certain neurodegenerative disorders, such as Parkinson's disease and Huntington's disease (Brandstadter and Oertel 2003; Rickards 2005). Other neurological diseases in which depression is common are tumors (particularly those of the orbitofrontal and temporoparietal cortex), multiple sclerosis, Wilson's disease, HIV encephalopathy, Alzheimer's disease, vascular dementia, and Lewy body dementia (Cummings 1994). At least 30% of stroke patients experience depression at some time (Paradiso et al. 1997; Singh et al. 2000). Factors that appear to determine the presence of depression include the location of the brain injury and its recency, the degree of disability, and the patient's level of social activity (Gustafson et al. 1995; Robinson 1998).

As computers have become valuable aids in many fields, interest in using computerized testing procedures has been increasing (Bleiberg et al. 2000; Wild et al. 2008). This technology offers the possibility of obtaining test data under highly standardized conditions with minimal time expenditure by the examiner.

The Nature of Neuropsychological Tests

An important component of neuropsychological evaluations is psychological testing, in which an individual's cognitive and often emotional status and executive functioning are assessed using standardized formats. The neuropsychological assessment of an adult relies on comparisons of the patient's present level of functioning with the known or estimated level of premorbid functioning based on demographically similar individuals and with the patient's current performance on tests of functions less likely to be affected by brain disorders.

Thus, much of clinical neuropsychological assessment involves *intraindividual* comparisons of the abilities and skills under consideration.

Most tests of cognitive abilities are designed with the expectations that very few persons will obtain a perfect score and that most scores will cluster in a middle range. For these tests, scores are conceptualized as continuous variables. The scores of many persons taking the test can be plotted as a distribution curve. Most scores on tests of complex learned behaviors fall into a characteristic bell-shaped curve called a normal distribution curve (Figure 1–1). The statistical descriptors of the curve are the *mean* or average score; the degree of spread of scores about the mean, expressed as the *standard deviation;* and the *range,* or the distance from the highest to the lowest scores.

The levels of competence in different cognitive functions, as well as other behaviors, vary from individual to individual and also within the same individual at different times. This variability also has the characteristics of a normal curve, as seen in Figure 1–1. Because of the normal variability of performance on cognitive tests, *any single score can be considered only as representative of a normal performance range and must not be taken as a precise value.*

An individual's score is compared with the normative data, often by calculating a standard or *z* score, which describes the individual's performance in terms of statistically regular distances from the normative mean (i.e., standard deviations). In this framework, scores within ±0.66 standard deviation are considered average, because 50% of subjects in a normative sample score within this range. The *z* scores are used to describe the probability that a deviant response occurs by chance or because of an impairment. A performance in the below-average direction that is greater than two standard deviations from the mean is usually described as falling in the impaired range, because 98% of subjects in the normative sample taking the test achieve better scores.

Psychological tests should be constructed to satisfy both reliability and validity criteria (Urbina 2004). Tests also should be constructed with large normative samples of individuals with similar demographic characteristics, particularly with regard to age and education (Heaton et al. 2003; Steinberg and Bieliauskas 2005).

Some psychological tests detect subtle deficits better than others. A simple signal detection test of attention, such as crossing out each letter *A* on a page, is a less sensitive test of attention than is a divided attention task, such as crossing out each of the letters *A* and *C.* Tests involving complex tasks, such as prob-

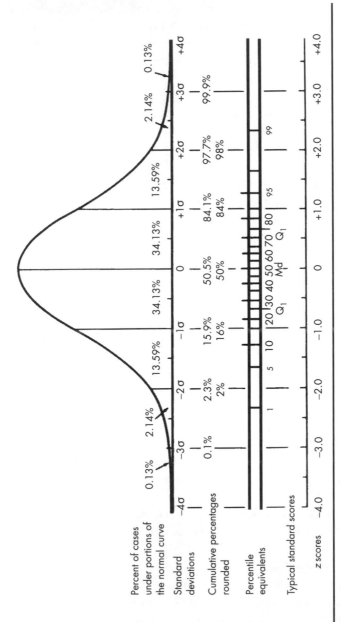

Figure 1–1. A normal distribution curve, showing the percentage of cases between −4 standard deviations (−σ) and +4 standard deviations (+σ).

The average range is defined as −0.6 to +0.6 standard deviation or the 25th to the 75th percentile.

Source. Adapted from the Test Service Bulletin of The Psychological Corporation, 1955. Reprinted from Howieson DB, Lezak MD: "The Neuropsychological Evaluation," in *Essentials of Neuropsychiatry and Behavioral Neurosciences*, 2nd Edition. Edited by Yudofsky SC, Hales RE. Washington, DC, American Psychiatric Publishing, 2010, pp. 29–54. Used with permission. Copyright © 2010 American Psychiatric Association.

lem solving requiring abstract thinking and cognitive flexibility, are more sensitive than many other cognitive tests in reflecting brain dysfunction, because a wide variety of brain disorders, mood disorders, and medication side effects can easily disrupt test performance. Therefore, these tests are sensitive to cognitive disruption but are not specific to one type of cognitive disturbance. The specificity of a test in detecting a disorder depends on the overlap between the distributions of the scores of persons with intact cognition and of the scores of persons who have the disorder. The less overlap there is, the better the test can differentiate normal from abnormal performances. Many neuropsychological tests offer a trade-off between sensitivity and specificity.

Indications of brain dysfunction come from qualitative features of the patient's performance as well as from test scores (Lezak et al. 2011; Malloy et al. 2003). A test can be failed for many reasons, and a poor score does not tell the means to the end (Darby and Walsh 2005). Some features of behavioral disturbance are best recognized by the manner in which the patient approaches the testing situation or behaves with the examiner. Brain-injured patients are prone to a short attention span, distractibility, impulsivity, poor self-monitoring, disorganization, irritability, perplexity, and suspiciousness.

Interpretation: Principles and Cautions

The interpretation of test performance is based on an assumption that the patient is expected to perform in a particular way on tasks; deviations from expectation require evaluation (Lezak 1986; Lezak et al. 2011). Most healthy people perform within a statistically definable range on cognitive tests, and this range of performance levels is considered to be characteristic of normality. Deviations below this expected range raise the question of impairment.

Interpretations of test performance also must take into account demographic variables. In the estimates of premorbid ability levels necessary for making intraindividual comparisons, a patient's educational and occupational background, sex, and race must be considered along with his or her level of test performance (Lezak et al. 2011; Vanderploeg et al. 1996). Some tests are fairly resistant to disruption by brain damage and may offer the best estimates of premorbid ability. Good examples are tests that assess fund of information and reading vocabulary, such as the National Adult Reading Test (Nelson 1982), developed in the United Kingdom, and a revision of this test for American English, the North American Adult Reading Test (Strauss et al. 2006).

For meaningful interpretations of neuropsychological test performance, examiners not only rely on many tests but also search for a performance pattern (test scores plus qualitative features) that makes neuropsychological sense. Because pathognomonic findings are rare in neuropsychology, and in most other branches of medical science for that matter (Hertzman et al. 2001; Sox et al. 1988), a performance pattern often can suggest several diagnoses. For example, a cluster of documented deficits, including slowed thinking and mild impairment of concentration and memory, is a nonspecific finding associated with a number of conditions: very mild dementia, a mild postconcussion syndrome, mild toxic encephalopathy, depression, and fatigue, to name a few. Other patterns may be highly specific for certain conditions. The finding of left-sided neglect and visuospatial distortions is highly suggestive of brain dysfunction and specifically occurs with right hemisphere damage. For many neuropsychological conditions, typical deficit patterns are known, allowing the examiner to evaluate the patient's performances in light of these known patterns for a possible match.

Major Test Categories

In this section, we present a brief review of tests used for assessment of major areas of cognition and personality. Many useful neuropsychological tests are not described in this summary. Please refer to *Neuropsychological Assessment,* 5th Edition (Lezak et al. 2011), for a relatively complete review and to *A Compendium of Neuropsychological Tests,* 3rd Edition (Strauss et al. 2006), for more detailed normative data on many frequently used tests.

Mental Ability

The most commonly used set of tests of general intellectual function in adults in the Western world is contained in the various versions and translations of the Wechsler Adult Intelligence Scale (WAIS; Psychological Corporation 2008; Wechsler 1997a). These batteries of brief subtests provide scores on a variety of cognitive tasks covering a range of skills. The individual subtests were designed to assess relatively distinct areas of cognition, such as arithmetic, abstract thinking, and visuospatial organization, and thus are differentially sensitive to dysfunction of various areas of the brain. Therefore, this test is often used to screen for specific areas of cognitive deficits.

When the WAIS is administered to persons with neuropsychological impairments, the summary IQ scores can be very misleading because the averaging of individual subtest scores that are lowered by specific cognitive deficits with scores that are relatively unaffected by the brain dysfunction can result in IQ scores that are associated with ability levels that represent neither the severity of deficits nor the patient's residual competencies (Lezak 1988b). Therefore, neuropsychologists focus on the pattern of the Wechsler scores rather than the summed or average performance on all the subtests in the battery.

Language

Lesions to the hemisphere dominant for speech and language, which is the left hemisphere in 95%–97% of right-handed persons and in 60%–70% of left-handed ones (Corballis 1991; Strauss and Goldsmith 1987), can produce any of a variety of disorders of symbol formation and use—namely, the aphasias (Spreen and Risser 2003). Although many aphasiologists argue against attempting to classify all patients into one of the standard aphasia syndrome groups because of so many individual differences, persons with aphasia tend to be grouped according to whether the main disorder is in language comprehension (receptive aphasia), expression (expressive aphasia), repetition (conduction aphasia), or naming (anomic aphasia).

Test selection may be based on whether the information is to be used for diagnostic, prognostic, or rehabilitation purposes. For example, the Boston Diagnostic Aphasia Examination, 3rd Edition (Goodglass et al. 2000), might be selected as an aid for treatment planning because of its wide scope and sensitivity to different aphasic characteristics.

Attention and Mental Tracking

A frequent consequence of brain disorders is slowed mental processing and impaired ability for focused behavior (Duncan and Mirsky 2004; Leclercq and Zimmermann 2002). Damage to the brain stem or diffuse damage involving the cerebral hemispheres, especially the white matter interconnections, can produce a variety of attentional deficits. Because attentional deficits are very common in neuropsychiatric disorders, most neuropsychological assessments include measures of attentional abilities. The Wechsler scales contain several relevant subtests. Digit Span measures attention span or short-term memory for numbers in two ways: forward and backward digit repetition. Backward digit repetition is a more demanding task because it requires concentration and mental tracking plus the short-term memory component. It is not uncommon for patients with moderate to severe brain damage to perform poorly only on the backward repetition portion of this test.

The Arithmetic subtest in the Wechsler battery is very sensitive to attentional disorders because it requires short-term auditory memory and rapid mental juggling of arithmetic problem elements. Poor performance on this subtest must be evaluated for the nature of the failures. Another commonly used measure of concentration and mental tracking is the Trail Making Test (Armitage 1946). In the first part of this test (Part A), the patient is asked to draw rapidly and accurately a line connecting in sequence a random display of numbered circles on a page. The level of difficulty is increased in the second part (Part B) by having the patient again sequence a random display of circles, this time alternating numbers and letters. This test requires concentration, visual scanning, and flexibility in shifting cognitive sets (Cicerone and Azulay 2002). It shares with many attention tests vulnerability to other kinds of deficits, such as motor slowing, which could be based on peripheral factors such as nerve or muscle damage, and diminished visual acuity.

In cases of subtle brain injury, the examiner can increase assessment sensitivity by selecting a more difficult measure of concentration and mental tracking, in which the patient must hold material in mind while manipulating information for the performance of such complex cognitive activities as comprehension, learning, and reasoning. The ability to hold information in mind while performing a mental task is called *working memory* (Baddeley 1994). Working memory requires both attention and short-term memory. An example of a difficult attentional task is the Paced Auditory Serial Addition Task (Gronwall 1977), in which the patient is required to add consecutive pairs of numbers rapidly under an interference condition.

Memory

Memory is another cognitive function frequently impaired by brain disorders. Many diffuse brain injuries produce general impairments in abilities for new learning and retention. Many focal brain injuries also produce memory impairment; left hemisphere lesions are more likely to produce primarily verbal memory deficits, whereas right hemisphere lesions are more likely to produce visuospatial memory impairments (Abrahams et al. 1997; Wagner et al. 1998), although not all visuospatial tests show a right hemisphere advantage (Raspall et al. 2005). Memory impairment often is a prominent feature of herpes encephalitis, Huntington's chorea, Korsakoff's syndrome, hypoxia, closed head injury, and a variety of neurological degenerative diseases, such as Alzheimer's disease (Baddeley et al. 2002; Bauer et al. 2003; Mayes 2000).

In most cases of brain injury, memory for information learned before the injury is relatively preserved compared with new learning. For this reason, many patients with memory impairment perform relatively well on tests of fund of information or recall of remote events. However, amnestic disorders can produce a retrograde amnesia, affecting memory from weeks, months, or years before the onset of the injury. Electroconvulsive therapy can also produce retrograde amnesia (Squire et al. 1975). Cases of isolated amnesia for personal identity often have a psychogenic cause (Hodges 1991).

In the United States, the Wechsler Memory Scale (WMS; Wechsler 1997b; Wechsler et al. 2009) is the most commonly used battery of subtests of new learning and retention. The WMS comprises a variety of subtests measuring free recall or recognition of both verbal and visual material. In addition, these subtests include measures of concentration, mental tracking, and recall of personal information and attention. Several of the subtests provide measures of both immediate and delayed (approximately 30 minutes) recall.

Other memory tests frequently used include word-list learning tasks, such as the Rey Auditory Verbal Learning Test (Lezak et al. 2011; Rey 1964; Schmidt 1996) and the California Verbal Learning Test, 2nd Edition (Delis et al. 2000), and visuospatial tasks, such as the Complex Figure Test (Lezak et al. 2011; Mitrushina et al. 2005).

Perception

Perception in any of the sensory modalities can be affected by brain disease. Perceptional inattention (sometimes called *neglect*) is one of the major perceptual syndromes because of its frequency of occurrence with focal brain damage (Heilman et al. 2000b; Lezak 1994; Rafal 2000). Perceptional neglect involves diminished or absent awareness of stimuli in one side of personal space by a patient with an intact sensory system. Unilateral inattention is often most prominent immediately after acute-onset brain injury such as stroke. Most commonly seen is left-sided inattention associated with right hemisphere lesions.

Several techniques can be used to detect unilateral inattention. Visual inattention can be assessed, for example, by using a line bisection test (Schenkenberg et al. 1980), in which the patient is asked to bisect a series of uneven lines on a page, or by using a cancellation task, which requires the patient to cross out a designated symbol distributed among other similar symbols over a page (Mitrushina et al. 2005).

Another important area of perceptual assessment is recognition of familiar visual stimuli. A brain injury can produce an inability to recognize visually familiar objects (visual object agnosia) and faces (prosopagnosia), although these syndromes are rare and often occur independently of each other (Barton et al. 2004; Bauer and Demery 2003). Assessment involves testing the recognition—often in the form of naming—of real objects or representations of objects, sometimes in a masked or distorted form.

Praxis

Many patients with left hemisphere damage have at least one form of apraxia, and this loss of ability is common in progressed stages of Alzheimer's disease, Parkinson's disease, Pick's disease, and progressive supranuclear palsy (Dobigny-Roman et al. 1998; Leiguarda et al. 1997). In patients with apraxia, the inability to perform a desired sequence of motor activities is not based on motor weakness. Rather, the deficit is in planning and carrying out the required activities (De Renzi et al. 1983; Heilman et al. 2000a) and is associated with disruption of neural representations for extrapersonal (e.g., spatial location) and intrapersonal (e.g., hand position) features of movement (Haaland et al. 1999). Tests for apraxia assess the patient's ability to reproduce learned movements of the face or limbs. These learned movements can include the use of objects (usually pantomime of object use) and gestures (Goodglass et al. 2000; Rothi et al. 1997) or sequences of movements demonstrated by the examiner (Haaland and Flaherty 1984).

Constructional Ability

Although problems with constructional ability were once considered a form of apraxia, more recent analysis has shown that the underlying deficits involve impaired appreciation of one or more aspects of spatial relationships. These impairments can include distortions in perspective, angulation, size, and distance judgment. The problem is not an inability to organize a motor response for drawing lines or assembling constructions, as in apraxia, but rather involves misperceptions and misjudgments of spatial relationships. Neuropsychological assessments may include any of a number of measures of visuospatial processing. Patients may be asked to copy geometric designs, such as in the Complex Figure Test (Lezak et al. 2011; Mitrushina et al. 2005). The WAIS battery includes constructional tasks involving copying pictured designs with blocks and assembling puzzle pieces (Psychological Corporation 2008; Wechsler 1981, 1997a). Lesions of the posterior cerebral cortex are associated with the greatest difficulty with constructions, and right hemisphere lesions produce greater deficits than left hemisphere lesions (Benton and Tranel 1993).

Conceptual Functions

Tests of concept formation measure aspects of thinking that include reasoning, abstraction, and problem solving. Conceptual dysfunction tends to occur with serious brain injury regardless of site. Most neuropsychological tests require that simple conceptual functioning be intact. For example, reasoning skills are required for the successful performance of most WAIS subtests (e.g., the Comprehension subtest assesses commonsense verbal reasoning and interpretation of proverbs; the Similarities subtest measures ability to make verbal abstractions by asking for similarities between objects or concepts).

Other commonly used tests of concept formation include the Category Test (Halstead 1947), Wisconsin Card Sorting Test (Berg 1948; Strauss et al. 2006), and California Sorting Test (Hartman et al. 2004). These tests measure concept formation, hypothesis testing, problem solving, flexibility of thinking, and short-term memory.

Executive Functions

Executive functions include abilities to formulate a goal, to plan, to carry out goal-directed plans effectively, and to monitor and self-correct spontaneously and reliably (Lezak 1982). Open-ended tests that permit the patient to decide how to perform the task and when it is complete are difficult for many patients with frontal lobe or diffuse brain injuries (Lezak 1982; Luria 1980). The abilities these tasks test are essential, however, for fulfilling most adult responsibilities and maintaining socially appropriate conduct. The Tower of London (Shallice 1982) and Tower of Hanoi tests also assess planning and foresight, because disks are moved from stack to stack to reach a stated goal. Few neuropsychological tests are specifically designed to assess these aspects of behavior, yet many complex tasks depend on this analysis. An exception is a set of real-world tasks developed for this purpose called the Behavioural Assessment of the Dysexecutive Syndrome (Wilson et al. 1996), which has been shown to detect problems with flexibility, planning, and priority setting in patients with brain injury (Norris and Tate 2000) or schizophrenia (Krabbendam et al. 1999).

Adaptive behavior often requires changing behavior according to new demands. The Wisconsin Card Sorting Test also measures adaptive decision making in that the patient must be able to recognize the changed sorting principle and adjust responses accordingly. Many patients with dorsolateral frontal lobe lesions recognize that a change has occurred but either are unable to alter their responses according to the new demands or are slow at making the change (Stuss et al. 2000).

Inertia presents one of the most difficult assessment problems for neuropsychologists. Few open-ended tests measure initiation or ability to carry out purposeful behavior. By their very nature, most tests are structured and require little initiation by the patient (Lezak 1982).

Personality and Emotional Status

Numerous questionnaires have been devised to measure symptoms of physical and emotional distress in patients with neurological or medical problems (Fischer et al. 2004; Lezak 1989). As examples, the Neurobehavioral Rating Scale (Levin et al. 1987) is an examiner-rated measure of problems commonly associated with traumatic brain injury, and the Mayo-Portland Adaptability Inventory provides for ratings from clinicians, the patient, and the patient's family members (Malec et al. 2000).

Many attempts have been made to use the second edition of the Minnesota Multiphasic Personality Inventory (MMPI-2; Butcher 1989; Butcher and Pope 1990; Butcher et al. 1989) to differentiate diagnoses of psychiatric and neurological illness. Results generally have been unsatisfactory, probably because of the extreme variety of brain disorders and their associated problems (Glassmire et al. 2003; Lezak et al. 2011). Not surprisingly, the MMPI-2 also has been an inefficient instrument for localizing cerebral lesions (Lezak et al. 2011).

Neuropsychologists are frequently asked to evaluate "psychological overlay" or functional complaints. The diagnostic problem occurs because some individuals may be financially motivated to establish injuries related to work or accidents for which financial compensation may be sought. In addition, some individuals receive emotional or social rewards for invalidism, leading to malingering and functional disabilities. It is difficult to establish with complete certainty that a person's complaints are functional. Adding to the complexity of the diagnosis, patients with established brain injury sometimes embellish their symptoms, wittingly or unwittingly, so that the range of problems may represent a combination of true deficits and exaggeration. The clinician usually must search for a combination of factors that would support or discredit a functional diagnosis (Lezak et al. 2011). General factors include evidence of inconsistency in history, reporting of symptoms, or test performance; the individual's emotional predisposition; the probability of secondary gain; and the patient's emotional reactions to his or her complaints, such as the classic *belle indifférence*.

Treatment and Planning

Examination findings are used to assess an individual's strengths and weaknesses and to formulate treatment interventions (Christensen and Uzzell 2000; Lezak 1987; Wilson et al. 2002). Clinical interventions vary according to the individual's specific needs. Many patients with brain disorders have primary or secondary emotional problems for which psychotherapy or counseling is advisable. However, patients with brain injuries frequently have problems that require special consideration. Foremost among these problems are cognitive rigidity, impaired learning ability, and diminished self-awareness, any one of which may limit the patient's adaptability and capacity to benefit from rehabilitation. Therefore, neuropsychological evaluations provide important information about treatment possibilities and strategies. These evaluations are also used to consider patients' capability for independence in society and their educational or vocational potential.

Recommended Readings

Heilman K, Valenstein E (eds): Clinical Neuropsychology, 4th Edition. New York, Oxford University Press, 2003

Lezak M, Howieson D, Bigler ED, et al: Neuropsychological Assessment, 5th Edition. New York, Oxford University Press, 2011

References

Abbruzzese M, Bellodi L, Ferri S, et al: Frontal lobe dysfunction in schizophrenia and obsessive-compulsive disorder: a neuropsychological study. Brain Cogn 27:202–212, 1995

Abrahams S, Pickering A, Polkey CE, et al: Spatial memory deficits in patients with unilateral damage to the right hippocampal formation. Neuropsychologia 35:11–24, 1997

Adler CM, McDonough-Ryan P, Sax KW, et al: fMRI of neuronal activation with symptom provocation in unmedicated patients with obsessive compulsive disorder. J Psychiatr Res 34:317–324, 2000

Ali SO, Denicoff KD, Altshuler LL, et al: A preliminary study of the relation of neuropsychological performance to neuroanatomic structures in bipolar disorder. Neuropsychiatry Neuropsychol Behav Neurol 13:20–28, 2000

Armitage SG: An analysis of certain psychological tests used for the evaluation of brain injury. Psychol Monogr (No 277) 60:1–48, 1946

Baddeley A: Working memory: the interface between memory and cognition, in Memory Systems 1994. Edited by Schacter DL, Tulving E. Cambridge, MA, MIT Press, 1994, pp 351–367

Baddeley A, Kopelman M, Wilson B (eds): The Handbook of Memory Disorders, 2nd Edition. West Sussex, UK, Wiley, 2002

Barton JJ, Cherkasova MV, Press DZ, et al: Perceptual functions in prosopagnosia. Perception 33:939–956, 2004

Basso MR, Bornstein RA: Relative memory deficits in recurrent versus first-episode major depression on a word-list learning task. Neuropsychology 13:557–563, 1999

Bauer R, Demery J: Agnosia, in Clinical Neuropsychology, 4th Edition. Edited by Heilman K, Valenstein E. New York, Oxford University Press, 2003, pp 236–295

Bauer R, Grande L, Valenstein E: Amnesic disorders, in Clinical Neuropsychology, 4th Edition. Edited by Heilman K, Valenstein E. New York, Oxford University Press, 2003, pp 495–573

Bennett T, Raymond M: Utilizing neuropsychological assessment in disability determination and rehabilitation planning, in Handbook of Forensic Neuropsychology. Edited by Horton AJ, Hartlage L. New York, Springer, 2003, pp 237–257

Benton AL, Tranel D: Visuoperceptual, visuospatial, and visuoconstructive disorders, in Clinical Neuropsychology, 3rd Edition. Edited by Heilman KM, Valenstein E. New York, Oxford University Press, 1993, pp 461–497

Berg EA: A simple objective test for measuring flexibility in thinking. J Gen Psychol 39:15–22, 1948

Bleiberg J, Kane RL, Reeves DL, et al: Factor analysis of computerized and traditional tests used in mild brain injury research. Clin Neuropsychol 14:287–294, 2000

Boone KB, Lesser IM, Miller BL, et al: Cognitive functioning in older depressed outpatients: relationship of presence and severity of depression to neuropsychological test scores. Neuropsychology 9:390–398, 1995

Brandstadter D, Oertel WH: Depression in Parkinson's disease. Adv Neurol 91:371–381, 2003

Butcher JN: User's Guide for the MMPI-2 Minnesota Report: Adult Clinical System. Minneapolis, MN, National Computer Systems, 1989

Butcher JN, Pope KS: MMPI-2: a practical guide to clinical, psychometric, and ethical issues. Independent Practitioner 10:20–25, 1990

Butcher JN, Dahlstrom WG, Graham JR, et al: Minnesota Multiphasic Personality Inventory (MMPI-2): Manual for Administration and Scoring. Minneapolis, University of Minnesota Press, 1989

Chamberlain SR, Blackwell AD, Fineberg NA, et al: The neuropsychology of obsessive compulsive disorder: the importance of failures in cognitive and behavioural inhibition as candidate endophenotypic markers. Neurosci Biobehav Rev 29:399–419, 2005

Christensen A-L, Uzzell B (eds): International Handbook of Neuropsychological Rehabilitation. Dordrecht, The Netherlands, Kluwer Academic Publishers, 2000

Cicerone K, Azulay J: Diagnostic utility of attention measures in postconcussion syndrome. Clin Neuropsychol 16:280–289, 2002

Corballis MC: The Lopsided Ape. New York, Oxford University Press, 1991

Cummings JL: Depression in neurologic diseases. Psychiatr Ann 24:525–531, 1994

Dalgleish T, Cox SG: Mood and memory, in Memory Disorders in Psychiatric Practice. Edited by Berrios GE, Hodges JR. New York, Cambridge University Press, 2000, pp 34–46

Damasio H, Damasio A: The lesion method in behavioral neurology and neuropsychology, in Behavioral Neurology and Neuropsychology. Edited by Feinberg T, Farah M. New York, McGraw-Hill, 2003, pp 71–84

Darby D, Walsh K: Walsh's Neuropsychology, 5th Edition. Edinburgh, Elsevier/Churchill Livingstone, 2005

Deckersbach T, Otto MW, Savage CR, et al: The relationship between semantic organization and memory in obsessive-compulsive disorder. Psychother Psychosom 69:101–107, 2000

Delis DC, Kaplan E, Kramer JH, et al: California Verbal Learning Test—Second Edition (CVLT-II) Manual. San Antonio, TX, Harcourt Brace, 2000

Deouell L, Ivry R, Knight R: Electrophysiologic methods and transcranial magnetic stimuluation in behavioral neurology and neuropsychology, in Behavioral Neurology and Neuropsychology. Edited by Feinberg T, Farah M. New York, McGraw-Hill, 2003, pp 105–134

De Renzi E, Faglioni P, Lodesani M, et al: Performance of left brain–damaged patients on imitation of single movements and motor sequences. Cortex 19:333–343, 1983

Dikmen S, Machamer J, Savoie T, et al: Life quality outcome in head injury, in Neuropsychological Assessment of Neuropsychiatric Disorders, 2nd Edition. Edited by Grant I, Adams KM. New York, Oxford University Press, 1996, pp 552–576

Diller L: Poststroke rehabilitation practice guidelines, in International Handbook of Neuropsychological Rehabilitation. Edited by Christensen A-L, Uzzell BP. New York, Kluwer Academic/Plenum, 2000, pp 167–182

Dobigny-Roman N, Dieudonne-Moinet B, Verny M, et al: Ideomotor Apraxia Test: a new test of imitation of gestures for elderly people. Eur J Neurol 5:571–578, 1998

Duncan C, Mirsky A: The Attention Battery for Adults: a systematic approach to assessment, in Comprehensive Handbook of Psychological Assessment, Vol 1: Intellectual and Neuropsychological Assessment. Edited by Goldstein G, Beers S, Hersen M. Hoboken, NJ, Wiley, 2004, pp 263–276

Farah MJ, Feinberg TE (eds): Patient-Based Approaches to Cognitive Neuroscience. Cambridge, MA, MIT Press, 2000

Fischer J, Hannay J, Loring D, et al: Observational methods, rating scales, and inventories, in Neuropsychological Assessment. Edited by Lezak M, Howieson D, Loring D. New York, Oxford University Press, 2004, pp 698–737

Gainotti G: Emotional disorders in relation to unilateral brain damage, in Behavioral Neurology and Neuropsychology. Edited by Feinberg T, Farah M. New York, McGraw-Hill, 2003, pp 725–734

Glassmire DM, Kinney DI, Greene RL, et al: Sensitivity and specificity of MMPI-2 neurologic correction factors: receiver operating characteristic analysis. Assessment 10:299–309, 2003

Goldman RS, Axelrod BN, Taylor SF: Neuropsychological aspects of schizophrenia, in Neuropsychological Assessment of Neuropsychiatric Disorders. Edited by Grant I, Adams KM. New York, Oxford University Press, 1996, pp 504–528

Goodglass H, Kaplan E, Barresi B: Boston Diagnostic Aphasia Examination, 3rd Edition. Philadelphia, PA, Lippincott Williams & Wilkins, 2000

Grafman J, Wassermann E: Transcranial magnetic stimulation can measure and modulate learning and memory. Neuropsychologia 37:159–167, 1999

Greisberg S, McKay D: Neuropsychology of obsessive-compulsive disorder: a review and treatment implications. Clin Psychol Rev 23:95–117, 2003

Gronwall DMA: Paced Auditory Serial-Addition Task: a measure of recovery from concussion. Percept Mot Skills 44:367–373, 1977

Gustafson Y, Nilsson I, Mattsson M, et al: Epidemiology and treatment of post-stroke depression. Drugs Aging 7:298–309, 1995

Haaland KY, Flaherty D: The different types of limb apraxia errors made by patients with left vs. right hemisphere damage. Brain Cogn 3:370–384, 1984

Haaland KY, Harrington DL, Kneight RT: Spatial deficits in ideomotor limb apraxia: a kinematic analysis of aiming movements. Brain 122:1169–1182, 1999

Halstead WC: Brain and Intelligence. Chicago, IL, University of Chicago Press, 1947

Hartman M, Nielsen C, Stratton B: The contributions of attention and working memory to age differences in concept identification. J Clin Exp Neuropsychol 26:227–245, 2004

Heaton RK, Taylor M, Manly J: Demographic effects and use of demographically corrected norms with the WAIS-III and WMS-III, in Clinical Interpretation of the WAIS-III and WMS-III. Edited by Tulsky D, Saklofske D. San Diego, CA, Academic Press, 2003, pp 181–210

Heilman KM, Watson RT, Rothi LJG: Disorders of skilled movement, in Patient-Based Approaches to Cognitive Neuroscience. Edited by Farah MJ, Feinberg TE. Cambridge, MA, MIT Press, 2000a, pp 335–343

Heilman KM, Watson RT, Valenstein E: Neglect, I: clinical and anatomic issues, in Patient-Based Approaches to Cognitive Neuroscience. Edited by Farah MJ, Feinberg TE. Cambridge, MA, MIT Press, 2000b, pp 115–123

Heilman K, Blonder L, Bowers D, et al: Emotional disorders associated with neurological diseases, in Clinical Neuropsychology, 4th Edition. Edited by Heilman K, Valenstein E. New York, Oxford University Press, 2003, pp 447–478

Heinrichs RW, Zakzanis KK: Neurocognitive deficit in schizophrenia: a quantitative review of the evidence. Neuropsychology 12:426–445, 1998

Hertel PT: Relation between rumination and impaired memory in dysphoric moods. J Abnorm Psychol 107:166–172, 1998

Hertzman PA, Clauw DJ, Duffy J, et al: Rigorous new approach to constructing a gold standard for validating new diagnostic criteria, as exemplified by the eosinophilia-myalgia syndrome. Arch Intern Med 161:2301–2306, 2001

Hill SK, Ragland JD, Gur RC, et al: Neuropsychological differences among empirically derived clinical subtypes of schizophrenia. Neuropsychology 15:492–501, 2001

Hodges JR: Transient Amnesia: Clinical and Neuropsychological Aspects. London, WB Saunders, 1991

Kalechstein AD, Newton TF, van Gorp WG: Neurocognitive functioning is associated with employment status: a quantitative review. J Clin Exp Neuropsychol 25:1186–1191, 2003

Kalska H, Punamaki RL, Makinen-Belli T, et al: Memory and metamemory functioning among depressed patients. Appl Neuropsychol 6:96–107, 1999

Kamitani Y, Tong F: Decoding the visual and subjective contents of the human brain. Nat Neurosci 8:679–685, 2005

Knopman D, Selnes O: Neuropsychology of dementia, in Clinical Neuropsychology, 4th Edition. Edited by Heilman K,Valenstein E. New York, Oxford University Press, 2003, pp 574–616

Krabbendam L, de Vugt ME, Derix MM, et al: The behavioural assessment of the dysexecutive syndrome as a tool to assess executive functions in schizophrenia. Clin Neuropsychol 13:370–375, 1999

Kramer JH, Jurik J, Sha SJ, et al: Distinctive neuropsychological patterns in frontotemporal dementia, semantic dementia, and Alzheimer disease. Cogn Behav Neurol 16:211–218, 2003

Leclercq M, Zimmermann P (eds): Applied Neuropsychology of Attention: Theory, Diagnosis, and Rehabilitation. New York, Psychology Press, 2002

Leiguarda RC, Pramstaller PP, Merello M, et al: Apraxia in Parkinson's disease, progressive supranuclear palsy, multiple system atrophy and neuroleptic-induced parkinsonism. Brain 120:75–90, 1997

Levin HS, High WM, Goethe KE, et al: The Neurobehavioral Rating Scale assessment of behavioural sequelae of head injury by the clinician. J Neurol Neurosurg Psychiatry 50:183–193, 1987

Levin JM, Ross MH, Harris G, et al: Applications of dynamic susceptibility contrast magnetic resonance imaging in neuropsychiatry. Neuroimage 4:S147–S162, 1996

Lezak MD: The problem of assessing executive functions. Int J Psychol 17:281–297, 1982

Lezak MD: An individual approach to neuropsychological assessment, in Clinical Neuropsychology. Edited by Logue PE, Schear JM. Springfield, IL, Charles C Thomas, 1986, pp 29–49

Lezak MD: Assessment for rehabilitation planning, in Neuropsychological Rehabilitation. Edited by Meier M, Benton AL, Diller L. Edinburgh, Churchill Livingstone, 1987, pp 41–58

Lezak MD: Brain damage is a family affair. J Clin Exp Neuropsychol 10:111–123, 1988a

Lezak MD: IQ: R.I.P. J Clin Exp Neuropsychol 10:351–361, 1988b

Lezak MD: Assessment of psychosocial dysfunctions resulting from head trauma, in Assessment of the Behavioral Consequences of Head Trauma, Vol 7: Frontiers of Clinical Neuroscience. Edited by Lezak MD. New York, Alan R Liss, 1989, pp 113–144

Lezak MD: Domains of behavior from a neuropsychological perspective: the whole story, in Integrative Views of Motivation, Cognition, and Emotion. Nebraska Symposium on Motivation. Edited by Spaulding WD. Lincoln, University of Nebraska Press, 1994, pp 23–55

Lezak MD, Howieson DB, Bigler ED, et al: Neuropsychological Assessment, 5th Edition. New York, Oxford University Press, 2011

Luria AR: Higher Cortical Functions in Man, 2nd Edition. New York, Basic Books, 1980

Malec JF, Moessner AM, Kragness M, et al: Refining a measure of brain injury sequelae to predict postacute rehabilitation outcome: rating scale analysis of the Mayo-Portland Adaptability Inventory. J Head Trauma Rehabil 15:670–682, 2000

Malloy P, Belanger H, Hall S, et al: Assessing visuoconstructional performance in AD, MCI and normal elderly using the Beery Visual-Motor Integration Test. Clin Neuropsychol 17:544–550, 2003

Markova IS, Berrios GE: Insight into memory deficits, in Memory Disorders in Psychiatric Practice. Edited by Berrios GE, Hodges JR. New York, Cambridge University Press, 2000, pp 34–46

Mayes AR: Selective memory disorders, in The Oxford Handbook of Memory. Edited by Tulving E, Craik FIM. Oxford, UK, Oxford University Press, 2000, pp 427–440

Mesulam M-M (ed): Principles of Behavioral and Cognitive Neurology, 2nd Edition. New York, Oxford University Press, 2000

Mitrushina M, Boone K, Razani J, et al: Handbook of Normative Data for Neuropsychological Assessment, 2nd Edition. New York, Oxford University Press, 2005

Nelson HE: The National Adult Reading Test (NART): Test Manual. Windsor, UK, NFER-Nelson, 1982

Norris G, Tate RL: The Behavioural Assessment of the Dysexecutive Syndrome (BADS); ecological, concurrent and construct validity. Neuropsychol Rehabil 10:33–45, 2000

Ochoa E, Erhan H, Feinberg T: Emotional disorders in relation to nonfocal brain damage, in Behavioral Neurology and Neuropsychology. Edited by Feinberg T, Farah M. New York, McGraw-Hill, 2003, pp 735–742

Paradiso S, Ohkubo T, Robinson RG: Vegetative and psychological symptoms associated with depressed mood over the first two years after stroke. Int J Psychiatry Med 27:137–157, 1997

Post RM: Neural substrates of psychiatric syndromes, in Principles of Behavioral and Cognitive Neurology, 2nd Edition. Edited by Mesulam M-M. New York, Oxford University Press, 2000, pp 406–438

Prigatano GP, Schacter DL (eds): Awareness of Deficit After Brain Injury. New York, Oxford University Press, 1991

Psychological Corporation: WAIS-IV Technical and Interpretive Manual. San Antonio, TX, Pearson Assessment, 2008

Rafal RD: Neglect, II: cognitive neuropsychological issues, in Patient-Based Approaches to Cognitive Neuroscience. Edited by Farah MJ, Feinberg TE. Cambridge, MA, MIT Press, 2000, pp 115–123

Raspall T, Donate M, Boget T, et al: Neuropsychological tests with lateralizing value in patients with temporal lobe epilepsy: reconsidering material-specific theory. Seizure 14:569–576, 2005

Rey A: L'examen clinique en psychologie. Paris, Presses Universitaries de France, 1964

Rickards H: Depression in neurological disorders: Parkinson's disease, multiple sclerosis, and stroke. J Neurol Neurosurg Psychiatry 76 (suppl 1):I48–I52, 2005

Robinson RG: The Clinical Neuropsychiatry of Stroke. New York, Cambridge University Press, 1998

Rothi LJG, Raymer AM, Heilman KM: Limb praxis assessment, in Apraxia: The Neuropsychology of Action. Edited by Rothi LJG, Heilman KM. Hove, UK, Psychology Press, 1997, pp 61–73

Savage CR, Deckersbach T, Wilhelm S, et al: Strategic processing and episodic memory impairment in obsessive compulsive disorder. Neuropsychology 14:141–151, 2000

Sbordone RJ: The assessment interview in clinical neuropsychology, in Neuropsychological Assessment in Clinical Practice. Edited by Groth-Marnat G. New York, Wiley, 2000, pp 94–126

Schenkenberg T, Bradford DC, Ajax ET: Line bisection and unilateral visual neglect in patients with neurologic impairment. Neurology 30:509–517, 1980

Schmidt M: Rey Auditory Verbal Learning Test (RAVLT): A Handbook. Los Angeles, CA, Western Psychological Services, 1996

Shallice T: Specific impairments of planning. Philos Trans R Soc Lond B Biol Sci 298:199–209, 1982

Singh A, Black SE, Herrmann N, et al: Functional and neuroanatomic correlations in poststroke depression: the Sunnybrook Stroke Study. Stroke 31:637–644, 2000

Sloan S, Ponsford J: Assessment of cognitive difficulties following TBI, in Traumatic Brain Injury: Rehabilitation for Everyday Adaptive Living. Edited by Ponsford J. Hillsdale, NJ, Erlbaum, 1995, pp 65–101

Sox HC, Blatt MA, Higgins MC, et al: Medical Decision Making. Boston, MA, Butterworths, 1988

Spreen O, Risser AH: Assessment of Aphasia. New York, Oxford University Press, 2003

Squire LR, Slater PC, Chace PM: Retrograde amnesia: temporal gradient in very long term memory following electroconvulsive therapy. Science 187:77–79, 1975

Steinberg B, Bieliauskas L: Introduction to the special edition: IQ-based MOANS norms for multiple neuropsychological instruments. Clin Neuropsychol 19:277–279, 2005

Stern E, Silbersweig DA: Advances in functional neuroimaging methodology for the study of brain systems underlying human neuropsychological function and dysfunction. J Clin Exp Neuropsychol 23:3–18, 2001

Strakowski SM, Del Bello MP, Sax KW, et al: Brain magnetic resonance imaging of structural abnormalities in bipolar disorder. Arch Gen Psychiatry 56:254–260, 1999

Strauss E, Goldsmith SM: Lateral preferences and performance on non-verbal laterality tests in a normal population. Cortex 23:495–503, 1987

Strauss E, Sherman MS, Spreen O: A Compendium of Neuropsychological Tests: Administration, Norms, and Commentary, 3rd Edition. New York, Oxford University Press, 2006

Stuss DT, Levine B, Alexander MP, et al: Wisconsin Card Sorting Test performance in patients with focal frontal and posterior brain damage: effects of lesion location and test structure on separable cognitive processes. Neuropsychologia 38:388–402, 2000

Urbina S: Essentials of Psychological Testing. New York, Wiley, 2004

Vanderploeg RD, Schinka JA, Axelrod BN, et al: Estimation of WAIS-R premorbid intelligence: current ability and demographic data used in a best-performance fashion. Psychol Assess 8:404–411, 1996

Veiel HO: A preliminary profile of neuropsychological deficits associated with major depression. J Clin Exp Neuropsychol 19:587–603, 1997

Wagner AD, Poldrack RA, Eldridge LL, et al: Material-specific lateralization of prefrontal activation during episodic encoding and retrieval. Neuroreport 9:3711–3717, 1998

Wechsler D: Wechsler Adult Intelligence Scale Manual. New York, Psychological Corporation, 1981

Wechsler D: Wechsler Adult Intelligence Scale, 3rd Edition (WAIS-III): Administration and Scoring Manual. San Antonio, TX, Psychological Corporation, 1997a

Wechsler D: Wechsler Memory Scale, 3rd Edition (WMS-III): Administration and Scoring Manual. San Antonio, TX, Psychological Corporation, 1997b

Wechsler D, Holdnack JA, Drozdick LW: Wechsler Memory Scale—Fourth Edition (WMS-IV) Technical and Interpretive Manual. San Antonio, TX, Pearson Assessment, 2009

Weiland-Fiedler P, Erickson K, Waldeck T, et al: Evidence for continuing neuropsychological impairments in depression. J Affect Disord 82:253–258, 2004

Wild K, Howieson D, Webbe F, et al: Status of computerized cognitive testing in aging: a systematic review. Alzheimers Dement 4:428–437, 2008

Wilson BA, Alderman N, Burgess PW, et al: Behavioural Assessment of the Dysexecutive Syndrome. Bury St Edmunds, UK, Thames Valley Test Co, 1996

Wilson BA, Evans JJ, Keohane C: Cognitive rehabilitation: a goal-planning approach. J Head Trauma Rehabil 17:542–555, 2002

2

Clinical and Functional Imaging in Neuropsychiatry

Robin A. Hurley, M.D., F.A.N.P.A.

Ronald E. Fisher, M.D., Ph.D.

Katherine H. Taber, Ph.D., F.A.N.P.A.

Modern medicine has embraced technology in almost every field. Although adapting the marvels of engineering and physics to emotion and behavior is slightly more challenging, psychiatry has seen the influence of technology. Neuropsychiatry, as a subspecialty, developed to assess and treat cognitive or emotional disturbances caused by brain dysfunction. This conceptual focus could not have evolved without the influence of brain imaging, engineering, and physics. In the short time span of one century, imaging technology advanced from a primitive skull X ray to real-time pictures of brain changes as a person performs a task or feels an emotion such as sadness or happiness. Cutting-edge imaging contributions are found not only in the diagnostic arena but also in estimating the course of illness and the expected treatment response and in the development of new neurotransmitter-specific medications.

Currently, brain imaging is divided into two categories: structural and functional (Table 2–1). *Structural imaging* is defined as information regarding the physical appearance of the brain that is independent of thought, neuronal or motor activity, or mood. Computed tomography (CT) and magnetic resonance imaging (MRI) are the standard tools. *Functional imaging* of the brain measures changes related to neuronal activity. The most common functional imaging techniques use indirect measures such as blood flow and glucose metabolism. Functional imaging techniques currently used in clinical practice include single-photon emission computed tomography (SPECT), positron emission tomography (PET), and magnetic resonance spectroscopy (MRS). Other functional imaging techniques under development for clinical use or for research include functional magnetic resonance imaging (fMRI), xenon-enhanced computed tomography (Xe/CT), and magnetoencephalography (MEG).

In the first section of this chapter, we review structural imaging concepts and basic technologies. We then discuss the functional techniques most used in psychiatric patients and conclude with a brief discussion of functional neuroanatomy. We do not summarize the imaging findings of all neuropsychiatric diseases or all of the potential research applications. We do, however, review the basics of how and why to image and how to understand the findings; thus, this chapter provides the reader with a knowledge base for using neuroimaging in clinical practice.

Structural Imaging

Early studies in the 1980s promoted limited use of CT scanning in psychiatric patients only after focal neurological findings had been developed (Larson et al. 1981). Studies in the late 1980s and the 1990s encouraged a broader use of diagnostic CT in psychiatric patients (Beresford et al. 1986; Kaplan et al. 1994; Rauch and Renshaw 1995; Weinberger 1984). With the advent of utilization review and cost containment in the late 1990s, more narrow criteria were again proposed, and CT was recommended only when reversible pathology was suspected (Branton 1999; Erhart et al. 2005). Diagnostic imaging has advanced considerably in the last decade, with multiple new brain imaging techniques

Table 2–1.   Brain imaging modalities

Type of imaging	Parameter measured
Structural	
Computed tomography (CT)	Tissue density
Magnetic resonance imaging (MRI)	Many properties of tissue (T1 and T2 relaxation times, spin density, magnetic susceptibility, water diffusion, blood flow)
Functional[a]	
Positron emission tomography (PET)	Radioactive tracers in blood or tissue
Single-photon emission computed tomography (SPECT)	Radioactive tracers in tissue
Xenon-enhanced computed tomography (Xe/CT)	Xenon concentration in blood
Functional magnetic resonance imaging (fMRI)	Deoxyhemoglobin levels in blood
Magnetoencephalography (MEG)	Magnetic fields induced by neuronal discharges
Magnetic resonance spectroscopy (MRS)	Metabolite concentrations in tissue

[a]Resting brain activity, brain activation, neurotransmitter receptors.
Source.   Adapted from Hurley RA, Fisher RE, Taber KH: "Clinical and Functional Imaging in Neuropsychiatry," in *Essentials of Neuropsychiatry and Behavioral Neurosciences,* 2nd Edition. Edited by Yudofsky SC, Hales RE. Washington, DC, American Psychiatric Publishing, 2010, pp. 55–93. Used with permission. Copyright © 2010 American Psychiatric Association.

coming into common clinical use. In addition, the understanding of functional anatomy, as it relates to psychiatric conditions, has increased enormously. For example, a study of psychiatric patients without dementia found that treatment was changed in 15% of patients as a result of imaging examinations (Erhart et al. 2005).

Clinical indications for neuroimaging include sustained confusion or delirium, subtle cognitive deficits, unusual age at symptom onset or evolution, atypical clinical findings, and abrupt personality changes with accompanying neurological signs or symptoms (Erhart et al. 2005; Hurley et al. 2002). In addition,

Table 2–2.　Indications for imaging

Diagnosis or medical condition

Traumatic brain injury

Significant alcohol abuse

Seizure disorders with psychiatric symptoms

Movement disorders

Autoimmune disorders

Eating disorders

Poison or toxin exposure

Delirium

Clinical signs and symptoms

Dementia or cognitive decline

New-onset mental illness after age 50

Initial psychotic break

Presentation at an atypical age for diagnosis

Focal neurological signs

Catatonia

Sudden personality changes

Source. Reprinted from Hurley RA, Fisher RE, Taber KH: "Clinical and Functional Imaging in Neuropsychiatry," in *Essentials of Neuropsychiatry and Behavioral Neurosciences,* 2nd Edition. Edited by Yudofsky SC, Hales RE. Washington, DC, American Psychiatric Publishing, 2010, pp. 55–93. Used with permission. Copyright © 2010 American Psychiatric Association.

neuroimaging is recommended following poison or toxin exposures (including significant alcohol abuse) and brain injuries of any kind (traumatic or "organic") (Table 2–2). The information obtained from brain imaging studies may assist with differential diagnosis, alter a treatment plan, and inform prognosis.

Practical Considerations

Ordering the Examination

The neuroradiologist needs very clear clinical information on the imaging request form (not just "rule out pathology" or "new-onset mental status changes").

If a lesion is suspected in a particular location, the neuroradiologist should be informed of this conjecture or given enough clinical data for selection of the best imaging method and parameters to view suspicious areas. The clinician should ask the neuroradiologist about any special imaging techniques that may enhance visualization of the limbic circuits (see subsection "Common Pulse Sequences" later in this chapter). The neuroradiologist and technical staff also need information on the patient's current condition (e.g., delirious, psychotic, easily agitated, paranoid). This knowledge may eliminate difficulties with patient management during the scan.

Contrast-Enhanced Studies

When ordering CT or MRI, the physician can request that an additional set of images be gathered after intravenous administration of a contrast agent. Although different physical principles are used for CT and MRI (see later sections for full discussion), contrast enhancement is required for identification of lesions that are the same signal intensity as surrounding brain tissue. Contrast agents travel in the vascular system and normally do not cross into the brain parenchyma because they cannot pass through the blood-brain barrier. The blood-brain barrier is formed by tight junctions in the capillaries that serve as a structural barrier and function like a plasma membrane. The ability of a substance to pass through these junctions depends on several factors, including the substance's affinity for plasma proteins, its lipophilic nature, and its size. (An excellent review of the physiology of the blood-brain barrier and the basics of contrast enhancement can be found in Sage et al. 1998.) In some disease processes, the blood-brain barrier is broken or damaged. As a result, contrast agents can diffuse into brain tissue. Pathological processes in which the blood-brain barrier is disrupted include autoimmune diseases, infections, and tumors. Contrast enhancement also can be useful in the case of vascular abnormalities (e.g., arteriovenous malformations and aneurysms), although the contrast agent remains intravascular. When ordering the imaging procedure, the psychiatrist should be mindful to request a study with contrast enhancement if one of the above disease states is suspected.

Patient Preparation

The psychiatrist should always explain the procedure to the patient shortly beforehand, being mindful to mention the loud noises of the scanner (MRI), the tightly enclosing imaging coil (MRI), and the requirement for absolute immobility during the test (MRI and CT). If the psychiatrist suspects that the patient may become agitated or be unable to remain still for the length of the examination, then sedation may be necessary. A clinician may select a regimen with which he or she is familiar and comfortable. We have found that for patients with agitation and psychosis, a sedating antipsychotic with lorazepam 1–2 mg intramuscularly 30 minutes before scanning usually works well in a physically healthy nongeriatric adult.

Understanding the Scan

The psychiatrist should review the scan and radiology report with the neuroradiologist. It is important to remember that the radiographic view places the patient's right on the reader's left and the patient's left on the reader's right. The first points to observe on a scan are the demographics: the hospital name; the date; the scanner number; and the patient's name, age, sex, and identification number. The clinician should note whether the scan was done with or without contrast enhancement. If a magnetic resonance image has been obtained, the weighting parameters are important. Next, the psychiatrist should ask the neuroradiologist to point out the normal anatomical markers and any pathology observed on the films. Prior understanding of limbic system anatomy is essential.

Neuropsychiatry Knowledge Gained From Structural Imaging

Soon after the advent of CT and MRI, scientists began to image patients with psychotic and mood disorders, hoping to demonstrate concrete proof that these illnesses are indeed brain disorders and not conditions of "weak personalities" or "poor parenting." Initial studies in the classic conditions of bipolar disorder, major depression, and schizophrenia met with disappointing results—with, at most, nonspecific findings that occur in many disease states (e.g., ventricular enlargement or generalized atrophy). As neuropsychiatry has matured, so has the knowledge that can be obtained from structural images. Researchers studying conditions such as cerebrovascular accidents, ruptured aneurysms, traumatic brain injury, and multiple sclerosis were among the first to document that psychiatric symptoms do occur as a result of brain injury; that emotion, memory, and thought processing happen by way of tracts or circuits (Mega and Cummings

1994); and that indeed many patients do have subtle lesions that account for their symptoms. Not only has this information led to a further understanding of brain function, but it has provided prognostic information for patients and has led to treatment plan changes (Diwadkar and Keshavan 2002; Erhart et al. 2005; Gupta et al. 2004; Symms et al. 2004).

Computed Tomography

The first CT image, obtained in 1972, required 9 days for data collection and more than 2 hours for processing on a mainframe computer (Orrison and Sanders 1995). The multiple detector scanners of today can capture multiple slices in less than 0.5 second, with the entire brain scanned in about 5 seconds.

Technical Considerations

Like a conventional radiograph, CT uses an X-ray tube as a source of photons. When a conventional radiograph is acquired, the photons directly expose X-ray film. When a CT image is acquired, the photons are collected by detectors. The latest-generation CT scanners split the X-ray beam and add multiple detectors, allowing collection of multiple slices simultaneously ("multislice scanners"). These data are relayed to a computer that places the data in a two-dimensional grid to form the image (Rauch and Renshaw 1995). Many hospitals now display and store the resultant images digitally via a picture archiving and communication system, although some still print to X-ray film (De Backer et al. 2004a, 2004b).

CT scans deliver a radiation dose of about 5 rads to the lens of the eye. Although a minimum of 200 rads is thought to be necessary to induce cataracts, many patients receive multiple scans, and pediatric patients are more sensitive than are adults (Hopper et al. 2001). To help prevent even this small dose of radiation to the lens of the eye, some institutions use a line drawn between the orbit and the external auditory meatus (referred to as the *orbitomeatal line*) as the inferior boundary of brain CT scans, thereby avoiding most of the exposure to the lens. The dose to the brain is about 7 rads in adults and about 10 rads in infants; although this amount was long believed to be quite safe, some controversy has arisen regarding data suggesting a possible long-term decrease in cognitive function following this level of radiation to the brain in infants (Hall et al. 2004). Although no appreciable radiation is deposited outside the head, a lead apron is often placed over the abdomen of a pregnant woman during a

Table 2–3. Relative gray-scale appearance on a noncontrast computed tomography scan

Tissue	Appearance
Bone	White
Calcified tissue	White
Clotted blood	White[a]
Gray matter	Light gray
White matter	Medium gray
Cerebrospinal fluid	Nearly black
Water	Nearly black
Air	Black

[a]Becomes isointense to brain as clot ages approximately 1–2 weeks.
Source.   Reprinted from Hurley RA, Fisher RE, Taber KH: "Clinical and Functional Imaging in Neuropsychiatry," in *Essentials of Neuropsychiatry and Behavioral Neurosciences,* 2nd Edition. Edited by Yudofsky SC, Hales RE. Washington, DC, American Psychiatric Publishing, 2010, pp. 55–93. Used with permission. Copyright © 2010 American Psychiatric Association.

head CT scan. As the photons pass through the head, some are absorbed by the tissues of the head. Detectors located opposite the beam source measure the attenuation of the photons. Thus, the CT images of the brain record tissue density as measured by the variable attenuation of X-ray photons. High-density tissues such as bone appear white, indicating an almost complete absorption of the X rays (high attenuation). Air has the lowest rate of attenuation (or absorption of radiation) and appears black. The appearance of other tissues is described in Table 2–3.

Contrast Agents

Administration of an intravenous iodinated contrast agent immediately before obtaining a CT scan greatly improves the detection of many brain lesions that are isodense on noncontrast CT. Contrast agents are useful when a breakdown of the blood-brain barrier occurs. Under normal circumstances, the blood-brain barrier does not allow passage of the contrast medium into the extravascular spaces of the brain. When a break in this barrier occurs, the contrast agent enters the damaged area and collects in or around the lesion. The increased density of the contrast agent will appear as a white area on the scan. Without a companion noncontrast CT scan, preexisting dense areas (calcified or hemorrhagic) might be mistaken for contrast-enhanced lesions. In difficult cases, a double dose of contrast agent may be used to improve detection of lesions with minimal blood-brain barrier impairment. Contrast agents, when administered as a fast bolus, can also be used to measure several aspects of cerebral perfusion, including cerebral blood flow, cerebral blood volume, and mean transit time (Halpin 2004).

Currently, two types of iodinated CT contrast agents are used: ionic or high osmolality and nonionic or low osmolality. Both types are associated with allergic reactions, and contraindications exist for both. Allergic reactions to contrast agents are defined by two types—anaphylactoid or nonanaphylactoid (chemotoxic)—in two time frames—immediate or delayed (Detre and Alsop 2005; Federle et al. 1998; Jacobs et al. 1998; Oi et al. 1997; Yasuda and Munechika 1998). Anaphylactoid reactions include hives, rhinitis, bronchospasm, laryngeal edema, hypotension, and death. Chemotoxic reactions include nausea, vomiting, warmth or pain at the injection site, hypotension, tachycardia, and arrhythmias (Cohan et al. 1998; Federle et al. 1998; Mortelé et al. 2005). Immediate reactions occur within 1 hour of injection; delayed reactions occur within 7 days but usually within 24 hours. The overall mortality rate from any contrast dye is reported to be 1 per 100,000. Data suggest that ionic contrast reactions occur at a rate of 4%–12% (most commonly mild) and nonionic reactions occur at a rate of 1%–3% (Cochran 2005; Cochran et al. 2002). One study reviewed approximately 20,000 contrast-enhanced CT examinations and found the rate of mild and moderate ionic dye reactions to be 2.2% and 0.08%, respectively, and the rate of mild and moderate nonionic dye reactions to be 0.59% and 0.05%, respectively (Valls et al. 2003).

The ionic agents are significantly less expensive, but they are less often used because of the greater risk of allergic reactions. The American College of Radiology standards recommend the use of nonionic dye in patients with histories of significant contrast media reactions; any previous serious allergic reaction to any material; asthma; sickle cell disease; diabetes; renal insufficiency (creatinine ≥1.5 mg/dL); cardiac diseases; inability to communicate; geriatric age; or other debilitating health problems (including myasthenia gravis, multiple myeloma, and pheochromocytoma) (Cohan et al. 1998; Halpern et al. 1999; Konen et al. 2002). Patients who are receiving dialysis or who have histories of milder reactions to shellfish require the use of nonionic dyes when contrast CT is unavoidable. The older ionic agents are not used in these patients.

Extravasation (leakage of the contrast dye at the injection site) is generally a mild problem associated with some stinging or burning. However, in infrequent cases, patients have developed tissue ulceration or necrosis. If a patient has had a previous episode of extravasation, then nonionic dye should be used because it is associated with fewer reactions. Caution is also necessary for patients with histories of anaphylaxis. These patients should be considered for types of imaging other than contrast-enhanced CT. If contrast-enhanced CT is necessary, then premedication with steroids and antihistamines and the use of nonionic dye are recommended. In patients taking metformin, an oral antihyperglycemic agent, the medication must be withheld before iodinated dye is given. It can be restarted after 48 hours with laboratory evidence of normal renal function. Metformin can cause lactic acidosis, especially in patients with a history of renal or hepatic dysfunction, alcohol abuse, or cardiac disease (Cohan et al. 1998).

Magnetic Resonance Imaging

In 1946, the phenomenon of nuclear magnetic resonance was discovered. The discovery led to the development of a powerful new technique for studying matter by using radio waves together with a static magnetic field. This development, combined with other important insights and emerging technologies in the 1970s, led to the first magnetic resonance image of a living patient. By the 1980s, commercial MRI scanners were becoming more common. Although the physics that make MRI possible are complex, a grasp of the basic principles will help the clinician to understand the results of the imaging examination and to explain this procedure to anxious patients.

Physical Principles

Reconstructing an image.   Clinical MRI is based on manipulating the small magnetic field around the nucleus of the hydrogen atom (proton), a major component of water in soft tissue. Making a magnetic resonance image of a patient's soft tissues requires that the patient be placed inside a large magnet. The strength of the magnet is measured in teslas (T). Standard clinical magnets have a field strength of 1.5 or 3.0 T. (More powerful systems are occasionally used in research settings.) The magnetic field of the MRI scanner slightly magnetizes the hydrogen atoms in the body, changing their alignment. The stronger the magnetic field, the more magnetized the hydrogen atoms in tissue become and the more signal they produce. The stronger signal available with 1.5-T and 3.0-T systems allows images of higher resolution to be collected. Some patients feel uncomfortable or frankly claustrophobic while lying inside these huge enclosing magnets. Open-design magnets that help the patient feel less confined (Scarabino et al. 2003) are increasingly popular, constituting an estimated 40% of sales between 2000 and 2005, although the image quality is lower than in closed systems (Moseley et al. 2005).

The patient is placed in the center of the MRI scanner's powerful magnetic field. This strong magnetic field (usually 1.5 or 3.0 T) is always on and is perfectly uniform across the patient. The nuclei of the hydrogen atoms in the patient's body possess tiny magnetic fields, which instantly align with the strong magnetic field of the scanner. A series of precisely calculated radio frequency (RF) pulses is then applied. The hydrogen nuclei absorb this RF energy, which causes them to temporarily lose their alignment with the strong magnetic field. They gradually relax back into magnetic alignment, releasing the absorbed energy in a characteristic temporal pattern, depending on the nature of the tissue containing the hydrogen atoms. This electromagnetic energy is detected by the same coils used to generate the RF pulses and is converted into an electrical signal that is sent to a computer. For some body regions, such as the brain or knee, a coil is placed directly around the body region to improve delivery and reception of the electromagnetic pulses and signals. The scanner's computer converts these signals into a spatial map, the magnetic resonance image. The final output is a matrix consisting of a three-dimensional image composed of many small blocks, or voxels. The voxel size on a 1.5-T scan of the brain is variable but approximately 1 mm on each side.

Creation of a magnetic resonance image requires the application of small magnetic field gradients across the patient, in addition to the constant, more powerful field. This allows the scanner to tell which part of the body is emitting what signal. The magnetic field gradients needed to acquire the image are created by huge coils of wire embedded in the magnet. These are driven with large-current audio amplifiers similar to those used for musical concerts. The current in these coils must be switched on and off very rapidly; this causes the coils to vibrate and creates loud noises during the scan that may occasionally distress the unprepared patient, although patients are always given earplugs, which greatly dampen the noise.

Common pulse sequences.   The combination of RF and magnetic field pulses used by the computer to create the image is called the *pulse sequence* (Haller et al. 2009). Pulse sequences have been developed that result in images sensitive to different aspects of the hydrogen atom's behavior in a high magnetic field. Thus, each image type contains unique information about the tissue. A pulse sequence is repeated many times to form an image.

The pulse sequence used most commonly in clinical MRI is the *spin echo* (SE) sequence (Haller et al. 2009). Most centers now use a faster variant of this sequence, the *fast spin echo* (FSE). These pulse sequences emphasize different tissue properties by varying two factors. One is the time between applying each repetition of the sequence, referred to as the *repetition time* or *time to recovery* (TR). The other is the time at which the receiver coil collects signal after the RF pulses have been given; this is called the *echo time* or *time until the echo* (TE). Images collected using a short TR and short TE are most heavily influenced by the T1 relaxation times of the tissues and thus are called *T1 weighted*. Traditionally, this type of image is considered best for displaying anatomy because it shows sharply marginated boundaries between the gray matter of the brain (medium gray), the white matter of the brain (very light gray), and cerebrospinal fluid (CSF) (black). Images collected using a long TR and a long TE are most heavily influenced by T2 relaxation times of the tissues and thus are called *T2 weighted*. Boundaries between the gray matter of the brain (medium gray), the white matter of the brain (dark gray), and CSF (white) are more blurred than on T1-weighted images. The T2-weighted image is best for displaying pathology, which most commonly appears bright, often similar in intensity to CSF. A very useful variant on the T2-weighted scan, called a *fluid-attenuated inversion recovery* (FLAIR) image, allows the intense signal from CSF to be nullified (CSF appears dark), which makes pathology near CSF-filled spaces much easier to see (Arakia et al. 1999; Haller et al. 2009). FLAIR improves identification of subtle lesions, making it useful for neuropsychiatric imaging.

The next most commonly used pulse sequence in clinical imaging is the *gradient echo* (GE or GRE) sequence (Haller et al. 2009). In this type of image acquisition, a gradient-reversing RF pulse is used to generate the echo. This technique is very sensitive to anything in the tissue causing magnetic field inhomogeneity, such as hemorrhage or calcium. These images are sometimes called *susceptibility weighted* because differences in magnetic susceptibility between tissues cause localized magnetic field inhomogeneity and signal loss. As a result, gradient echo images have artifacts at the interfaces between tissues with very different magnetic susceptibility, such as bone and brain. The artifacts at the skull base are sometimes severe. A more recently developed method of MRI that is finding increasing clinical use is diffusion-weighted imaging (Haller et al. 2009). Diffusion-weighted MRI is sensitive to the speed of water diffusion and may be able to visualize areas of ischemic stroke in the critical first few hours after onset (Huisman 2003; Kuhl et al. 2005; Mascalchi et al. 2005; Nakamura et al. 2005; Symms et al. 2004). This procedure is also showing potential in the imaging of other conditions, such as hypoglycemic encephalopathy, infection, neurodegenerative conditions, traumatic brain injury, and metabolic diseases (Jung et al. 2005; Mascalchi et al. 2005; Symms et al. 2004).

New pulse sequences.   Two pulse sequences that are sensitive to other aspects of tissue state are being tested for clinical work. *Magnetization transfer imaging* is sensitive to interactions between free protons (unbound water in tissue) and bound protons (water bound to macromolecules such as those in myelin membranes) (Hanyu et al. 1999; Tanabe et al. 1999). This type of imaging may be able to differentiate white matter lesions of different causes and thus provide insight into pathological processes (Filippi and Rocca 2004; Hanyu et al. 1999; Hurley et al. 2003; Symms et al. 2004; Tanabe et al. 1999). *Diffusion tensor imaging* is a more complex version of diffusion-weighted imaging (Chanraud et al. 2010; Dong et al. 2004; Haller et al. 2009; Kubicki et al. 2002; Sundgren et al. 2004; Taber et al. 2002; Taylor et al. 2004). A set of images is collected that allows calculation of a multidimensional matrix (the diffusion tensor) that describes the diffusional speed in each direction for every voxel in the image. The speed of diffusion is similar in all directions in gray matter (isotropic diffusion) but is faster parallel to axons in white matter (anisotropic diffusion). This technique is sensitive to many processes that alter diffusion, including ischemia and gliosis. It can be used to identify areas of pathology or damage, such as those that occur in multiple sclerosis or following traumatic brain injury. It also has potential for studying very subtle structural changes, such as altered brain connectivity in neuropsychiatric disorders.

Another promising new magnetic resonance technique provides a method for imaging of cerebral blood flow by "tagging" water molecules in the carotid arteries with RF pulses (arterial spin labeling), which changes the signal intensity of the blood as it flows up into the brain (Detre and Alsop 2005; Haller et al. 2009). This technique has great potential because it does not require administration of a contrast agent or exposure to any form of radiation. In the future, a combination of some of these newer methods of MRI may provide important information for differential diagnosis.

Contrast Agents

The first experimental contrast-enhanced magnetic resonance image was made in 1982 using a gadolinium complex, gadolinium-diethylenetriamine pentaacetic acid (Gd-DTPA), now called gadopentetate dimeglumine. Six years later, gadopentetate dimeglumine was approved as an intravenous contrast agent for human clinical MRI scans (Wolf 1991). Metal ions such as gadolinium are quite toxic to the body if they are in a free state. To make an MRI contrast agent, the metal ion is attached to a very strong ligand (such as DTPA) that prevents any interaction with surrounding tissue. This allows the gadolinium complex to be excreted intact by the kidneys. Several gadolinium-based contrast agents are currently in common use for brain imaging, including gadopentetate dimeglumine (Magnevist, Berlex Laboratories), gadodiamide (Omniscan, Nycomed Amersham), gadoteridol (ProHance, Bracco Diagnostics), gadobenate dimeglumine (MultiHance, Bracco Diagnostics), and gadoversetamide (OptiMARK, Tyco Healthcare/Mallinckrodt) (Baker et al. 2004; Kirchin and Runge 2003; Runge 2001; Shellock and Kanal 1999). These agents are administered intravenously, whereupon they distribute to the vascular compartment and then diffuse throughout the extracellular compartment (Mitchell 1997).

Gadolinium is a metal ion that is highly paramagnetic, meaning that it generates its own small magnetic field when placed in a stronger magnetic field. This produces an inhomogeneous magnetic field in tissues that contain gadolinium. Unlike the iodinated contrast agents used in CT, the currently used clinical MRI contrast agents are not imaged directly. Rather, the presence of the contrast agent changes the T1 and T2 properties of hydrogen atoms (protons) in nearby tissue (Runge et al. 1997). Like CT contrast agents, MRI contrast agents do not enter the brain under normal conditions because they cannot pass through the blood-brain barrier. When the blood-brain barrier is damaged, these agents accumulate in tissue around the breakdown. The effect of this accumulation is most easily seen on a T1-weighted scan. This accumulation results in an increase in signal (seen as a white or bright area) (Runge et al. 1997). As in CT, cerebral blood flow can be assessed if images are acquired very quickly after administration of a contrast agent (this technique is variously called dynamic susceptibility contrast, first-pass perfusion MRI, or bolus perfusion MRI) (Latchaw 2004; Sunshine 2004).

The total incidence of adverse side effects from contrast enhancement in MRI appears to be less than 3%–5%, with any single type of side effect occurring in fewer than 1% of patients (Kirchin and Runge 2003; Runge 2001; Runge et al. 1997; Shellock and Kanal 1999). Immediate reactions at the injection site include warmth or a burning sensation, pain, and local edema. Delayed reactions (including erythema, swelling, and pain) appear 1–4 days after the injection. Immediate systemic reactions include nausea (sometimes vomiting) and headache. Anaphylactoid reactions have been reported, particularly in patients with a history of allergic respiratory disease. The incidence of these reactions appears to be somewhere between 1 and 5 in 500,000.

Nephrogenic systemic fibrosis (NSF) has been documented in patients with severe renal insufficiency or liver diseases after single or multiple administrations of gadolinium-based contrast agents (Kanal et al. 2008; Kuo et al. 2007). NSF can be quite debilitating and is potentially fatal. Pathological changes include fibrosis and thickening in the connective tissues (including around major organs) and skin. These changes can compromise organ function and may result in inability to move. Standard of care now requires appropriate screening procedures prior to contrast administration. Consultation with the radiologist is advised if contrast MRI is under consideration in patients with kidney or liver disease.

The presence of some of these contrast agents (Omniscan, OptiMARK) has been reported to interfere with colorimetric assays for serum calcium, resulting in an incorrect diagnosis of hypocalcemia in 15% of patients in one study (Kirchin and Runge 2003). (For a more extensive review of the biosafety aspects of MRI contrast agents, see Shellock and Kanal 1999.) Many new MRI contrast agents are under development (Bulte 2004). As new contrast agents become available for MRI of the brain, the range of applications in neuropsychiatry may well expand.

Safety and Contraindications

To date, no permanent hazardous effects appear to result from short-term exposure to magnetic fields and RF pulses generated in clinical MRI scanners (Hartwig et al. 2009; Price 1999; Shellock and Crues 2004). Volunteers scanned in systems with higher field strength (4 T) have reported effects such as headaches, dizziness, and nausea (Shellock 1991). Although peripheral nerves can be stimulated directly with very intense gradients, this does not occur at clinical field strengths (Bourland et al. 1999; Hartwig et al. 2009; Hoffmann et al. 2000; Shellock and Crues 2004).

There are, however, important contraindications to the use of MRI (see Table 2–4 for summary). The magnetic field can damage electrical, mechanical, or magnetic devices implanted in or attached to the patient. Pacemakers can be damaged by programming changes, possibly inducing arrhythmias. Currents can develop within the wires, leading to burns, fibrillation, or movement of the wires or the pacemaker unit itself. Cochlear implants, dental implants, magnetic stoma plugs, bone-growth stimulators, and implanted medication-infusion pumps can all be demagnetized or injure the patient by movement during exposure to the scanner's magnetic field. In addition, metallic implants, shrapnel, or bullets, or metal shavings within the eye (e.g., from welding), can conduct a current and/or move, injuring the eye. All of these devices distort the magnetic resonance image locally and may decrease diagnostic accuracy. Metallic objects near the magnet can be drawn into the magnet at high speed, injuring the patient or staff (Hartwig et al. 2009; Price 1999; Shellock 1991, 2002; Shellock and Crues 2004).

Although no evidence has shown that MRI damages the developing fetus, most authorities recommend caution. Judgment should be exercised when considering MRI of a pregnant woman. When possible, the patient should be asked to provide express written consent, especially in the first trimester (Shellock 1991; Shellock and Crues 2004; Shellock and Kanal 1991; Wilde et al. 2005). Difficulties also have been encountered when a patient requires physiological monitoring during MRI. Several manufacturers have developed MRI-compatible respirators and monitors for blood pressure and heart rate. If these are not available, then the standard monitoring devices must be placed at least 8 feet from the magnet. Otherwise, the readout may be altered or the devices may interfere with obtaining the MRI scan.

Table 2–4.   Factors considered when choosing computed tomography (CT) or magnetic resonance imaging (MRI) examination

Clinical considerations	CT	MRI
Availability	Universal	Limited
Sensitivity	Good	Superior
Resolution	1.0 mm	1.0 mm
Average examination time	4–5 minutes	30–35 minutes
Plane of section	Axial only	Any plane of section
Conditions for which it is the preferred procedure	Screening examination Acute hemorrhage Calcified lesions Bone injury	All subcortical lesions Poison or toxin exposure Demyelinating disorders Eating disorders Examination requiring anatomical detail, especially temporal lobe or cerebellum Any condition best viewed in nonaxial plane
Contraindications	History of anaphylaxis or severe allergic reaction (contrast-enhanced CT) Creatinine ≥1.5 mg/dL (contrast-enhanced CT) Metformin administration on day of scan (contrast-enhanced CT)	Any magnetic metal in the body, including surgical clips and sutures Implanted electrical, mechanical, or magnetic devices Claustrophobia History of welding (requires skull films before MRI) Pregnancy (legal contraindication)

Source.   Adapted from Hurley RA, Fisher RE, Taber KH: "Clinical and Functional Imaging in Neuropsychiatry," in *Essentials of Neuropsychiatry and Behavioral Neurosciences,* 2nd Edition. Edited by Yudofsky SC, Hales RE. Washington, DC, American Psychiatric Publishing, 2010, pp. 55–93. Used with permission. Copyright © 2010 American Psychiatric Association.

Magnetic Resonance Imaging Versus Computed Tomography

The choice of imaging modality should be based on the anatomy and/or pathology that one desires to view (see "Conditions for Which It Is the Preferred Procedure" in Table 2–4). CT is used as an inexpensive screening examination. Also, a few conditions are best viewed with CT, including calcification, acute hemorrhage, and any bone injury, because these pathologies are not yet reliably imaged with MRI (Coles 2007). In the vast majority of cases, however, MRI is the preferred modality. This is mainly because most brain pathologies are more easily seen on MRI. In addition, gray-white contrast is clearer, and anatomical detail is often better. For example, demyelination resulting from poison exposure or autoimmune disease (e.g., multiple sclerosis) is far better seen on MRI than CT, especially when many small lesions are present. MRI does not produce the artifacts from bone that are seen in CT, so all lesions near bone (e.g., brain stem, posterior fossa, pituitary, hypothalamus) are better visualized with MRI.

Functional Imaging

Functional brain imaging techniques provide several ways of assessing brain physiology (McArthur et al. 2011; Otte and Halsband 2006). Regional cerebral blood flow (rCBF) and regional cerebral metabolic rate (rCMR) are the most broadly used measures (SPECT and PET, respectively). These both provide an indirect measure of brain activity. Neuronal activity consumes oxygen and metabolites and induces vasodilation of the nearby muscular arterioles, leading to a prompt increase in blood flow. A close coupling occurs between neuronal activity, rCBF, and rCMR, although the increase in blood flow, for unknown reasons, is more than is necessary to supply the increased demand for oxygen and glucose.

If acquired under resting conditions, rCMR and rCBF each provide a way to assess the baseline functional state of brain areas. Many functional brain imaging techniques can also be used as a patient performs a mental or physical task designed to activate specific neuronal pathways or structures; thus, brain activity under specific cognitive or affective conditions can be measured. Pharmacological challenges are also used. Neuronal activity can be directly assessed during activation tasks via measures of electrical activity (electroencephalography [EEG]) or magnetic activity (MEG). In addition, functional imaging techniques are available to measure various neurotransmitter receptor systems and regional brain metabolites. These techniques have been immensely helpful in laboratory study of multiple aspects of cognitive and emotional functioning, including learning, memory, emotional regulation, control of attention, and modulation of behavior. Differences between specific patient groups and healthy individuals have provided important insights into functional impairments that occur in some psychiatric diseases. Many research studies have been done of common psychiatric conditions such as major depressive disorder, schizophrenia, obsessive-compulsive disorder, and attention-deficit/hyperactivity disorder. Results have been quite variable, and therefore, clinical applications of functional imaging have been limited by the translation of this understanding to the individual patient.

Unlike structural imaging, functional imaging is dynamic and state dependent. Many factors can influence scan results of a particular individual on a particular day. Thus, the penetration of functional imaging into the clinical arena has been slower to evolve. Functional imaging is particularly useful for identification of "hidden" lesions, areas that are dysfunctional but do not look abnormal on structural imaging. Evaluation of the resting state also has shown potential for prediction of treatment response in some conditions. In general, patients whose clinical symptoms do not fit the classic historical picture for the working diagnosis should be considered for some form of functional imaging.

Nuclear Brain Imaging: Positron Emission Tomography and Single-Photon Emission Computed Tomography

Both PET and SPECT involve intravenous injection of a radioactive compound that distributes in the brain and emits (indirectly, in the case of PET) photons that are detected and used to form an image (McArthur et al. 2011; Otte and Halsband 2006). The tracer is a molecule whose chemical properties determine its distribution in the body (e.g., fluorodeoxyglucose distributes in cells in proportion to their glucose metabolic rate) and which contains one radioactive atom, called a *radionuclide*. Depending on the compound injected, the distribution of radioactivity indicates regional blood flow, metabolism, number of available neurotransmitter receptors, and so forth. Regional cerebral metabolism and cerebral perfusion are tightly linked under most physiological and pathophysiological conditions (Raichle 2003). Both types of imaging studies provide very similar functional information. Notably, in principle, almost any cellular function can be imaged by synthesizing a radioactive compound that crosses the blood-brain barrier and binds to a component of the relevant cellular machinery. For example, this has already been accomplished for adenylyl cyclase, protein kinase C, more than a dozen neurotransmitter receptors and transporters, and many other components of cellular biochemistry and physiology. Although these tracers are most useful in research, clinical applications for some are under development (McArthur et al. 2011; Otte and Halsband 2006).

Practical Considerations

Ordering the examination.   The nuclear medicine physician needs very clear clinical information on the imaging request form (not just "rule out pathology" or "new-onset mental status changes"). If a lesion is suspected in a particular location, the request form should include this suspicion. The imaging physician and technical staff also need information on the patient's current condition (e.g., delirious, psychotic, easily agitated, paranoid); this awareness may eliminate difficulties with patient management during tracer administration or scanning.

Patient preparation.   The psychiatrist should always explain the procedure to the patient shortly beforehand, being mindful to mention the requirement for absolute immobility during the approximately 30 minutes of scanning. Nuclear cameras are not nearly as confining as magnetic resonance scanners and very rarely cause claustrophobic reactions. Nonetheless, the scanning table is quite hard and can be uncomfortable for patients with back pain; pain medication may be worthwhile in some patients. If the psychiatrist suspects that the patient may become agitated or be unable to remain still for the length of the examination, then sedation may be necessary. Because of unknown effects on cerebral activity and blood flow, antianxiety medications and other sedative medications are best given after the tracer distribution in the brain has become fixed (approximately 5–10 minutes after injection for SPECT and 20–30 minutes after injection for PET). Such medications can be critical to achieving a successful scan in selected patients. A clinician may select a regimen with which he or she is familiar and comfortable. We have found that for patients with agitation and psychosis, a sedating antipsychotic with lorazepam 1–2 mg intramuscularly 30 minutes before scanning usually works well in a physically healthy nongeriatric adult. During imaging, the patient's head is generally held still with support from a head-holder attachment on the imaging table, sometimes with additional support from light taping.

In preparation for scanning, an intravenous line is inserted, and the patient is placed in a quiet and darkened room. Ten to 20 minutes later, a technologist enters the room quietly and injects the radioactive tracer. This procedure allows for decreased visual and auditory stimulation during tracer uptake. The patient typically remains in the room for 30–60 minutes, although the darkness and quiet are essential only during the tracer uptake period. For clinical SPECT, uptake occurs within 1–2 minutes of injection; for clinical PET, uptake requires 20–30 minutes. During the uptake period, the tracer distributes and is trapped in the tissue of interest. Theoretically, the patient could be imaged immediately following the uptake period; however, if the scan is delayed for at least 30 minutes, for tracer washout from adjacent facial and scalp areas, background activity is decreased and image quality is improved. The patient is then transported to the scanner, where the patient lies on the imaging table for about 30 minutes for the scan. If clinically necessary, scanning can be delayed for up to about 4 hours, although the activity in the brain gradually decreases from radioactive decay, resulting in gradually worsening image quality.

Understanding the scan.   Cerebral blood flow and cerebral metabolism are high in gray matter, where synapses and cell bodies are located. These measures are lower in white matter, composed of axons. Thus, tracer uptake is high in cellular areas, such as the thalami, basal ganglia, and cortex, and lower in white matter. Consequently, SPECT and PET are not good for evaluating white matter diseases.

The psychiatrist should review the images and radiology report with the nuclear medicine physician. It is important to remember that the radiographic view places the patient's right on the reader's left and the patient's left on the reader's right. After confirmation of patient identification, the psychiatrist should ask the nuclear medicine physician to point out normal anatomical markers and any pathology observed on the images. Note that PET and SPECT scans are always interpreted as digital images. Reasonable copies can be printed on photographic paper. However, paper reproductions are often quite suboptimal for image interpretation. Images printed on X-ray film are rarely diagnostically useful and should be avoided. Three-dimensional renderings are sometimes available.

SPECT Imaging

Technical considerations.   The two SPECT tracers approved for clinical use in the United States are technetium Tc 99m d,l-hexamethylpropyleneamine oxime (^{99m}Tc-HMPAO; Ceretec) and technetium Tc 99m ethyl cysteinate dimer (^{99m}Tc-ECD; Neurolite). Both tracers provide very comparable measures of cerebral blood flow (perfusion), with regional uptake roughly proportional to flow (McArthur et al. 2011; Otte and Halsband 2006). Uptake occurs during the first 1–2 minutes after injection. After that, the tracer is "fixed" in the brain. These tracers are lipophilic compounds that diffuse across the blood-brain barrier and into neurons and glia, where they are converted into hydrophilic compounds that cannot diffuse out of the cell. Abnormalities in intracellular esterase or glutathione metabolism, in neurons or glia, might lead to SPECT abnormalities independent of blood flow changes. In fact, evidence suggests that most tracer uptake, at least for HMPAO, may be in glial cells rather than in neurons (Slosman et al. 2001). An important fact to remember is that the uptake of tracer does not have to be within neurons to be useful. Uptake is used as an indirect indicator of neuronal electrochemical activity. Even if the uptake is mainly in glia, it has been shown to clearly reflect local cerebral blood flow, which is tightly linked to neuronal activity (Magistretti and Pellerin 1996). Although several differences between these two tracers have been described (Inoue et al. 2003), the two remain very comparable in terms of their clinical utility. A previously used perfusion tracer, N-isopropyl-p-[^{123}I]-iodoamphetamine, is no longer commercially available in the United States and is infrequently used elsewhere. SPECT tracers are commonly available for imaging the dopamine transporter in Europe and Asia, but this technique has not been approved by the U.S. Food and Drug Administration (Warwick 2004).

Safety and contraindications.   The only contraindication to a nuclear medicine scan is pregnancy, and even this is only a relative indication. If the brain scan can be postponed until after delivery, a small radiation dose to the fetus can be avoided. Although very rarely necessary, the study can be performed in uncommon situations in which the scan result is critical. It is important to recognize that the tracers used in all diagnostic nuclear medicine examinations are 1,000 to 1 million times too low a concentration to have any pharmacological effects or allergenic side effects (other than placebo effects). They disappear by radioactive decay, so renal and hepatic function tests are irrelevant. The radiation dose to the patient as a result of a nuclear brain scan is comparable to that of a CT scan and is generally considered to be without long-term consequences, although some controversy over this issue has arisen (see discussion in the "Technical Considerations" subsection of "Computed Tomography" earlier in this chapter).

PET Imaging

Technical considerations.   PET is based on imaging the distribution of a short-lived radioactive tracer (radiotracer) that has been introduced into the bloodstream (Cherry 2001; Fahey 2002; Otte and Halsband 2006; Paans et al. 2002; Turner and Jones 2003; Van Heertum et al. 2004). Several positron-emitting radionuclides are available for incorporation into tracers, but virtually all current clinical PET tracers use fluorine-18 (^{18}F). The most important PET tracer, and the only one approved for clinical use in the United States, is [^{18}F]fluorodeoxyglucose (FDG), which provides a map of glucose metabolism. This tracer is taken up into cells much as glucose is and undergoes metabolism to FDG-6-phosphate. It does not undergo further metabolism and is trapped within these cells, providing a measure of cerebral metabolic activity (rCMR glucose). Glucose uptake in PET images is likely to reside predominantly in glial cells, which convert glucose into lactate and provide the lactate to neurons as a key energy source for neurons (Magistretti and Pellerin 1996). It must be remembered that the uptake of tracer does not have to be within neurons; uptake is used as an indirect indicator of neuronal electrochemical activity. Even if the uptake is mainly in glia, it has been shown to clearly reflect local cerebral glucose metabolism, which is tightly linked to neuronal activity.

Safety and contraindications.   The safety considerations and contraindications are the same as for SPECT (see prior section).

Clinical Applications

SPECT versus PET.   Nuclear brain imaging is coming into increasing use for the clinical evaluation and case formulation of psychiatric patients (Malhi and Lagopoulos 2008; Otte and Halsband 2006). SPECT and PET can contribute to differential diagnosis, assist in treatment planning, and provide information for prognostic decisions. PET has the advantages of higher spatial resolution and true attenuation correction (nearly eliminating attenuation artifacts). SPECT has the advantages of being more widely available, less expensive, and reimbursable for most conditions. Reimbursement for brain PET in the United States is currently limited to distinguishing frontotemporal dementia from Alzheimer's disease, doing presurgical evaluation of intractable epilepsy (seizure focus localization), and distinguishing radiation necrosis from recurrent brain tumors. SPECT imaging is considered a standard clinical investigative tool for neuropsychiatric evaluation. However, PET scanners are rapidly becoming more commonplace, and reimbursement for other indications is likely to occur in the near future. The old requirement for an on-site cyclotron has been obviated by the establishment of numerous commercial cyclotrons throughout the United States, many of which can deliver an ^{18}F tracer (110-minute half-life) great distances by airplane. Virtually any hospital in the United States with a PET scanner can have [^{18}F]-FDG delivered to it relatively inexpensively. Tracers that use carbon-11 (20-minute half-life), oxygen-15 (2-minute half-life), or nitrogen-13 (10-minute half-life) require an on-site cyclotron facility.

SPECT and PET in neuropsychiatry.   In neuropsychiatry, perfusion SPECT and glucose metabolism PET are used primarily in the diagnostic workup of patients with dementia. Both types of imaging have reasonably high diagnostic accuracy in distinguishing Alzheimer's disease from frontotemporal dementia (currently the only reimbursable indication for brain PET in patients with dementia) and in distinguishing neurodegenerative disease from other causes of dementia and from pseudodementia. PET is generally superior to SPECT because of higher resolution and better attenuation correction. PET is more expensive and less widely available than SPECT, although both of these issues are rapidly improving. Both modalities have a clearly defined role in the preoperative evaluation of patients with medically refractory epilepsy, with ictal perfusion SPECT showing the best results. There is currently much excitement over new PET tracers that directly bind to amyloid in the brain. These tracers recently have been shown to accurately distinguish Alzheimer's disease from other dementias and to fairly accurately predict which patients with mild cognitive impairment will progress rapidly to Alzheimer's disease (Vallabhajosula 2011). They have not yet, however, been proven superior to standard FDG PET imaging, which is quite good for both purposes.

Both SPECT and PET are sensitive and reasonably specific for vascular disease, but a specific clinical role has yet to be defined. Acetazolamide stress perfusion SPECT shows promise for determining clinical significance of borderline vascular obstructions and for selecting patients who need intervention. Clinical benefit for these potential indications, however, has yet to be proven. Both modalities are very sensitive in detecting neuronal injury in patients with mild traumatic brain injuries. However, false-positive scans are a concern, and the clinical significance of positive scans in patients with brain trauma has yet to be fully determined. The routine clinical application of nuclear imaging to patients with mood disorders, attention-deficit/hyperactivity disorder, schizophrenia, obsessive-compulsive disorder, and other psychiatric disorders has been disappointing, despite numerous abnormalities reported in research studies. Perhaps more promising for these disorders is the use of neurotransmitter SPECT and PET. Such studies, particularly dopamine transporter SPECT, have already shown excellent accuracy and clinical utility in patients with movement disorders, especially Parkinson's disease and related disorders. DaTscan, a tracer that binds to the dopamine transporter, was approved by the FDA for clinical use in patients with suspected Parkinson's disease in 2011 and now is available for routine clinical use in the United States. Imaging of receptors and transporters may eventually play an important role in the diagnosis and management of many neuropsychiatric illnesses.

Functional Magnetic Resonance Imaging

fMRI is based on the modulation of image intensity by the oxygenation state of blood. Deoxygenated hemoglobin (deoxyhemoglobin) is highly paramagnetic. It distorts the local magnetic field in its immediate vicinity. This causes a loss of magnetic resonance signal, particularly on gradient echo and other susceptibility-weighted pulse sequences. Thus, deoxyhemoglobin is a natural magnetic resonance contrast agent. Image intensity is dependent on the local balance between oxygenated and deoxygenated hemoglobin; this is the origin of the acronym BOLD (blood oxygen level dependent) for the fMRI technique (Otte and Halsband 2006; Sava and Yurgelun-Todd 2008; Taber et al. 2003; Turner and Jones 2003).

An area of brain suddenly becomes more active when it is participating in a cognitive task. The increase in local blood flow is larger than is required to meet the activity-related increase in oxygen consumption. As a result, the venous blood becomes slightly *more* oxygenated. This decrease in local deoxyhemoglobin concentration causes a slight (1%–5%) increase in signal intensity in the activated area of brain on the magnetic resonance image. The change is too small to see by eye. It is measured by comparing signal intensity under a baseline (resting or control) condition with signal intensity under an activated condition. Unlike PET or SPECT, all fMRI measures depend on comparison of two conditions (e.g., baseline and activated).

A problem with the most commonly used fMRI methods is the presence of susceptibility-related artifacts in areas of magnetic field inhomogeneity, such as the interfaces between brain, bone, and air. Thus, regions of importance to neuropsychiatry that are adjacent to bone, such as the orbitofrontal cortex and the inferior temporal region, may be difficult to assess. It is also important to differentiate areas of increased signal within activated tissue itself from increased signal in the veins that drain the activated area. Motion artifacts can also be a problem. Any movement (minor head movement, respiration, speech-related movement) can create spurious areas of activation and mask areas of true activation. Head restraints and postprocessing are both important in this regard (Bizzi et al. 1993; Desmond and Annabel Chen 2002; Matthews and Jezzard 2004; Taber et al. 2003; Turner and Jones 2003).

fMRI has several advantages over other methods of imaging brain activity. Most important, it is totally noninvasive and requires no ionizing radiation or radiopharmaceuticals. Minimal risk makes it appropriate for use in both children and adults and for use in longitudinal studies requiring multiple scanning sessions for each subject. High-resolution structural images are acquired in the same session, providing much better localization of areas of interest than is possible with PET or SPECT. In addition, most clinical MRI scanners can be modified without great expense to enable fMRI. However, fMRI is neither simple nor easy to implement and analyze, which may limit its clinical usefulness. At present, it should be considered a research technique (Sava and Yurgelun-Todd 2008).

Normal Imaging Anatomy

The practicing psychiatrist needs to have a basic understanding of the cortical and subcortical anatomy involved in thought, memory, and emotion if he or she is to use information gathered from imaging. The psychiatrist must have sufficient knowledge to identify these structures on neuroimaging in the various planes of section. In addition, the psychiatrist must have the ability to identify clinical scenarios that warrant imaging investigation for lesions (e.g., traumatic brain injury, stroke, poison and toxin exposure). Thought, memory, and emotion are believed to occur by way of complicated circuits or networks of interconnected areas of brain. Lesions at any point in a circuit can potentially give rise to identical symptoms (Burruss et al. 2000; Dalgleish 2004; Filley 2010; Naumescu et al. 1999; Taber et al. 2004; Tekin and Cummings 2002). A comprehensive review of these circuits is beyond the scope of this chapter. With the advent of graphic programs and computer technology, many three-dimensional models are available that make these circuits easier to understand.

Recommended Readings

Anderson KE, Taber KH, Hurley RA: Functional imaging, in Textbook of Traumatic Brain Injury. Edited by Silver JM, McAllister TW, Yudofsky SC. Washington, DC, American Psychiatric Publishing, 2005, pp 107–133

Coles JP: Imaging after brain injury. Br J Anaesth 99:49–60, 2007

Dalgleish T: The emotional brain. Nat Rev Neurosci 5:583–589, 2004

Erhart SM, Young AS, Marder SR, et al: Clinical utility of magnetic resonance imaging radiographs for suspected organic syndromes in adult psychiatry. J Clin Psychiatry 66:968–973, 2005

Gupta A, Elheis M, Pansari K: Imaging in psychiatric illness. Int J Clin Pract 58:850–858, 2004

Schmahmann JD: Disorders of the cerebellum: ataxia, dysmetria of thought, and the cerebellar cognitive affective syndrome. J Neuropsychiatry Clin Neurosci 16:367–378, 2004

Tekin S, Cummings JL: Frontal-subcortical neuronal circuits and clinical neuropsychiatry—an update. J Psychosom Res 53:647–654, 2002

References

Arakia Y, Ashikaga R, Fujii K, et al: MR fluid-attenuated inversion recovery imaging as routine brain T2-weighted imaging. Eur J Radiol 32:136–143, 1999

Baker JF, Kratz LC, Stevens GR, et al: Pharmacokinetics and safety of the MRI contrast agent gadoversetamide injection (OptiMARK) in healthy pediatric subjects. Invest Radiol 39:334–339, 2004

Beresford TP, Blow FC, Hall RCW, et al: CT scanning in psychiatric inpatients: clinical yield. Psychosomatics 27:105–112, 1986

Bizzi A, Righini A, Turner R, et al: MR of diffusion slowing in global cerebral ischemia. AJNR Am J Neuroradiol 14:1347–1354, 1993

Bourland JD, Nyenhuis JA, Schaefer DJ: Physiologic effects of intense MR imaging gradient fields. Neuroimaging Clin N Am 9:363–377, 1999

Branton T: Use of computerized tomography by old age psychiatrists: an examination of criteria for investigation of cognitive impairment. Int J Geriatr Psychiatry 14:567–571, 1999

Bulte JW: MR contrast agents for molecular and cellular imaging (editorial). Curr Pharm Biotechnol 5:483, 2004

Burruss JW, Hurley RA, Taber KH, et al: Functional neuroanatomy of the frontal lobe circuits. Radiology 214:227–230, 2000

Chanraud S, Zahr N, Sullivan EV, et al: MR diffusion tensor imaging: a window into white matter integrity of the working brain. Neuropsychol Rev 20:209–225, 2010

Cherry S: Fundamentals of positron emission tomography and applications in preclinical drug development. J Clin Pharmacol 41:482–491, 2001

Cochran ST: Anaphylactoid reactions to radiocontrast media. Curr Allergy Asthma Rep 5:28–31, 2005

Cochran ST, Bomyea K, Sayre JW: Trends in adverse events after IV administration of contrast media. AJR Am J Roentgenol 178:1385–1388, 2002

Cohan RH, Matsumoto JS, Quagliano PV: ACR Manual on Contrast Media, 4th Edition. Reston, VA, American College of Radiology, 1998

Coles JP: Imaging after brain injury. Br J Anaesth 99:49–60, 2007

Dalgleish T: The emotional brain. Nat Rev Neurosci 5:583–589, 2004

De Backer AI, Mortelé KJ, De Keulenaer BL: Considerations for planning and implementation. JBR-BTR 87:241–246, 2004a

De Backer AI, Mortelé KJ, De Keulenaer BL: Picture archiving and communication system, part 1: filmless radiology and distance radiology. JBR-BTR 87:234–241, 2004b

Desmond JE, Annabel Chen SH: Ethical issues in the clinical application of fMRI: factors affecting the validity and interpretation of activations. Brain Cogn 50:482–497, 2002

Detre JA, Alsop DC: Arterial spin labeled perfusion magnetic resonance imaging, in Imaging of the Nervous System. Edited by Latchaw RE, Kucharczyk J, Moseley ME. Philadelphia, PA, Elsevier Mosby, 2005, pp 323–331

Diwadkar VA, Keshavan MS: Newer techniques in magnetic resonance imaging and their potential for neuropsychiatric research. J Psychosom Res 53:677–685, 2002

Dong Q, Welsh RC, Chenevert TL, et al: Clinical applications of diffusion tensor imaging. J Magn Reson Imaging 19:6–18, 2004

Erhart SM, Young AS, Marder SR, et al: Clinical utility of magnetic resonance imaging radiographs for suspected organic syndromes in adult psychiatry. J Clin Psychiatry 66:968–973, 2005

Fahey FH: Data acquisition in PET imaging. J Nucl Med Technol 30:39–40, 2002

Federle MP, Willis LL, Swanson DP: Ionic versus nonionic contrast media: a prospective study of the effect of rapid bolus injection on nausea and anaphylactoid reaction. J Neurol Sci 22:341–345, 1998

Filippi M, Rocca MA: Magnetization transfer magnetic resonance imaging in the assessment of neurological diseases. J Neuroimaging 14:303–313, 2004

Filley CM: White matter: organization and functional relevance. Neuropsychol Rev 20:158–173, 2010

Gupta A, Elheis M, Pansari K: Imaging in psychiatric illness. Int J Clin Pract 58:850–858, 2004

Hall P, Adami HO, Trichopoulos D, et al: Effect of low doses of ionising radiation in infancy on cognitive function in adulthood: Swedish population based cohort study. BMJ 328:19, 2004

Haller S, Pereira VM, Lazeyras F, et al: Magnetic resonance imaging techniques in white matter disease. Top Magn Reson Imaging 20:301–312, 2009

Halpern JD, Hopper KD, Arredondo MG, et al: Patient allergies: role in selective use of nonionic contrast material. Radiology 199:359–362, 1999

Halpin SF: Brain imaging using multislice CT: a personal perspective. Br J Radiol 77:S20–S26, 2004

Hanyu H, Asano T, Sakurai H, et al: Magnetization transfer ratio in cerebral white matter lesions of Binswanger's disease. J Neurol Sci 1:87–89, 1999

Hartwig V, Giovannetti G, Vanello N, et al: Biological effects and safety in magnetic resonance imaging: a review. Int J Environ Res Public Health 6:1778–1798, 2009

Hoffmann A, Faber SC, Werhahn KJ, et al: Electromyography in MRI—first recordings of peripheral nerve activation caused by fast magnetic field gradients. Magn Reson Med 43:534–539, 2000

Hopper KD, Neuman JD, King SH, et al: Radioprotection to the eye during CT scanning. AJNR Am J Neuroradiol 22:1194–1198, 2001

Huisman TAGM: Diffusion-weighted imaging: basic concepts and application in cerebral stroke and head trauma. Eur Radiol 13:2283–2297, 2003

Hurley RA, Hayman LA, Taber KH: Clinical imaging in neuropsychiatry, in The American Psychiatric Publishing Textbook of Neuropsychiatry and Clinical Neurosciences, 4th Edition. Edited by Yudofsky SC, Hales RE. Washington, DC, American Psychiatric Publishing, 2002, pp 245–283

Hurley RA, Ernst T, Khalili K, et al: Identification of HIV associated progressive multifocal leukoencephalopathy: magnetic resonance imaging and spectroscopy. J Neuropsychiatry Clin Neurosci 15:1–6, 2003

Inoue E, Nakagawa M, Goto R, et al: Regional differences between 99mTC-ECD and 99mTc-HMPAO SPET in perfusion changes with age and gender in healthy adults. Eur J Nucl Med Mol Imaging 30:489–497, 2003

Jacobs JE, Birnbaum BA, Langlotz CP: Contrast media reactions and extravasation: relationship to intravenous injection rates. Radiology 209:411–416, 1998

Jung SL, Kim BS, Lee KS, et al: Magnetic resonance imaging and diffusion-weighted imaging changes after hypoglycemic coma. J Neuroimaging 15:193–196, 2005

Kanal E, Broome DR, Martin DR, et al: Response to the FDA's May 23, 2007, nephrogenic systemic fibrosis update. Radiology 246:11–14, 2008

Kaplan H, Sadock B, Grebb J: The brain and behavior, in Kaplan and Sadock's Synopsis of Psychiatry: Behavioral Sciences, Clinical Psychiatry, 7th Edition. Edited by Kaplan H, Sadock BJ, Graff JA. Baltimore, MD, Williams & Wilkins, 1994, pp 112–125

Kirchin MA, Runge VM: Contrast agents for magnetic resonance imaging: safety update. Top Magn Reson Imaging 14:426–435, 2003

Konen E, Konen O, Katz M, et al: Are referring clinicians aware of patients at risk from intravenous injection of iodinated contrast media? Clin Radiol 57:132–135, 2002

Kubicki M, Westin CF, Maier SE, et al: Uncinate fasciculus findings in schizophrenia: a magnetic resonance diffusion tensor imaging study. Am J Psychiatry 159:813–820, 2002

Kuhl CK, Textor J, Gieseke J, et al: Acute and subacute ischemic stroke at high-field-strength (3.0-T) diffusion-weighted MR imaging: intraindividual comparative study. Radiology 234:509–516, 2005

Kuo PH, Kanal E, Abu-Alfa AK, et al: Gadolinium-based MR contrast agents and nephrogenic systemic fibrosis. Radiology 242:647–649, 2007

Larson EB, Mack LA, Watts B, et al: Computed tomography in patients with psychiatric illnesses: advantage of a "rule-in" approach. Ann Intern Med 95:360–364, 1981

Latchaw RE: Cerebral perfusion imaging in acute stroke. J Vasc Interv Radiol 15:S29–S46, 2004

Magistretti PL, Pellerin L: The contribution of astrocytes to the 18F-2-deoxyglucose signal in PET activation studies. Mol Psychiatry 1:445–452, 1996

Malhi GS, Lagopoulos J: Making sense of neuroimaging in psychiatry. Acta Psychiatr Scand 117:100–117, 2008

Mascalchi M, Filippi M, Floris R, et al: Diffusion-weighted MR of the brain: methodology and clinical application. Radiol Med 109:155–197, 2005

Matthews PM, Jezzard P: Functional magnetic resonance imaging. J Neurol Neurosurg Psychiatry 75:6–12, 2004

McArthur C, Jampana R, Patterson J, et al: Applications of cerebral SPECT. Clin Radiol 66:651–661, 2011

Mega MS, Cummings JL: Frontal-subcortical circuits and neuropsychiatric disorders. J Neuropsychiatry Clin Neurosci 6:358–370, 1994

Mitchell DG: MR imaging contrast agents—what's in a name? J Magn Reson Imaging 7:1–4, 1997

Mortelé KJ, Olivia MR, Ondategui S, et al: Universal use of nonionic iodinated contrast medium for CT: evaluation of safety in a large urban teaching hospital. AJR Am J Roentgenol 184:31–34, 2005

Moseley ME, Sawyer-Glover A, Kucharczyk J: Magnetic resonance imaging principles and techniques, in Imaging of the Nervous System. Edited by Latchaw RE, Kucharczyk J, Moseley ME. Philadelphia, PA, Elsevier Mosby, 2005, pp 3–30

Nakamura H, Yamada K, Kizu O, et al: Effect of thin-section diffusion-weighted MR imaging on stroke diagnosis. AJNR Am J Neuroradiol 26:560–565, 2005

Naumescu I, Hurley RA, Hayman LA, et al: Neuropsychiatric symptoms associated with subcortical brain injuries. International Journal of Neuroradiology 5:51–59, 1999

Oi H, Yamazaki H, Matsushita M: Delayed vs. immediate adverse reactions to ionic and non-ionic low-osmolality contrast media. Radiat Med 15:23–27, 1997

Orrison WW Jr, Sanders JA: Clinical brain imaging: computerized axial tomography and magnetic resonance imaging, in Functional Brain Imaging. Edited by Orrison WW Jr, Lewine JD, Sanders JA, et al. St Louis, MO, Mosby–Year Book, 1995, pp 97–144

Otte A, Halsband U: Brain imaging tools in neurosciences. J Physiol Paris 99:281–292, 2006

Paans AMJ, van Waarde A, Elsinga PH, et al: Positron emission tomography: the conceptual idea using a multidisciplinary approach. Methods 27:195–207, 2002

Price RR: The AAPM/RSNA physics tutorial for residents: MR imaging safety considerations. Radiological Society of North America. Radiographics 19:1641–1651, 1999

Raichle ME: Functional brain imaging and human brain function. J Neurosci 23:3959–3962, 2003

Rauch S, Renshaw PF: Clinical neuroimaging in psychiatry. Harv Rev Psychiatry 2:297–312, 1995

Runge VM: Safety of magnetic resonance contrast media. Top Magn Reson Imaging 12:309–314, 2001

Runge VM, Lawrence RM, Wells JW: Principles of contrast enhancement in the evaluation of brain diseases: an overview. J Magn Reson Imaging 7:5–13, 1997

Sage MR, Wilson AJ, Scroop R: Contrast media and the brain: the basis of CT and MR imaging enhancement. Neuroimaging Clin N Am 8:695–707, 1998

Sava S, Yurgelun-Todd DA: Functional magnetic resonance imaging in psychiatry. Top Magn Reson Imaging 19:71–79, 2008

Scarabino T, Nemore F, Giannatempo GM, et al: 3.0 T magnetic resonance in neuroradiology. Eur J Radiol 48:154–164, 2003

Shellock FG: Bioeffects and safety considerations, in Magnetic Resonance Imaging of the Brain and Spine. Edited by Atlas SW. New York, Raven, 1991, pp 87–107

Shellock FG: Magnetic resonance safety update 2002: implants and devices. J Magn Reson Imaging 16:485–496, 2002

Shellock FG, Crues JV: MR procedures: biologic effects, safety, and patient care. Radiology 232:635–652, 2004

Shellock FG, Kanal E: Policies, guidelines, and recommendations for MR imaging safety and patient management. SMRI Safety Committee. J Magn Reson Imaging 1:97–101, 1991

Shellock FG, Kanal E: Safety of magnetic resonance imaging contrast agents. J Magn Reson Imaging 10:477–484, 1999

Slosman DO, Ludwig C, Zerarka S, et al: Brain energy metabolism in Alzheimer's disease: 99mTc-HMPAO SPECT imaging during verbal fluency and role of astrocytes in the cellular mechanism of 99mTc-HMPAO retention. Brain Res Brain Res Rev 36:230–240, 2001

Sundgren PC, Dong Q, Gomez-Hassan DM, et al: Diffusion tensor imaging of the brain: review of clinical applications. Neuroradiology 46:339–350, 2004

Sunshine JL: CT, MR imaging, and MR angiography in the evaluation of patients with acute stroke. J Vasc Interv Radiol 15:S47–S55, 2004

Symms M, Jäger HR, Schmierer K, et al: A review of structural magnetic resonance neuroimaging. J Neurol Neurosurg Psychiatry 75:1235–1244, 2004

Taber KH, Pierpaoli C, Rose SE, et al: The future for diffusion tensor imaging in neuropsychiatry. J Neuropsychiatry Clin Neurosci 14:1–5, 2002

Taber KH, Rauch SL, Lanius RA, et al: Functional magnetic resonance imaging: application to post traumatic stress disorder. J Neuropsychiatry Clin Neurosci 15:125–129, 2003

Taber KH, Wen C, Khan A, et al: The limbic thalamus. J Neuropsychiatry Clin Neurosci 16:127–132, 2004

Tanabe JL, Ezekiel F, Jagust WJ, et al: Magnetization transfer ratio of white matter hyperintensities in subcortical ischemic vascular dementia. AJNR Am J Neuroradiol 20:839–844, 1999

Taylor WD, Hsu E, Krishnan KRR, et al: Diffusion tensor imaging: background, potential, and utility in psychiatric research. Biol Psychiatry 55:201–207, 2004

Tekin S, Cummings JL: Frontal-subcortical neuronal circuits and clinical neuropsychiatry—an update. J Psychosom Res 53:647–654, 2002

Turner R, Jones T: Techniques for imaging neuroscience. Br Med Bull 65:3–20, 2003

Vallabhajosula S: Positron emission tomography radiopharmaceuticals for imaging brain beta-amyloid. Semin Nucl Med 41:283–299, 2011

Valls C, Andria E, Sanchez A, et al: Selective use of low-osmolality contrast media in computed tomography. Eur Radiol 13:2000–2005, 2003

Van Heertum RL, Greenstein FA, Tikofsky RS: 2-Deoxy-fluoroglucose-positron emission tomography imaging of the brain: current clinical applications with emphasis on the dementias. Semin Nucl Med 34:300–312, 2004

Warwick JM: Imaging of brain function using SPECT. Metab Brain Dis 19:113–123, 2004

Weinberger DR: Brain disease and psychiatric illness: when should a psychiatrist order a CAT scan? Am J Psychiatry 141:1521–1527, 1984

Wilde JP, Rivers AW, Price DL: A review of the current use of magnetic resonance imaging in pregnancy and safety implications for the fetus. Prog Biophys Mol Biol 87:335–353, 2005

Wolf GL: Paramagnetic contrast agents for MR imaging of the brain, in MR and CT Imaging of the Head, Neck, and Spine. Edited by Latchaw RE. St Louis, MO, Mosby–Year Book, 1991, pp 95–108

Yasuda R, Munechika H: Delayed adverse reactions to nonionic monomeric contrast-enhanced media. Invest Radiol 33:1–5, 1998

3

Delirium

Paula T. Trzepacz, M.D.
David J. Meagher, M.D., M.R.C.Psych.

Delirium is a commonly occurring neuropsychiatric syndrome primarily, but not exclusively, characterized by impairment in cognition, which causes a "confusional state." Delirium is an altered state of consciousness between normal alertness and awakeness and stupor or coma. Delirium may have a rapid, forceful onset with many symptoms, or it may be preceded by a subsyndromal delirium with gradual changes over the course of a few days, such as alterations in sleep pattern or aspects of cognition. Emergence from coma usually involves a period of delirium before normal consciousness is achieved, except in drug-induced comatose states (Ely and Dittus 2004; McNicoll et al. 2003).

Because delirium has a wide variety of underlying etiologies—identification of which is part of clinical management—it is considered a syndrome. Delirium may, however, represent dysfunction of a final common neural pathway that leads to its characteristic symptoms. Table 3–1 lists signs and symptoms of delirium that affect nearly every neuropsychiatric domain, including charac-

Table 3–1. Signs and symptoms of delirium

Diffuse cognitive deficits

Attention

Orientation (time, place, person)

Memory (short- and long-term; verbal and visual)

Visuoconstructional ability

Executive functions

Temporal course

Acute or abrupt onset

Fluctuating severity of symptoms over 24-hour period

Usually reversible

Subclinical syndrome may precede and/or follow the episode

Psychosis

Perceptual disturbances (especially visual), including illusions, hallucinations, metamorphopsia

Delusions (usually paranoid and poorly formed)

Thought disorder (tangentiality, circumstantiality, loose associations)

Sleep-wake disturbance

Fragmented throughout 24-hour period

Reversal of normal cycle

Sleeplessness

Psychomotor behavior

Hyperactive

Hypoactive

Mixed

Language impairment

Word-finding difficulty/dysnomia/paraphasia

Dysgraphia

Altered semantic content

Severe forms can mimic expressive or receptive aphasia

Table 3–1. Signs and symptoms of delirium *(continued)*

Altered or labile affect

Any mood can occur, usually incongruent to context

Anger or increased irritability common

Hypoactive delirium often mislabeled as depression

Lability (rapid shifts) common

Unrelated to mood preceding delirium

Source. Reprinted from Trzepacz PT, Meagher DJ: "Neuropsychiatric Aspects of Delirium," in *Essentials of Neuropsychiatry and Behavioral Neurosciences*, 2nd Edition. Edited by Yudofsky SC, Hales RE. Washington, DC, American Psychiatric Publishing, 2010, pp. 149–221. Used with permission. Copyright © 2010 American Psychiatric Association.

teristic features that help differentiate delirium from other psychiatric disorders. Its broad constellation of symptoms includes not only the diffuse cognitive deficits implicit for its diagnosis but also delusions, perceptual disturbances, affective lability, language abnormalities, disordered thought processes, sleep-wake cycle disturbance, and psychomotor changes.

Unlike symptoms of most other psychiatric disorders, those of delirium typically fluctuate in intensity over a 24-hour period, during which relatively lucid or quiescent periods often occur. In a study by Rudberg et al. (1997), daily Delirium Rating Scale (DRS) ratings of postoperative patients showed patterns in which symptoms diminished but reappeared consistent with either serial short episodes or diminution to subsyndromal levels.

Delirium can occur at any age, and the less mature neural pathways of children may put them at high risk. Although delirium in children is vastly understudied, descriptions indicate that symptoms are essentially identical to those in adults (Platt et al. 1994b; Prugh et al. 1980; Turkel et al. 2003, 2006).

Delirium is the accepted term to denote acute disturbances of global cognitive function, encompassing a unitary syndrome with multiple possible different etiologies, as defined in both DSM-IV (American Psychiatric Association 1994, 2000) and ICD-10 (World Health Organization 1992) research classification systems. Unfortunately, multiple synonyms, based on the etiology or setting in which delirium is encountered, persist both in the literature and between disciplines in clinical practice. Examples include *acute confusional state, intensive care unit (ICU) psychosis, hepatic encephalopathy, toxic psychosis, acute brain fail-*

ure, and *posttraumatic amnesia.* The term *reversible cognitive deficit* is used in geriatric literature but is poorly defined and is not synonymous with *delirium;* it could instead represent subclinical delirium or cognitive impairment related to many other causes (e.g., pain, poor sleep, medication adverse events). Research shows that DSM-IV delirium occurs after traumatic brain injury (Sherer et al. 2005), despite misnomers and poor recognition by nonpsychiatrists. Consistent and proper use of the term *delirium* will greatly enhance medical communication, diagnosis, and research.

Diagnosis

Diagnostic Criteria Systems

Diagnostic criteria for delirium first appeared in DSM-III (American Psychiatric Association 1980). Symptom rating scales for delirium began to appear around the time of DSM-III.

DSM-IV (as well as its text revision, DSM-IV-TR) has five categories of delirium: delirium due to 1) a general medical condition, 2) substance intoxication, 3) substance withdrawal, or 4) multiple etiologies, and 5) delirium not otherwise specified. This notation of etiology in DSM-IV is reminiscent of the first DSM (American Psychiatric Association 1952). The criteria are the same for each category (see Table 3–2) except Criterion D for multiple etiologies.

DSM-III through DSM-IV (and DSM-IV-TR) include the major criterion that describes altered state of consciousness, considered as either inattention or "clouding of consciousness." The elements of consciousness that are altered are not specified, nor is it clear how "clouding" differs from "level" of consciousness. Attentional disturbance distinguishes delirium from dementia, for which the first criterion is memory impairment. Attentional disturbances in delirium range from general, nonspecific reduction in alertness (typically associated with nicotinic, cholinergic, histaminergic, or adrenergic actions) to decreased selective focusing or sustaining of attention (which may be related to muscarinic cholinergic dysfunction). The contribution of attentional deficits to the altered awareness that occurs in delirium is insufficient by itself to account for other prominent symptoms—formal thought disorder, language and sleep-wake cycle disturbances, and other cognitive-perceptual deficits. Motor activity changes are also prominent but not required in DSM-IV.

Table 3–2. DSM-IV-TR criteria for delirium due to a general medical condition

A. Disturbance of consciousness (i.e., reduced clarity of awareness of the environment) with reduced ability to focus, sustain, or shift attention.

B. A change in cognition (such as memory deficit, disorientation, language disturbance) or the development of a perceptual disturbance that is not better accounted for by a preexisting, established, or evolving dementia.

C. The disturbance develops over a short period of time (usually hours to days) and tends to fluctuate during the course of the day.

D. There is evidence from the history, physical examination, or laboratory findings that the disturbance is caused by the direct physiological consequences of a general medical condition.

Source. Reprinted from the *Diagnostic and Statistical Manual of Mental Disorders,* 4th Edition, Text Revision. Washington, DC, American Psychiatric Association, 2000. Copyright © 2000 American Psychiatric Association. Used with permission.

The characteristic features of the temporal course of delirium—acute onset and fluctuation of symptoms—have constituted a separate criterion in DSM-III, DSM-III-R (American Psychiatric Association 1987), and DSM-IV. Temporal features assist in distinguishing delirium from most types of dementia.

Dysexecutive symptoms (impairment of prefrontal executive cognition) are not mentioned in any DSM edition, despite the importance of prefrontal involvement in delirium (Trzepacz 1994). Psychosis has not received much attention except in DSM-II (American Psychiatric Association 1968), despite the occurrence of delusions in about one-third of patients with delirium and hallucinations in slightly more (Meagher 2005; Morita et al. 2004; Webster and Holroyd 2000). Characteristic features of delusions (which are usually paranoid and poorly formed) and hallucinations (often visual) have not been specified in DSM criteria, despite their usefulness to the clinician.

The ICD-10 research diagnostic criteria for delirium are similar to DSM-IV criteria but diverge from them in that cognitive dysfunction is manifested by both memory impairment and disorientation, and also by a disturbance in sleep.

Less diagnostic emphasis on disorganized thinking in DSM-IV accounts for the greater sensitivity and inclusivity (but lower specificity) of the diagnosis in comparison to the earlier DSM systems and ICD-10.

Prodromal and Subsyndromal Symptoms

Although delirium is usually characterized by an acute onset replete with many symptoms, it may be subsyndromal. Matsushima et al. (1997) prospectively studied 10 cardiac care unit patients who met DSM-III-R criteria for delirium and 10 nondelirious control subjects and found that the former group had prodromal changes of background slowing on electroencephalography (EEG) (theta/alpha ratio) and sleep disturbance associated with changing consciousness. Duppils and Wikblad (2004) studied elderly hip surgery patients and found that in 62%, delirium was preceded by prodromal symptoms, including disorientation, calls for assistance, and anxiety, 2 days before full delirium. de Jonghe et al. (2005) studied delirium symptoms daily with the Delirium Rating Scale—Revised–98 (DRS-R-98) in elderly hip surgery patients. Disorientation, short- and long-term memory disturbance, and inattention occurred during the 3 days before emergence of full delirium, whereas sleep-wake cycle disturbance, hallucinations, and thought process disorder occurred 1 day before, suggesting that cognitive impairments precede sleep-wake and psychotic symptoms. Kaneko et al. (1999) found a close correlation between development of postoperative delirium and decreased nocturnal and excessive daytime sleep. Fann et al. (2005) found that both psychobehavioral and cognitive disturbances predated onset of full delirium by 4 days in patients undergoing bone marrow stem cell transplantation.

In a study of the relationship between cognitive status at admission and incident delirium in older medical inpatients, Franco et al. (2010) found many symptoms at intermediate severity in subsyndromal delirium. However, the following were comparable to full syndromal delirium: sleep-wake cycle; perceptual, motor, and short-term memory disturbances; affective lability; and acute onset. The best brief tool to assess for subsyndromal symptoms with a high degree of predictability has not been determined. Nonspecific symptoms such as anxiety or calls for assistance may be less useful than cognitive and sleep-wake items.

Subsyndromal Outcomes

Subsyndromal delirium symptoms in elderly persons may be associated with poorer prognosis, approaching that of the full syndrome. Cole et al. (2003) prospectively studied subsyndromal delirium in 164 elderly medical patients with one or more of four symptoms: clouding of consciousness, inattention, disorientation, and perceptual disturbances. More symptoms predicted worse prognosis, as evidenced by longer inpatient stays, poorer cognitive and functional status, and greater subsequent mortality at 12-month follow-up. Bourdel-Marchasson et al. (2004) found that subsyndromal delirium (equivalently to full syndromal delirium) predicted postdischarge need for institutional care among elderly patients admitted to medical facilities. Marcantonio et al. (2002) found that reduced independent-living status in elderly postoperative hip surgery patients with subsyndromal delirium was similar to that of patients with mild delirium when both groups were assessed at 6-month follow-up. Moreover, in postacute skilled nursing facilities, mortality rates for patients with subsyndromal delirium (18%) were lower than rates for patients with full delirium (25%) but significantly higher than rates for nondelirious patients (5%) (Marcantonio et al. 2005). Research is lacking in children and nongeriatric adults, in whom frailty, diminished cognitive reserve, and dementia are not confounding issues.

Misdiagnosis

Delirium frequently goes undetected in clinical practice. Between one-third and two-thirds of cases are missed across a range of therapeutic settings and by various specialists, including psychiatrists and neurologists (Johnson et al. 1992). Nonrecognition of delirium results in poorer outcomes, including increased mortality (Kakuma et al. 2003; Rockwood et al. 1994). Altered mental status was noted in only 16% of elderly emergency department patients with delirium (Hustey et al. 2003).

Misdiagnosis of delirium is more likely in patients who are older; who have sensory impairments, preexisting dementia, or a hypoactive presentation; or who are referred from surgical or intensive care settings (Armstrong et al. 1997; Inouye et al. 2001). Delirium is commonly misdiagnosed as depression by nonpsychiatrists (Farrell and Ganzini 1995; Nicholas and Lindsey 1995; Trzepacz et al. 1985). ICU populations have delirium prevalence rates ranging from 40% to 87% (Ely et al. 2001), but delirium is unfortunately understudied and neglected, either because it is "expected" to happen during severe illness or because medical resources are preferentially dedicated to managing more immediate, "life-threatening" problems.

The stereotyped image of delirium as an agitated psychotic state misrepresents most patients with delirium, who may not have psychotic symptoms or may have a hypoactive presentation (Meagher and Trzepacz 2000). Detection can be improved by assessing cognitive function, improving awareness of the varied presentations of delirium, and routinely using a screening tool (O'Keeffe et al. 2005; Rockwood et al. 1994).

Differential Diagnosis

Because delirium encompasses so many domains of higher cortical functions, its differential diagnosis is broad, and it can be mistaken for dementia, depression, primary or secondary psychosis, anxiety and somatoform disorders, and, particularly in children, behavioral disturbance (Table 3–3). Accurate diagnosis requires close attention to symptoms, temporal onset, results of tests (e.g., cognitive and laboratory measures, EEG), and charts, including medication lists and anesthesia records. Given that delirium can be the presentation for serious medical illness, any patient experiencing a sudden deterioration in cognitive function should be assessed for possible delirium. Urinary tract infections in nursing home patients commonly present as delirium. Delirium occurs commonly in stroke patients (Caeiro et al. 2004; Ferro et al. 2002) and is frequently the first indication of cerebrovascular accident (Wahlund and Bjorlin 1999).

Delirium Versus Dementia

The most difficult differential diagnosis for delirium is distinguishing it from dementia, the other cause of generalized cognitive impairment. Lewy body dementia has a more aggressive temporal course than Alzheimer's disease and mimics delirium, with fluctuation of symptom severity, visual hallucinations, attentional impairment, alteration of consciousness, and delusions (Robinson 2002). Dementia is a potent predisposing factor for the development of delirium and is often comorbid with delirium in elderly patients.

Despite this substantial overlap, delirium and dementia can be reliably distinguished by a combination of careful history taking for onset of characteristic symptoms and clinical investigation. Abrupt onset and fluctuating course are highly characteristic of delirium. In addition, attention is markedly disturbed in delirium but relatively intact in uncomplicated dementia, in which memory im-

Table 3–3. Differential diagnosis of delirium

	Delirium	Dementia	Depression	Schizophrenia
Onset	Acute	Insidious[a]	Variable	Variable
Course	Fluctuating	Often progressive	Diurnal variation	Variable
Reversibility	Usually[b]	Not usually	Usually but can be recurrent	No, but has exacerbations
Level of consciousness	Impaired	Unimpaired until late stages	Generally unimpaired	Unimpaired (perplexity in acute stage)
Attention and memory	Inattention is primary with poor memory	Poor memory without marked inattention	Mild attention problems, inconsistent pattern, memory intact	Poor attention, inconsistent pattern, memory intact
Hallucinations	Usually visual; can be auditory, tactile, gustatory, olfactory	Can be visual or auditory	Usually auditory	Usually auditory
Delusions	Fleeting, fragmented, usually persecutory	Paranoid, often fixed	Complex and mood congruent	Frequent, complex, systematized, often paranoid

[a]Except for large strokes, which can be abrupt, and Lewy body dementia, which can be subacute.
[b]Can be chronic (as in paraneoplastic syndrome, central nervous system adverse effects of medications, or severe brain damage).
Source.   Reprinted from Trzepacz PT, Meagher DJ: "Neuropsychiatric Aspects of Delirium," in *Essentials of Neuropsychiatry and Behavioral Neurosciences,* 2nd Edition. Edited by Yudofsky SC, Hales RE. Washington, DC, American Psychiatric Publishing, 2010, pp. 149–221. Used with permission. Copyright © 2010 American Psychiatric Association.

pairment is instead the cardinal feature. Dementia patients often awaken at night, mistaking it as daytime, whereas disruption of the sleep-wake cycle, including fragmentation throughout 24 hours or even sleeplessness, is more characteristic in patients with delirium.

Only a few studies have investigated differences in symptom profiles between patients with delirium and patients with dementia (O'Keeffe 1994; Trzepacz and Dew 1995). Trzepacz et al. (2002), using the DRS-R-98, noted significant differences (after Bonferroni correction) between delirium and dementia groups (who had been blindly evaluated) for sleep-wake cycle disturbances, thought process abnormalities, motor agitation, attention, and visuospatial ability, which were more impaired in delirium, but no differences for delusions, affective lability, language, motor retardation, orientation, or short- or long-term memory. Careful assessment can distinguish groups of patients with these two disorders, but more work is needed to clarify features that differentiate delirium and dementia and that can be considered in individual cases in clinical practice.

Even more challenging is distinguishing delirium from comorbid delirium-dementia. Most studies have found few differences between groups (Cole et al. 2002; Liptzin et al. 1993; Trzepacz et al. 1998; Voyer et al. 2006). Thus, it appears that when delirium and dementia are comorbid, the phenomenology of delirium generally overshadows that of the dementia, but when delirium and dementia are assessed as individual conditions, more symptoms can distinguish them, at least by mean scores. These research findings are consistent with the clinical rule of thumb for preventing misattribution of delirium to dementia— namely, that "altered cognition reflects delirium until proven otherwise."

Most tools used for delirium assessment have not been validated for their ability to distinguish delirium from dementia, although three have been—DRS (Trzepacz and Dew 1995), DRS-R-98 (Trzepacz et al. 2001, 2002), and Cognitive Test for Delirium (CTD; Hart et al. 1996). A simple visual attention span task differentiated patients with delirium from those with dementia (Meagher et al. 2010).

Although electroencephalographic abnormalities are common to both delirium and dementia, diffuse slowing occurs more frequently (81% vs. 33%) in delirium and favors its diagnosis. In contrast, electroencephalographic slowing occurs later in the course of most degenerative dementias, although slowing occurs sooner with viral and prion dementias. The percentage of theta activity on quantitative electroencephalograms allows differentiation of delirium from dementia (Jacobson and Jerrier 2000).

Delirium Versus Mood Disorders

Hypoactive delirium is frequently mistaken for depression (Nicholas and Lindsey 1995). Farrell and Ganzini (1995) found that more than half of delirious patients referred to a consultation-liaison service for "depression" had thoughts of death, and almost one-quarter had suicidal thoughts. Although some symptoms of major depression occur in delirium (e.g., psychomotor slowing, sleep disturbances, irritability), in patients with major depression, symptom onset tends to be less acute and mood disturbances tend to be more sustained and typically dominate the clinical picture.

The distinction of delirium from depression is particularly important because in addition to delayed treatment, use of antidepressants can aggravate delirium. The more widespread and profound cognitive changes of delirium, along with the etiological backdrop and differing clinical course, usually enable a firm distinction, and EEG can be diagnostic.

Delirium Versus Psychotic Disorders

Abnormalities of thought process and content and misperceptions can occur in both delirium and schizophrenia but manifest differently in these two disorders. Delusions in delirium are rarely as fixed or stereotyped as in schizophrenia, and first-rank symptoms are uncommon (Cutting 1987). Delusions are usually persecutory, and sometimes grandiose or somatic, and fragmented because they incorporate aspects of the environment that are poorly comprehended. Paranoid concerns about immediate well-being or perceived danger in the environment are common. Unlike in schizophrenia, hallucinations in delirium are more often visual and, on occasion, olfactory, tactile, or gustatory. Tactile hallucinations (including formications) often suggest a hyperdopaminergic or hypocholinergic state. Illusions are common in delirium, whereas depersonalization, derealization, and delusional misidentification are less common.

Level of consciousness, attention, and memory are generally unimpaired in schizophrenia. Careful physical examination, coupled with EEG and/or use of a delirium-specific instrument, distinguishes delirium or allows diagnosis of superimposed delirium in medically ill patients with schizophrenia.

Reversibility of a Delirium Episode

Delirium traditionally has been distinguished from dementia by delirium's potential for reversal and its transient neurobiological state. Bedford's (1959) study of delirium found that only 5% of the patients were still "confused" at 6-month follow-up. Elderly patients may not have full resolution of symptoms at hospital discharge. Levkoff et al. (1992) found that only 4% of the elderly patients with delirium had complete resolution of symptoms at discharge, 20.8% at 6 weeks, and 17.7% at 6 months, but the researchers did not exclude patients with comorbid dementia. McCusker et al. (2003) found that 12 months after diagnosis of delirium in elderly medical inpatients, inattention, disorientation, and poor memory were the most persistent individual symptoms both in those with and in those without concomitant dementia (see next subsection, "Persistent Cognitive Deficits").

One explanation for persisting impairments may be incomplete treatment or the recurring course of delirium (Meagher 2001a). The ever-increasing financial pressures to shorten hospital stays have resulted in many patients being discharged from the hospital before delirium has resolved, even though families and nursing homes are not resourced to manage delirium to its resolution. Kiely et al. (2004) studied 2,158 patients from seven Boston-area skilled nursing facilities and found that 16% of these patients had full-blown delirium. They warned of the adverse effect of delirium persisting in subacute care settings. Marcantonio et al. (2005) assessed 1,248 elderly patients soon after admission to postacute facilities and found that 15% had delirium and another 51% had subsyndromal delirium. Ongoing efforts to resolve delirium are important.

Persistent Cognitive Deficits

The term *persistent cognitive impairment* is used to describe the condition of an elderly patient in the weeks or months following a delirium episode during a medical-surgical hospitalization; however, the neuropsychological pattern and etiology of this impairment are not clear and are highly confounded by comorbid pathophysiologies that are difficult to measure. Possible causes of persistent cognitive difficulties in patients who have experienced delirium are shown in Figure 3–1.

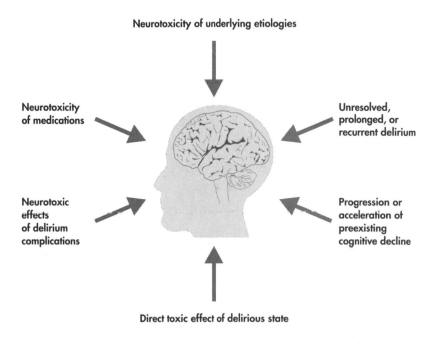

Figure 3–1. Possible reasons for persistent cognitive impairment in patients after an episode of delirium.

Source. Adapted from Trzepacz PT, Meagher DJ: "Neuropsychiatric Aspects of Delirium," in *Essentials of Neuropsychiatry and Behavioral Neurosciences,* 2nd Edition. Edited by Yudofsky SC, Hales RE. Washington, DC, American Psychiatric Publishing, 2010, pp. 149–221. Used with permission. Copyright © 2010 American Psychiatric Association.

The increased diagnosis of dementia in patients who have had an episode of delirium suggests a preexisting dementia heralded by the delirium. Kolbeinsson and Jonsson (1993) found that delirium was complicated by dementia at follow-up in 70% of patients. Rahkonen et al. (2000) found that when the index episode of delirium resolved, a new diagnosis of dementia was made in 27% of 51 prospectively studied community-dwelling elderly individuals, and during the 2-year follow-up, another 27% of the 51 individuals had a new diagnosis of dementia. Rockwood et al. (1999) reported an 18% annual incidence of dementia in patients with delirium—a more than three times higher risk than in nondelirious patients after the researchers adjusted for the confounding effects of comorbid illness severity and age.

Persistent cognitive deficits appear to indicate a previously undiagnosed dementia that progresses after delirium resolution. Among 252 community-dwelling older people, 64% had a new diagnosis of dementia that had gone previously undetected (Sternberg et al. 2000). Koponen et al. (1994), in a 5-year longitudinal study of delirium in elderly patients, attributed persistence and progression of symptoms more to the underlying dementia than to the previous delirium episode. Similarly, in a cross-sectional study of consecutive psychogeriatric admissions, the only factor significantly linked to incomplete symptom resolution in delirium was the presence of preexisting cognitive impairment (Camus et al. 2000). Cognitive impairment, even subtle, at hospitalization increases risk of delirium (Franco et al. 2010). Kasahara et al. (1996) compared delirium and dementia in two groups of alcoholic patients—adults ages 35–45 and adults age 60 and older—and found similar frequency of delirium in the two groups but no cases of dementia in the younger group, compared with 62% in the older group. Therefore, younger adults with delirium either have better brain recovery than do older adults or are at less risk for degenerative and vascular dementias that can be misattributed to delirium persistence and often go undetected on admission.

Assessment

Assessment Instruments

On the basis of issues such as instrument design, purpose, available translations, and breadth of use, we recommend a few of the various available instruments for the assessment of delirium (Table 3–4). These instruments can be used together or separately, depending on the clinical or research need. For example, a screening tool can be used for case detection, followed by a more thorough assessment for meeting DSM or ICD criteria and symptom severity.

Electroencephalography

In the 1940s, Engel and Romano (1944, 1959; Romano and Engel 1944) began a series of now-classic papers that described the relationship of delirium, as

Table 3–4. Recommended delirium assessment instruments

Instrument[a]	Type	Rater
Confusion Assessment Method (Inouye et al. 1990)	4-item diagnostic screener	Nonpsychiatric clinician
Confusion Assessment Method for ICU (Ely et al. 2001)	4-item diagnostic screener anchored by objective tests	ICU nurses
Delirium Rating Scale[b] (Trzepacz et al. 1988)	10-item severity/ diagnostic scale	Psychiatrically trained clinician
Memorial Delirium Assessment Scale (Breitbart et al. 1997)	10-item severity scale	Clinician
Delirium Rating Scale— Revised–98 (Trzepacz et al. 2001)	16-item scale (severity and diagnostic subscales)	Psychiatrically trained clinician
Cognitive Test for Delirium (Hart et al. 1996)	5 cognitive domains as bedside test	Trained technician or clinician

Note. ICU=intensive care unit.
[a]See text for descriptions of the instruments.
[b]Has been used in children.
Source. Reprinted from Trzepacz PT, Meagher DJ: "Neuropsychiatric Aspects of Delirium," in *Essentials of Neuropsychiatry and Behavioral Neurosciences,* 2nd Edition. Edited by Yudofsky SC, Hales RE. Washington, DC, American Psychiatric Publishing, 2010, pp. 149–221. Used with permission. Copyright © 2010 American Psychiatric Association.

measured by cognitive impairment, to electroencephalographic slowing. In their seminal work, they showed an association between abnormal electrical activity of the brain and the psychiatric symptoms of delirium; the reversibility of both conditions; the ubiquity of electroencephalographic changes in different underlying disease states; and an improvement in electroencephalographic background rhythm that paralleled clinical improvement. The thalamus drives the normal awake, resting alpha rhythm, and cholinergic activity is necessary such that anticholinergic agents cause slowing of the dominant posterior rhythm. Abnormalities in evoked potentials support a role for the thalamus in delirium (Trzepacz et al. 1989).

Electroencephalographic characteristics in delirium include slowing or dropping out of the dominant posterior rhythm, diffuse theta or delta waves (i.e., slowing), poor organization of background rhythm, and loss of reactivity on EEG to eye opening and closing (Jacobson and Jerrier 2000). Similarly, quantitative EEG (QEEG) in patients with delirium shows parallel findings affecting slowing of power bands' mean frequency as compared with nondelirious control subjects.

Different electroencephalographic patterns, from a variety of causes, can be seen clinically in patients with delirium. These include diffuse slowing, low-voltage fast activity, spikes/polyspikes (frontocentral), left/bilateral slowing or delta bursts, frontal intermittent rhythmic delta, and epileptiform activity (frontotemporal or generalized). Although diffuse slowing is the most common presentation, false-negative results occur when a person's characteristic dominant posterior rhythm does not slow sufficiently to drop from the alpha to the theta range, thereby being read as normal despite the presence of abnormal slowing for that individual. (Generally, a change of more than 1 Hz from an individual's baseline is considered abnormal.) Comparison with prior baseline electroencephalograms is often helpful to document that slowing has in fact occurred. Less commonly, but nonetheless important, EEG may detect focal problems, such as ictal and subictal states or a previously unsuspected tumor that presents with prominent confusion. These problems include toxic ictal psychosis, nonconvulsive status, and complex partial status epilepticus (Drake and Coffey 1983; Trzepacz 1994) or focal lesions (Jacobson and Jerrier 2000). New-onset complex partial seizures, related to ischemic damage, are underappreciated in elderly people (Sundaram and Dostrow 1995). Jacobson and Jerrier (2000) warned that it can be difficult to distinguish delirium from drowsiness and light sleep unless the technologist includes standard alerting procedures during EEG. In most cases, EEG is not needed to make a clinical diagnosis of delirium and is used instead when seizures are suspected or differential diagnosis is difficult, such as in schizophrenic patients with medical illness.

More recent advances in electroencephalographic technologies have expanded knowledge about delirium. Koponen et al. (1989) used spectral analysis of elderly patients with delirium (about 75% of whom also had dementia) and found significant reductions in alpha percentage, increased theta and delta activity, and slowing of the peak and mean frequencies. All of these findings are consistent with electroencephalographic slowing. The authors also found a correlation between the severity of cognitive decline and length of the patient's hospital stay and the degree of electroencephalographic slowing. Jacobson et al. (1993a) found that QEEG could be used to distinguish delirious from nondelirious individuals with the relative power of the alpha frequency band and could distinguish delirious from patients with dementia according to theta activity and the relative power of the delta band. Serial electroencephalograms of delirious patients showed associations between the relative power of the alpha band and cognitive ability, whereas in patients with dementia, the absolute power of the delta band was associated with cognitive changes (Jacobson et al. 1993b). QEEG potentially could replace conventional EEG for delirium assessment in the future (Jacobson and Jerrier 2000).

Evoked potentials also may be abnormal in patients with delirium, suggesting thalamic or subcortical involvement in the production of symptoms. Metabolic causes of delirium precipitate abnormalities in visual, auditory, and somatosensory evoked potentials (Kullmann et al. 1995; Trzepacz et al. 1989), whereas somatosensory evoked potentials are abnormal in patients whose delirium is due to posttraumatic brain injury, suggesting damage to the medial lemniscus. In general, normalization of evoked potentials parallels clinical improvement, although evoked potentials are not routinely recorded for clinical purposes.

EEG and evoked potential testing in children with delirium result in patterns similar to those in adults, with diffuse slowing on electroencephalograms and increased latencies of evoked potentials (Katz et al. 1988; Okumura et al. 2005; Prugh et al. 1980; Ruijs et al. 1993, 1994). The degree of slowing on electroencephalograms and increased latencies of evoked potentials recorded serially over time in children and adolescents correlate with the severity of delirium and with recovery from delirium (Foley et al. 1981; Montgomery et al. 1991; Onofrj et al. 1991).

Phenomenology

Symptom Frequency

Wolff and Curran's (1935) classic descriptive report of 106 consecutive patients with "dysergastic reaction" is still consistent with modern-day notions of delirium symptoms. Inconsistent terminology, unclear definitions of symptoms, and underuse of standardized symptom assessment tools have hampered subsequent efforts to describe delirium phenomenology more carefully or to compare symptom incidences across studies and etiological populations (Meagher and Trzepacz 1998). Most studies are cross-sectional, so an understanding of how various symptoms change over the course of an episode is lacking.

More recent longitudinal research that included daily delirium ratings has focused on total scale scores and not the occurrence of individual symptoms and their pattern over time. Rudberg et al. (1997) used the DRS and DSM-III-R criteria for daily ratings of 432 medical-surgical patients age 65 years and older at a university hospital. They found that 63 of the patients (15%) experienced delirium; in 69% of these patients, the delirium lasted for only a day. Mean DRS scores on day 1 were significantly higher (i.e., worse) in those patients whose delirium occurred for multiple days than in those whose delirium lasted 1 day, suggesting a relation between severity and duration in delirium episodes. Marcantonio et al. (2003) studied delirium symptom progression measured with nursing staff ratings of minimum data set symptoms over the first week after admission to post–acute care facilities. The authors noted that all six symptoms measured (distractibility, altered perception, disorganized speech, restlessness, lethargy, and mental fluctuation) persisted in two-thirds of patients, with symptoms worsening in 12%. Fann et al. (2005) prospectively studied patients undergoing hematopoietic stem cell transplantation with thrice-weekly assessments with the DRS and Memorial Delirium Assessment Scale (MDAS) from pretransplantation to day 30 posttransplantation. They found that neuropsychiatric features (psychomotor changes, sleep-wake cycle disturbance, and psychotic symptoms) dominated in the early phases but that cognitive impairment peaked 1 week into delirium and dominated thereafter.

Despite across-study inconsistencies (see Table 3–5) for symptom frequencies, certain symptoms occur more often than others, consistent with the proposal that delirium has core symptoms irrespective of etiology (Trzepacz 1999, 2000). In the more recent studies, DRS-R-98 was used to assess more symptoms with greater consistency than was possible in prior studies. Only one study reported symptoms in children (Turkel et al. 2006) that differed significantly from those in adults: less frequent delusions, more fluctuation of symptoms, greater sleep-wake cycle disturbance, more affective lability, and more agitation. However, none of those adult studies used the DRS-R-98, and generally symptom collection was neither well standardized nor comprehensive. In contrast, Turkel et al.'s (2006) data in children showed frequencies more consistent with the adult DRS-R-98 studies.

Multiple etiologies for delirium may "funnel" into a final common neural pathway (Trzepacz 1999, 2000) so that the phenomenological expression becomes similar despite a breadth of different physiologies. This "funneling" implies, as well, that certain brain circuits and neurotransmitter systems are more affected (Trzepacz 1994, 1999, 2000).

Core Symptoms

Candidates for "core" symptoms of delirium include attentional deficits, memory impairment, disorientation, sleep-wake cycle disturbance, thought process abnormalities, language disturbances, and motor alterations, whereas "associated" or noncore symptoms would include perceptual disturbances (illusions, hallucinations), delusions, and affective changes (Trzepacz 1999). Analysis of DRS-R-98 blinded ratings supports this separation of so-called core from associated symptoms on the basis of their relative prevalence (Trzepacz et al. 2001). Occurrence of the less frequent associated symptoms might suggest involvement of particular etiologies and their specific pathophysiologies or individual differences in brain circuitry and vulnerability.

The severity of symptoms in delirium typically fluctuates over any 24-hour period, unlike that in most other psychiatric disorders. Symptom fluctuation is thus an important indicator of delirium and is emphasized in diagnostic classifications (American Psychiatric Association 1994, 2000; World Health Organization 1992). During this characteristic waxing and waning of symptoms, relatively lucid or quiescent periods pose challenges for accurate diagnosis and severity ratings. Some lucid periods may restore enough capacity for patients to communicate their management choices (Bostwick and Masterson 1998). The underlying reason for this fluctuation in symptom severity is not understood; it may relate to shifts between hypoactive and hyperactive periods or fragmentations of the sleep-wake cycle, including daytime rapid eye movement sleep and circadian disturbances.

Historically, delirium has been viewed by some neurologists primarily as a disturbance of attention; less importance has been attributed to its other cognitive deficits and behavioral symptoms. Attentional disturbance is the cardinal symptom required for diagnosis of delirium yet is unlikely to explain the breadth of delirium symptoms. The nondominant posterior parietal and pre-

Table 3–5.   Studies of delirium phenomenology

	Frequency (%) in children	Frequencies (%) from adult studies that used various classifications	Frequencies (%) from studies that used DRS-R-98
Disorientation	77	43, 70, 78, 80, 88, 94, 96, 100	76, 96
Attentional deficits	100	17, 62, 100, 100, 100	97, 100
Sustained attention		89	
Shifting attention		87	
Clouded consciousness	93	58, 65, 65, 87, 91, 100	
Memory impairment (unspecified)	52	64, 90, 95, 100	
Short-term memory			88, 92
Long-term memory			89, 96
Visuospatial impairment			87, 96
Language abnormalities		41, 47, 62, 76, 93	57, 67
Disorganized thinking/thought process abnormalities		57, 64, 76, 95	54, 79
Incoherence		77	
Sleep-wake cycle disturbance	98	25, 49, 77, 95, 96	92, 97
Perceptual disturbance/hallucinations	43	24, 35, 35, 41, 45, 46, 71	50, 63
Delusions		18, 19, 25, 37, 38, 45, 68	21, 31
Affective lability/emotional disturbance	79	43, 63, 97, 97	53, 54

Table 3–5. Studies of delirium phenomenology (*continued*)

	Frequency (%) in children	Frequencies (%) from adult studies that used various classifications	Frequencies (%) from studies that used DRS-R-98
Apathy	68	86	
Anxiety	61	55	
Irritability	86		
Psychomotor changes (general)		38, 53, 55, 83, 88, 92, 93	
Motor agitation	69	59	62, 79
Motor retardation		71	29, 62

Note.   DRS-R-98 = Delirium Rating Scale—Revised–98.
Source.   Reprinted from Trzepacz PT, Meagher DJ: "Neuropsychiatric Aspects of Delirium," in *Essentials of Neuropsychiatry and Behavioral Neurosciences,* 2nd Edition. Edited by Yudofsky SC, Hales RE. Washington, DC, American Psychiatric Publishing, 2010, pp. 149–221. Used with permission. Copyright © 2010 American Psychiatric Association.

frontal cortices, as well as the brain stem and anteromedial thalamus, play roles in subserving attention, but other brain regions are likely to be involved in other symptoms of delirium. Distractibility, inattention, and poor environmental awareness can be evident during interview and on formal testing. Attentional impairment was found in 100% of delirium patients in a blinded assessment with the DRS-R-98 (Trzepacz et al. 2001). O'Keeffe and Gosney (1997) found that attentional deficits discriminated delirium patients from either patients with dementia or elderly inpatients without psychiatric disorders when sensitive tests such as Digit Span Backward and the Digit Cancellation Test were used.

Memory impairment occurs often in delirium, affecting both short- and long-term memory, although most reports have not distinguished between types of memory impairment. In delirium due to posttraumatic brain injury, procedural and declarative memory are impaired, and procedural memory improves first (Ewert et al. 1985). Patients are usually amnestic for some or all of their delirium episodes, although recent studies have highlighted that many patients can recall some of the often distressing experiences of delirium. Breitbart et al. (2002a) found that about half of their patients with resolved delirium were amnestic for their episode and that more severe amnesia was associated with greater severity of delirium on the MDAS, suggesting a defect in new learning during delirium. Similarly, O'Keeffe (2005) found that about half of elderly delirious patients without dementia recalled their delirium, and many continued to be disturbed by their recollections 6 months later. Trzepacz et al. (2001) found a high correlation between the DRS-R-98 short- and long-term memory items ($r=0.51$, $P=0.01$) in patients with delirium, with attention correlating with short-term memory ($r=0.44$, $P=0.03$) but not with long-term memory. This outcome is consistent with adequate attention being a prerequisite for information to enter short-term (working) memory, followed by storage of selected data from working memory into long-term memory.

Disturbances of the sleep-wake cycle are especially common in patients with delirium. The DRS-R-98 identified sleep-wake cycle disturbances in 92%– 97% of delirious patients (Meagher et al. 2007; Trzepacz et al. 2001). Sleep disturbances range from napping and nocturnal disruptions to a more severe disintegration of the normal circadian cycle. The role of sleep disturbances in early or prodromal phases of delirium is uncertain; some authors have suggested that sleep disturbances may be a central feature of delirium evolution, possibly related to disturbed melatonin secretion (Charlton and Kavanau 2002; Shigeta et al. 2001). However, Harrell and Othmer (1987), in a study of postcardiotomy delirium, found that sleep disturbance mirrored reductions in Mini-Mental State Examination (MMSE) scores but did not predate them. Similarly, de Jonghe et al. (2005) found that the prodromal phase of delirium was characterized principally by cognitive disturbances rather than behavioral or sleep disturbances. In a retrospective study, Dautzenberg et al. (2004) measured treatment response and found that 2 or more consecutive nights of undisturbed sleep was equated with delirium resolution.

Visuospatial disturbances of patients with delirium have not been studied in detail, but Clock Drawing Test deficits and wandering behaviors indicate difficulties. Accuracy of both the overall shapes and the details of drawings is impaired, suggesting dysfunction of bilateral posterior parietal lobes and prefrontal cortex. Meagher et al. (2007) found disturbances of visuospatial function in 87% of patients with delirium and noted that these disturbances were moderate or severe in 64%.

Language disturbances in patients with delirium include dysnomia, paraphasias, impaired comprehension, dysgraphia, and word-finding difficulties. In extreme cases, language resembles a fluent dysphasia. Incoherent speech or speech disturbance is reported commonly. Dysgraphia was once believed to be specific to delirium (Chedru and Geschwind 1972), but comparisons of writing samples from patients with other psychiatric disorders revealed that dysgraphia was not specific to delirium (Patten and Lamarre 1989); rather, abnormal semantic content of language was more differentiating in delirium. The language item on the DRS-R-98 did not distinguish delirium and dementia patients, but the CTD comprehension item, which incorporates language and executive function, did (Trzepacz et al. 2002).

Disorganized thinking was found in 95% of patients with delirium in one study (Rockwood 1993) and was noted in another study to be different from schizophrenic thought processes (Cutting 1987). However, very little work has been done to characterize thought process disorder in patients with delirium, which clinically ranges from tangentiality and circumstantiality to loose associations. On the DRS-R-98, 21% of delirium patients had tangentiality or circumstantiality, whereas 58% had loose associations (Trzepacz et al. 2001). Greater severity of thought process disturbances can distinguish delirium when it occurs with concomitant dementia (Laurila et al. 2004), and thought disorder is significantly worse in delirium than in dementia (Trzepacz et al. 2002). Besides thought process abnormality, other indications of psychosis include abnormal thought content and perceptual disturbances, although these occur less often than do core symptoms (Trzepacz et al. 2001).

Treatment

Delirium is an example par excellence of a disorder requiring a multifaceted biopsychosocial approach to assessment and treatment. After delirium is diagnosed, the process of identifying and reversing suspected causes begins. Rapid treatment is important because of the high morbidity and mortality rates associated with delirium. Treatments include medication, environmental manipulation, and patient and family psychosocial support (American Psychiatric Association 1999), although no drug has a U.S. Food and Drug Administration (FDA) indication for the treatment of delirium. Placebo-controlled randomized double-blind, adequately powered efficacy trials are lacking. In "Practice Guideline for the Treatment of Patients With Delirium," the American Psychiatric Association (1999) Work Group noted the need for such research, and research is ever more necessary given the escalating range of therapeutic options available for delirium, including atypical antipsychotics, procholinergic agents, and melatonergic compounds. Most prospective drug studies have used open-label designs, although blinded randomized controlled efficacy and prophylaxis trials are growing in number (Table 3–6); more is published about atypical antipsychotics than about conventional neuroleptics in these studies. Trials using neuroleptics suggest their efficacy and good tolerability, although no neuroleptic agent has yet been shown to adequately target all core symptoms of delirium (Bourne et al. 2008). Cholinergic agents hold more promise in chronic than acute prophylactic dosing, although shorter-acting agents such as physostigmine, which offer faster onset of action in acute settings, have not been tried for non-drug-induced delirium. Conventional and atypical neuroleptics carry an FDA black box warning for increased risk of mortality and cerebrovascular accidents when used in agitated elderly dementia patients; this warning needs to be considered as part of the risk-benefit assessment when these drugs are used in elderly dementia patients who also have delirium. Some authors have proposed that short-term antipsychotic use for a condition that is an acute medical urgency associated with its own high morbidity and mortality may be warranted

(Elie et al. 2009; Herrmann et al. 2004; Insau and Lawley 2004). Medication choice should be guided by a careful consideration of the overall risk-benefit ratio (Schneider et al. 2005).

Prevention Strategies

Prevention of delirium can involve nonpharmacological and pharmacological methods. Preoperative patient education and preparation have been found to be helpful in reducing delirium symptom rates (Chatham 1978; Owens and Hutelmyer 1982; Schindler et al. 1989; Williams et al. 1985). However, studies that used caregiver education and environmental or risk factor interventions had mixed results, with two not finding any significant effect on delirium rate (Nagley 1986; Wanich et al. 1992) and one finding modest gains in delirium diagnosis (3%–9%) through special internal medicine house staff education efforts (Rockwood et al. 1994).

In contrast, Inouye et al. (1999) studied the effect on delirium of preventive measures that minimized six of the risk factors identified in their previous work with hospitalized elderly patients. They used standardized protocols in a prospective study of 852 elderly medical inpatients to address cognitive impairment, sleep deprivation, immobility, visual impairment, hearing impairment, and dehydration, and use of these protocols resulted in significant reductions in the number (62 vs. 90) and duration (105 vs. 161 days) of delirium episodes relative to control subjects. Effects of adherence to the delirium risk protocol were subsequently reported for 422 elderly patients during implementation (Inouye et al. 2003): adherence ranged from 10% for the sleep protocol to 86% for orientation. Higher levels of adherence by staff resulted in lower delirium rates up to a maximum of an 89% reduction, even after the investigators controlled for confounding variables such as medical comorbidity, functional status, and illness severity. At 6-month follow-up of 705 survivors from this intervention study of six risk factors, no differences were seen between groups for any of 10 outcome measures except for less frequent incontinence in the intervention group (Bogardus et al. 2003), suggesting that the intervention's effect was essentially during the index hospitalization, without longer-lasting benefits. When a subset of patients at high risk for delirium at baseline was compared to control subjects, however, patients who received the intervention had significantly better self-rated health and functional status at follow-up.

Table 3–6. Prospective pharmacological trials in delirium

Study	Agent	Population	Design	Purpose	Primary outcome scale
Conventional antipsychotics					
Platt et al. 1994a	Haloperidol vs. chlorpromazine	24 AIDS inpatients	Not stated	Efficacy for motor subtypes	DRS
Breitbart et al. 1996	Haloperidol vs. chlorpromazine vs. lorazepam	30 AIDS inpatients	Double-blind, randomized	Efficacy	DRS
Kaneko et al. 1999	Intravenous haloperidol vs. intravenous placebo	78 gastrointestinal postoperative inpatients	Randomized, not blinded	Prophylaxis (acute) and rescue	Clinical assessment
Kalisvaart et al. 2005	Haloperidol vs. placebo	430 elderly hip surgery inpatients	Double-blind, randomized	Prophylaxis (acute)	DRS-R-98
Atypical antipsychotics					
Sipahimalani and Masand 1998	Olanzapine vs. haloperidol	22 consultation-liaison referrals	Open label, not randomized	Efficacy	DRS
Kim et al. 2001	Olanzapine	20 medical-surgical patients	Open label	Efficacy	DRS
Breitbart et al. 2002b	Olanzapine	79 cancer inpatients	Open label	Efficacy	MDAS
Hill et al. 2002	Olanzapine vs. risperidone vs. haloperidol	50 general hospital patients	Open label, not randomized	Efficacy	DRS-R-98

Table 3–6. Prospective pharmacological trials in delirium *(continued)*

Study	Agent	Population	Design	Purpose	Primary outcome scale
Atypical antipsychotics (continued)					
Horikawa et al. 2003	Risperidone	10 consultation-liaison referrals	Open label	Efficacy	DRS
Kim et al. 2003	Quetiapine	12 geriatric medical patients	Open label	Efficacy	DRS
Sasaki et al. 2003	Quetiapine	12 patients	Open label	Efficacy	DRS
Han and Kim 2004	Risperidone vs. haloperidol	28 consultation-liaison referrals	Double-blind, randomized	Efficacy	MDAS
Mittal et al. 2004	Risperidone	10 medical-surgical admissions	Open label	Efficacy	DRS
Pae et al. 2004	Quetiapine	22 inpatients	Open label	Efficacy	DRS-R-98
Parellada et al. 2004	Risperidone	64 medical inpatients	Open label	Efficacy	DRS
Skrobik et al. 2004	Olanzapine vs. haloperidol	103 ICU patients	Randomized, not blinded	Efficacy	DI
Kim et al. 2005	Haloperidol vs. risperidone	42 medical-surgical patients	Open label, not randomized	Efficacy	DRS-R-98
Lee et al. 2005	Amisulpride vs. quetiapine	40 patients	Open label, randomized	Efficacy	DRS-R-98
Toda et al. 2005	Risperidone	10 elderly inpatients	Open label	Efficacy	DRS

Table 3–6.   Prospective pharmacological trials in delirium (continued)

Study	Agent	Population	Design	Purpose	Primary outcome scale
Atypical antipsychotics (continued)					
Hua et al. 2006	Risperidone vs. olanzapine vs. placebo	175 elderly inpatients	Double-blind, randomized	Efficacy	DRS
Straker et al. 2006	Aripiprazole	14 general hospital patients	Open label	Efficacy	DRS-R-98
Prakanrattana and Prapaitrakool 2007	Risperidone vs. placebo	126 elective cardiac by-pass surgery inpatients	Double-blind, randomized	Prophylaxis	CAM-ICU
Takeuchi et al. 2007	Perospirone	38 medical-surgical inpatients	Open label	Efficacy	DRS-R-98
Devlin et al. 2010	Quetiapine vs. placebo as an add-on to as-needed daily haloperidol	36 ICU patients	Double-blind, randomized	Acute adjunctive prophylaxisto haloperidol	ICDSC
Girard et al. 2010	Ziprasidone vs. haloperidol vs. placebo	101 mechanically ventilated ICU patients	Double-blind, randomized	Efficacy	CAM-ICU
Larsen et al. 2010	Olanzapine vs. placebo perioperatively	400 elderly joint replacement surgery patients	Double-blind, randomized	Acute prophylaxis	DRS-R-98, MMSE, CAM
Tahir et al. 2010	Quetiapine vs. placebo	42 medical-surgical inpatients	Double-blind, randomized	Efficacy	DRS-R-98

Table 3–6. Prospective pharmacological trials in delirium *(continued)*

Study	Agent	Population	Design	Purpose	Primary outcome scale
Procholinergics					
Díaz et al. 2001	Citicoline vs. placebo	81 elderly non-demented hip surgery patients	Randomized	Prophylaxis (acute)	CAM, AMT
Moretti et al. 2004	Rivastigmine vs. cardioaspirin	230 elderly vascular dementia outpatients	Case-control, not randomized	Prophylaxis (chronic)	CAM Index at 2 years
Liptzin et al. 2005	Donepezil vs. placebo perioperatively	80 elderly elective hip surgery patients	Double-blind, randomized	Prophylaxis (subacute)	DSI
Sampson et al. 2006	Donepezil vs. placebo perioperatively	33 postoperative elective hip surgery inpatients	Double-blind, randomized	Prophylaxis (acute)	DSI
Other					
Nakamura et al. 1994	Mianserin vs. haloperidol vs. oxypertine at bedtime	23 general hospital inpatients	Not specified	Efficacy	DRS
Nakamura et al. 1995	Mianserin vs. haloperidol	65 consultation-liaison referrals	Open label, not randomized	Efficacy	DRS
Uchiyama et al. 1996	Mianserin	62 psychogeriatric inpatients	Open label	Efficacy	DRS
Nakamura et al. 1997a	Mianserin vs. haloperidol	66 consultation-liaison referrals	Open label, not randomized	Efficacy	DRS

Table 3–6.   Prospective pharmacological trials in delirium *(continued)*

Study	Agent	Population	Design	Purpose	Primary outcome scale
Other (continued)					
Nakamura et al. 1997b	Mianserin suppositories at bedtime	16 consultation-liaison postoperative referrals	Open label	Efficacy	DRS
Bayindir et al. 2000	Ondansetron	35 postcardiotomy patients	Open label	Efficacy	4-point clinical scale
Gagnon et al. 2005	Methylphenidate, adjunctive to methotrimeprazine	14 cancer patients with hypoactive delirium	Open label	Efficacy	MMSE
Leung et al. 2006	Gabapentin vs. placebo as perioperative pain management	21 spine surgery patients	Double-blind, randomized	Prophylaxis	CAM
Pandharipande et al. 2007	Dexmedetomidine vs. lorazepam for sedation	106 mechanically ventilated ICU patients	Double-blind, randomized	Prophylaxis	CAM-ICU
Hudetz et al. 2009	Ketamine vs. placebo for anesthesia induction	52 elective cardiac surgery patients	Randomized	Prophylaxis	Neuropsychological test battery (memory and executive function)
Kain et al. 2009	Melatonin vs. midazolam preoperatively	148 pediatric patients	Randomized	Prophylaxis	Yale Preoperative Anxiety Scale (PAED scale secondary)

Table 3–6. Prospective pharmacological trials in delirium *(continued)*

Study	Agent	Population	Design	Purpose	Primary outcome scale
Other *(continued)*					
Katznelson et al. 2009	Statins preoperatively vs. none	1,059 cardiac bypass surgery patients	Observational	Prophylaxis	CAM-ICU
Maldonado et al. 2009	Dexmecetomidine vs. midazolam vs. propofol for postoperative sedation	90 elective cardiac valve surgery patients in ICU	Randomized, open label	Prophylaxis; add-on adjunctive to usual care	DRS
Riker et al. 2009	Dexmedetomidine vs. midazolam intravenous infusion	366 medical-surgical ICU patients	Double-blind, randomized	Prophylaxis	RASS (CAM-ICU secondary)
Al-Aama et al. 2011	Melatonin vs. placebo at bedtime	145 elderly medical inpatients	Double-blind, randomized	Efficacy	CAM, MDAS
Rubino et al. 2010	Clonidine vs. placebo for ventilator weaning	30 aortic dissection surgery patients	Randomized	Prophylaxis	DDS

Note. AMT = Abbreviated Mental Test; CAM = Confusion Assessment Method; DDS = Delirium Detection Score; DI = Delirium Index; DRS = Delirium Rating Scale; DRS-R-98 = Delirium Rating Scale—Revised-98; DSI = Delirium Symptom Inventory; ICDSC = Intensive Care Delirium Symptom Checklist; ICU = intensive care unit; MDAS = Memorial Delirium Assessment Scale; MMSE = Mini-Mental State Examination; PAED = Pediatric Anesthesia Emergence Delirium; RASS = Richmond Agitation Sedation Scale.

Source. Adapted from Trzepacz PT, Meagher DJ: "Neuropsychiatric Aspects of Delirium," in *Essentials of Neuropsychiatry and Behavioral Neurosciences,* 2nd Edition. Edited by Yudofsky SC, Hales RE. Washington, DC, American Psychiatric Publishing, 2010, pp. 149–221. Used with permission. Copyright © 2010 American Psychiatric Association.

Marcantonio et al. (2001) found that proactive geriatric consultation for patients undergoing hip surgery was associated with significantly reduced incidence and severity of delirium in the intervention group, who had received a mean of 10 recommendations regarding risk factor prevention and active treatment of emergent delirium. Interestingly, more than three-quarters of these recommendations were adhered to, but with relatively less adherence to suggestions regarding analgesia, nutritional inadequacies, and correction of sensory impairments. Young and George (2003) studied the effect of introducing consensus guidelines for delirium management in general hospital settings and found that management processes improved only when the intervention was reinforced by regular teaching sessions, but these effects did not reach statistical significance.

Milisen et al. (2001) compared delirium rates in two cohorts of elderly hip surgery patients (each $n=60$), before and after implementing an intervention composed of nurse education, cognitive screening, consultation by a nurse or physician geriatric/delirium specialist, and a scheduled pain protocol. They found no effect on delirium incidence but, instead, a shorter delirium duration (median = 1 vs. 4 days) and a lower delirium severity score in the intervention group as measured by a modified (not validated) Confusion Assessment Method (CAM). Marcantonio et al. (2001), using a different study design, randomly assigned 62 elderly hip fracture patients to either a perioperative geriatric consultation or usual care. Daily ratings on the MMSE, Delirium Symptom Inventory, CAM, and MDAS indicated a lower delirium rate (32% vs. 50%) and fewer severe delirium cases (12% vs. 29%) in the consultative group. Length of stay was not affected, and the effect of consultation was greatest in those patients without preexisting dementia or poor activities of daily living skills, in contrast to the subgroup analysis of Bogardus et al. (2003), in which most benefit accrued at follow-up for high-risk patients.

Comparing prophylactic intravenous treatments in gastrointestinal surgery patients, Kaneko et al. (1999) found a significantly lower incidence of delirium (10.5%) in the haloperidol group than in controls (32.5%). In a placebo-controlled randomized blinded trial, Kalisvaart et al. (2005) studied low dosages of perioperative haloperidol in 430 elderly hip surgery patients and found that the groups had no difference in incidence of postoperative delirium rates but the treatment group had significantly lower delirium severity and duration and shorter length of stay. Prakanrattana and Prapaitrakool (2007) similarly found a significantly reduced incidence of delirium using risperidone versus placebo in a double-blind randomized prophylaxis trial in post–cardiac surgery ICU patients. In a study with an unusual design in which quetiapine prophylaxis was compared with placebo in ICU patients who were also receiving as-needed haloperidol, Devlin et al. (2010) reported some advantages for quetiapine, although this trial altered neuroleptic characteristics more than the total neuroleptic dosing did. Larsen et al. (2010) performed a placebo-controlled randomized double-blind prophylaxis trial in 400 elderly joint replacement patients and reported that low-dose olanzapine significantly reduced delirium incidence and severity.

In contrast to favorable findings using neuroleptics for acute prophylaxis, data have not shown that acetylcholinesterase inhibitors have significant effects on delirium in placebo-controlled trials (Díaz et al. 2001; Liptzin et al. 2005; Sampson et al. 2006). However, these studies may have been underpowered: Sampson et al., for example, found a numerical difference favoring donepezil. Compared with cardioaspirin, chronic rivastigmine for delirium prevention over a 2-year period significantly reduced delirium incidence in patients with vascular dementia (Moretti et al. 2004).

Another strategy has been to prevent delirium by switching away from a more deliriogenic iatrogenic treatment to a lesser one. Several trials suggest that use of dexmedetomidine instead of lorazepam, midazolam, or propofol results in a lower incidence of delirium in postoperative and ICU patients (Maldonado et al. 2009; Pandharipande et al. 2007; Riker et al. 2009). Compared with midazolam, melatonin administered preoperatively resulted in lower postanesthesia emergence delirium incidence in children (Kain et al. 2009). In a comparison with placebo, ketamine for anesthesia induction resulted in less severe cognitive decline at 7 days in cardiac surgery patients (Hudetz et al. 2009). Cardiac bypass patients who had been taking statins had lower odds for postoperative delirium than did those who were not taking statins (Katznelson et al. 2009). Gabapentin for postoperative pain management (Leung et al. 2006) and clonidine for ventilator weaning (Rubino et al. 2010) have also been associated with lower delirium incidence and severity, respectively.

Nonpharmacological Treatment of a Delirium Episode

The principles of good ward management of patients with delirium include ensuring the safety of the patient and of those in his or her immediate surroundings (including sitters), achieving optimal levels of environmental stimulation, and minimizing the effects of any sensory impediments. The complications of delirium can be minimized by careful attention to the potential for falls and avoidance of prolonged hypostasis. The use of orienting techniques (e.g., calendars, night-lights, reorientation by staff) and familiarizing the patient with the environment (e.g., with photographs of family members) are sometimes comforting, although environmental manipulations alone do not reverse delirium (American Psychiatric Association 1999; Anderson 1995). Diurnal cues from natural lighting may reduce sensory deprivation and incidence of delirium (Wilson 1972), although sensory deprivation alone is insufficient to cause delirium (Francis 1993). Unfortunately, the routine implementation of nursing interventions occurs primarily in response to hyperactivity and behavioral management challenges rather than to the core cognitive disturbances of delirium (Meagher et al. 1996).

A variety of intensive delirium-focused techniques target delirium reduction. An alternative to hospitalization is home-based care ("hospital in the home"), which results in reduced incidence and duration of delirium and substantially reduced rehabilitation costs in elderly patients undergoing physical rehabilitation (Caplan et al. 2005). The "flying delirium team" uses a nurse-led coordinated approach to multidisciplinary care (psychiatry, geriatrics, and neurology) of hospitalized patients with delirium (Lemey et al. 2005). The "delirium room" (Flaherty et al. 2003) is a specialized four-bed unit for management and mobilization of disturbed elderly patients without the use of restraints (restraint use being a well-recognized risk factor for delirium [McCusker et al. 2001]). This model involves comprehensive delirium-oriented treatment to minimize risk and aggravating factors, medication use, and daily multidisciplinary reviews of progress. Preliminary investigation suggests that exposure to delirium risk factors and mortality rates are reduced in this model of care. McCaffrey and Locsin (2004) found a lower incidence of delirium in elderly postoperative patients provided with passive ("easy listening") music therapy via a bedside compact disc player, which also had a calming effect on the ward.

Supportive interaction with relatives and caregivers is fundamental to good management of delirium. During implementation of a psychoeducational intervention for family caregivers of terminally ill cancer patients, Gagnon et al. (2002) found that few caregivers were aware of the risk of delirium or of the fact that it could be treated. The intervention was associated with significant improvements in caregiver confidence. Lundstrom et al. (2005) found reduced delirium duration and mortality in patients receiving care on a ward where staff had received training in delirium assessment and treatment and where improved caregiver-patient interaction was emphasized. Although relatives can play an integral role in efforts to support and reorient patients with delirium, they can add to the burden if they are ill-informed, critical, or anxious, especially if medical staff members respond to their distress by inappropriately medicating patients. Recovered delirium patients reported that simple but firm communication, reality orientation, a visible clock, and the presence of a relative contributed to a heightened sense of control (Schofield 1997). Clarification of the cause and meaning of symptoms, combined with recognition of treatment goals, can allow better management of what is a distressing experience for both patients and loved ones (Breitbart et al. 2002a; Meagher 2001b).

Pharmacological Treatment of Delirium

Current delirium pharmacotherapies are borrowed from the treatment of primary psychiatric disorders. Pharmacological treatment with a neuroleptic agent (dopamine D_2 antagonist) is the clinical standard of delirium treatment, although other agents have been tried and are described in this section (see Table 3–6). Dosages need to be modified for elderly patients; however, Hally and Cooney (2005) found that these modifications were frequently overlooked for both haloperidol (62%) and lorazepam (47%) prescribing.

Benzodiazepines

Benzodiazepines are generally reserved for delirium due to ethanol or sedative-hypnotic withdrawal, for which they are first-line agents (Mayo-Smith et al. 2004). Lorazepam or clonazepam (the latter for alprazolam withdrawal) is often used. However, Klijn and van der Mast (2005) warn about overlooking other causes of delirium when patients have alcohol withdrawal, and contend that haloperidol should be the first-choice treatment in these patients as well.

Some clinicians use lorazepam as an adjunctive medication with haloperidol in the most severe cases of delirium or for patients who need extra assistance with sleep. Benzodiazepine monotherapy is generally not effective for non-substance-related delirium and may exacerbate the delirium, as shown in a controlled blinded study by Breitbart et al. (1996). None of the survey respondents from the American Geriatrics Society would use lorazepam alone to treat severe delirium in elderly postoperative patients (Carnes et al. 2003). In a retrospective study of 52 consecutive toxicology consultations, Burns et al. (2000) found that physostigmine controlled anticholinergic toxicity–induced delirium and reversed agitation in 87% and 96% of patients, respectively, whereas benzodiazepines controlled agitation in 24% of patients and were ineffective in treating delirium. Additionally, patients who received physostigmine rather than benzodiazepines had a lower incidence of complications (7% vs. 46%) and a shorter time to recovery (median = 12 vs. 24 hours). Pandharipande et al. (2006) found a significant deliriogenic effect, in medical ICU patients, only for benzodiazepines when compared with other commonly used medications (propofol, morphine, and fentanyl), even though higher dosages of all of these agents were used in delirious than in nondelirious ICU patients. A survey of ICU physicians found that 66% of the respondents treated delirium with haloperidol, 12% used lorazepam, and fewer than 5% used atypical antipsychotics. More than 55% administered haloperidol and lorazepam at daily dosages of 10 mg or less, but some physicians used more than 50 mg/day of either medication (Ely et al. 2004).

Cholinergic Enhancers

The cholinergic deficiency hypothesis of delirium suggests that treatment with a cholinergic enhancer—generally acetylcholinesterase inhibitors—could be therapeutic. Physostigmine reverses anticholinergic delirium (Stern 1983), but its side effects (seizures) and short half-life make it unsuitable for routine clinical treatment of delirium. Tacrine also was shown to reverse central anticholinergic syndrome (Mendelson 1977), but it has not been studied formally. In several case reports, donepezil was found to improve delirium in the postoperative state, comorbid Lewy body dementia, and comorbid alcohol dementia (Burke et al. 1999; Wengel et al. 1998, 1999). Physostigmine administered in the emergency department to patients suspected of having muscarinic toxicity resulted in reversal of delirium in 22 of 39 patients, including several in whom the cause could not be determined (Schneir et al. 2003); only 1 of the 39 patients had an adverse event (brief seizure). Kalisvaart et al. (2004) reported that three cases of prolonged delirium that was unresponsive to haloperidol or atypical antipsychotics rapidly resolved when treatment was switched to rivastigmine.

Neuroleptics

Haloperidol is the neuroleptic most often chosen for the treatment of delirium. It can be administered orally, intramuscularly, or intravenously (Adams 1984, 1988; Dudley et al. 1979; Gelfand et al. 1992; Moulaert 1989; Sanders and Stern 1993; Tesar et al. 1985), although the intravenous route has not been approved by the FDA. Intravenously administered haloperidol is twice as potent as that taken orally (Gelfand et al. 1992). Bolus intravenous doses usually range from 0.5 to 20 mg, although larger doses are sometimes given. In severe, refractory cases, continuous intravenous infusions of 15–25 mg/hour (up to 1,000 mg/day) can be given (Fernandez et al. 1988; Levenson 1995; Riker et al. 1994; Stern 1994). The specific brain effects of haloperidol in alleviating delirium are not known, but positron emission tomography scans show reduced glucose utilization in the limbic cortex, thalamus, caudate, and frontal and anterior cingulate cortices (Bartlett et al. 1994). These regions are important for behavior and cognition and have been implicated in the neuropathogenesis of delirium. Milbrandt et al. (2005) found in nearly 1,000 ICU patients that use of haloperidol was associated with reduced mortality.

Clinical use of haloperidol traditionally has been considered to be relatively safe in patients who are seriously medically ill (Gelfand et al. 1992; Moulaert 1989; Tesar et al. 1985). Haloperidol does not antagonize dopamine-induced increases in renal blood flow (Armstrong et al. 1986). Even when haloperidol is given intravenously at high dosages in delirium, extrapyramidal symptoms (EPS) are usually not a problem except in more sensitive patients (e.g., those with HIV infection or Lewy body dementia) (Fernandez et al. 1989; McKeith et al. 1992; Swenson et al. 1989). In a case series, five ICU patients receiving 250–500 mg/day of continuous or intermittent intravenous haloperidol had self-limited withdrawal dyskinesia following high-dose haloperidol (Riker et al. 1997). Intravenous lorazepam is sometimes combined with intravenous haloperidol in critically ill patients to lessen EPS and increase sedation.

Cases of prolonged QTc interval on electrocardiogram (ECG) and torsades de pointes tachyarrhythmia (multifocal ventricular tachycardia) have been increasingly recognized and attributed to intravenously administered haloperidol (Hatta et al. 2001; Huyse 1988; Kriwisky et al. 1990; Metzger and Friedman 1993; O'Brien et al. 1999; Perrault et al. 2000; Wilt et al. 1993; Zee-Cheng et al. 1985). In "Practice Guideline for the Treatment of Patients With Delirium," the American Psychiatric Association (1999) Work Group recommended that QTc prolongation greater than 450 milliseconds or greater than 25% over a previous ECG may warrant telemetry, cardiology consultation, dosage reduction, or discontinuation. They also recommended monitoring serum magnesium and potassium in critically ill delirious patients whose QTc is 450 milliseconds or greater, because of the common use of concomitant drugs and/or electrolyte disturbances that also can prolong the QTc interval.

Empirical evidence for neuroleptic benefits in treating delirium is substantial, and although most efficacy or prophylaxis trials are open label, the number of controlled randomized blinded trials is growing. In a controlled double-blind randomized design, Breitbart et al. (1996) found that delirium in patients with AIDS worsened with lorazepam but significantly improved with haloperidol or chlorpromazine, although DRS and MMSE scores still did not return to normal. In addition, both hypoactive and hyperactive subtypes responded to treatment with haloperidol or chlorpromazine, and improvement was noted within hours of treatment, even before the underlying medical causes were addressed (Platt et al. 1994a). Kaneko et al. (1999) found significantly lower rates of postoperative delirium in patients intravenously administered haloperidol rather than placebo. Kalisvaart et al. (2004) used perioperative haloperidol in elderly hip surgery patients in a placebo-controlled blinded randomized prophylaxis trial. Although the researchers did not find a difference for incidence of delirium, they reported that the haloperidol group had a significantly lower severity and duration of delirium and shorter length of stay. Prakanrattana and Prapaitrakool (2007) found significantly lower incidence of delirium using prophylactic risperidone than placebo in cardiac bypass patients. Larsen et al. (2010) reported a significantly lower incidence of postoperative delirium in elderly joint replacement patients taking perioperative olanzapine than in those taking placebo.

Haloperidol use in pediatric patients with delirium is not well documented, despite its use in adult delirium and in other childhood psychiatric disorders (Teicher and Glod 1990). Its efficacy in children for delusions, hallucinations, thought disorder, aggressivity, stereotypies, hyperactivity, social withdrawal, and learning disability (Teicher and Glod 1990) suggests that it may have a beneficial role in pediatric delirium. Clinical experience with haloperidol in pediatric delirium supports its beneficial effects, although no controlled studies have been done. A retrospective report of 30 children (mean age=7±1 years, range = 8 months to 18 years) with burn injuries supports the use of haloperidol for agitation, disorientation, hallucinations, delusions, and insomnia (Brown et al. 1996). The mean haloperidol dosage was 0.47 ± 0.002 mg/kg, with a mean maximum dosage in 24 hours of 0.46 mg/kg, administered intravenously, orally, or intramuscularly. Mean efficacy, as scored on a 0- to 3-point scale (3 = excellent), was 2.3 ± 0.21, but the drug was not efficacious in 17% of cases (four of five of these failures followed oral administration). EPS were not observed, and one episode of hypotension occurred with the intravenous route.

Atypical Antipsychotic Agents

Atypical antipsychotic agents differ from haloperidol and other conventional neuroleptics in a variety of neurotransmitter activities, especially serotonergic activities. In addition to presynaptic serotonin type 2 receptor ($5\text{-}HT_2$) antagonism, it is hypothesized that loose binding at the dopamine D_2 receptor may define atypicality (Kapur and Seeman 2001). Some atypical antipsychotics are being used routinely to treat delirium, and literature on their use is accumulating. Hally and Cooney (2005) surveyed general hospital medical staff regarding prescribing practices for delirium and noted that risperidone was the second most frequently prescribed antipsychotic agent (38%) after haloperidol. In several patients who had a poor response to haloperidol, delirium improved after treatment was switched to an atypical antipsychotic agent (Al-Samarrai et al. 2003; Leso and Schwartz 2002; Passik and Cooper 1999). Haloperidol is avoided in posttraumatic brain injury patients with delirium because dopamine blockade is thought to be deleterious to cognitive recovery; two traumatic brain injury patients with delirium who were given low-dose olanzapine showed remarkable improvement within a short time (Ovchinsky et al. 2002), suggesting a possible role for atypical antipsychotics in this population.

Because atypical antipsychotics differ in their chemical structures and are not a pharmacological class per se, they may differ in how they affect delirium. Receptor activities and adverse event profiles differ among the atypical agents, and their associated EPS, QTc prolongation, and effects on cognition are particularly relevant to any use in delirium. Ziprasidone was implicated in causing QTc prolongation in a patient with delirium (Leso and Schwartz 2002) and was temporally related to runs of torsades de pointes and QTc prolongation during rechallenge in a patient with delirium (Heinrich et al. 2006). In some case reports, risperidone, quetiapine, and olanzapine were implicated in causing delirium (Chen and Cardasis 1996; Karki and Masood 2003; Ravona-Springer et al. 1998; Samuels and Fang 2004; Sim et al. 2000).

Risperidone and haloperidol were found to be equally effective in a double-blind randomized trial (Han and Kim 2004). Skrobik et al. (2004) found similar efficacy for haloperidol and olanzapine in ICU patients, with more EPS in the haloperidol group, but standardized delirium ratings were not used and investigators were not blinded to drug. Kim et al. (2005) used the DRS-R-98 to compare haloperidol and risperidone in an open-label nonrandomized trial and found equivalent efficacy. Hua et al. (2006) compared haloperidol, olanzapine, and placebo in a randomized trial and found significant differences from placebo. Ziprasidone, haloperidol, and placebo were studied in a double-blind randomized trial of mechanically ventilated ICU patients (Girard et al. 2010) in which the number of delirium- and coma-free days was the outcome measure, but no differences were found; unfortunately, the primary measure was not incidence or severity of delirium using a sensitive rating scale. In a pilot double-blind randomized placebo-controlled study, Tahir et al. (2010) found more rapid improvement using quetiapine, although the study was not powered to detect an efficacy difference.

Atypical agents in intramuscular formulations are therapeutic options being tried by clinicians whose medically ill patients cannot take oral medications.

Psychostimulants

Psychostimulants can worsen delirium—probably via increased dopaminergic activity—and their use when a depressed mood is present is contentious (Levenson 1992; Rosenberg et al. 1991). Morita et al. (2000) reported improvement of hypoactive delirium in a terminally ill cancer patient due to disseminated intravascular coagulation and multiorgan failure when methylphenidate 10–20 mg/day was administered, which raised the arousal level within 1 day and improved MDAS and DRS scores. They attributed the improvement to amelioration of an overstimulated γ-aminobutyric acid (GABA) system. In an open-label study, Gagnon et al. (2005) administered 20–30 mg of adjunctive methylphenidate to 14 patients with advanced metastatic cancer and hypoactive delirium; median MMSE scores improved at 1-hour postdose. Cases with psychosis were excluded.

Anticonvulsant Agents

Anticonvulsant agents such as valproic acid may have a role in some cases of delirium, and they are first-line treatments when ictal states are the cause of delirium (Bourgeois et al. 2005; Schneider 2005).

Postdelirium Management

Treatment of delirium should continue until symptoms have fully resolved, but the role of continued treatment thereafter is uncertain. Alexopoulos et al. (2004) surveyed 52 experts on the treatment of older adults and found consensus that treatment of delirium should be continued for at least a week after response before tapering and discontinuation are attempted. However, many patients experiencing delirium are discharged before full resolution of symptoms, and, unfortunately, continued monitoring and management are often not part of postdischarge planning, whether the patient returns home or goes to an institutionalized setting. Problems with attention and orientation are especially persistent (McCusker et al. 2003). Further episodes may be prevented by addressing risk factors such as medication exposure and sensory impairments. Literature on the psychological aftermath of delirium is limited, but research suggests that approximately 50% of patients can recall the episode (Breitbart et al. 2002a; O'Keeffe 2005). Depression and posttraumatic stress disorder have been described, but most patients dismiss the episode once it has passed, often despite lingering concerns that the episode heralds a first step toward loss of mental faculties and independence (Schofield 1997). Other patients experience silent delirium and are ashamed or afraid to admit to symptoms. Explicit recognition and discussion of the meaning of delirium can facilitate adjustment but also can allow more detailed discussion of how best to minimize future risk. A follow-up visit can facilitate postdelirium adjustment by clarifying the transient nature of delirium symptoms in contrast to dementia (Easton and MacKenzie 1988) and by providing any ongoing medication adjustments.

Conclusion

Delirium is a common neuropsychiatric disorder affecting cognition, thinking, perception, sleep, language, and other behaviors. Mortality increases following an episode, but whether mortality can be attributed to delirium itself or underlying medical problems is unclear. Delirium affects persons of any age, although elderly patients may be particularly vulnerable, especially if they have dementia. Research in nongeriatric adults and children is sorely needed to avoid error in applying data from elderly to younger persons. Clinical assessment of delirium can be aided through the use of diagnostic criteria and rating scales, as well as by knowledge of which populations are at risk. Research could greatly benefit from consensus on using certain valid, specific, and sensitive instruments across studies. Underdetection and misdiagnosis are rampant, begging for valid, concise screening and monitoring tools.

Certain symptoms of delirium may represent "core" symptoms, whereas others may be associated symptoms that occur under various conditions, possibly more related to etiology or idiopathic features. Core symptoms may reflect dysfunction of certain brain regions and neurotransmitter systems that constitute a "final common neural pathway" that is responsible for the presentation of the syndrome of delirium. Regions implicated include prefrontal cortex, thalamus, basal ganglia, right temporoparietal cortex, and fusiform and lingual gyri. Diverse physiologies related to the wide variety of etiologies may funnel into a common neurofunctional expression for delirium via elevated brain dopaminergic and reduced cholinergic activity or a relative imbalance between these. Other neurochemical candidates include serotonin, melatonin, norepinephrine, GABA, glutamate, and cytokines, although these may interact to regulate or alter activity of acetylcholine and dopamine in key circuitry.

The clinical standard of treatment involves a dopamine antagonist medication—a neuroleptic—although, theoretically, procholinergic drugs should help. Findings from drug treatment studies for delirium, particularly double-blind randomized controlled studies, are increasingly reported and support the judicious use of neuroleptics for acute prophylaxis. They also indicate that treatment with atypical agents has some advantages over treatment with conventional agents. The risk-benefit ratio may still be favorable for time-limited delirium treatment using a neuroleptic in elderly patients with dementia. Chronic dosing with cholinesterase inhibitors or statins and avoidance of deliriogenic agents during anesthesia, analgesia, and ICU care have been shown to reduce delirium incidence, severity, or both in a growing number of studies. Benzodiazepines are particularly problematic and should be avoided whenever possible, unless alcohol withdrawal is involved. It is important to initiate treatment even before medical causes have been rectified and for both hypoactive and hyperactive motor presentations because target symptoms are cognition, thought, sleep, and language. (Both motor presentations respond to treatment.) That delirium is common yet inadequately detected; associated with increased morbidity, mortality, and length of hospitalization; and potentially caused by virtually anything from a textbook of medicine has been well substantiated. The travesty is the lack of an efficacious and well-tolerated treatment approved by a regulatory agency. Clearly, delirium needs to become a top priority for regulatory agencies and national research funding institutions.

Recommended Readings

Breitbart W, Gibson C, Tremblay A: The delirium experience: delirium recall and delirium-related distress in hospitalized patients with cancer, their spouses/caregivers, and their nurses. Psychosomatics 43:183–194, 2002

Engel GL, Romano J: Delirium, a syndrome of cerebral insufficiency. J Chronic Dis 9:260–277, 1959

Kalisvaart KJ, de Jonghe JFM, Bogaards MJ, et al: Haloperidol prophylaxis for elderly hip surgery patients at risk for delirium: a randomized placebo-controlled study. J Am Geriatr Soc 53:1658–1666, 2005

Marcantonio ER, Flacker JM, Wright RJ, et al: Reducing delirium after hip fracture: a randomized trial. J Am Geriatr Soc 49:516–522, 2001

Meagher D: Delirium: optimising management. BMJ 322:144–149, 2001

Trzepacz PT: Is there a final common neural pathway in delirium? Focus on acetylcholine and dopamine. Semin Clin Neuropsychiatry 5:132–148, 2000

References

Adams F: Neuropsychiatric evaluation and treatment of delirium in the critically ill cancer patient. Cancer Bull 36:156–160, 1984

Adams F: Emergency intravenous sedation of the delirious medically ill patient. J Clin Psychiatry 49(suppl):22–26, 1988

Al-Aama T, Brymer C, Gutmanis I, et al: Melatonin decreases delirium in elderly patients: a randomized, placebo-controlled trial. Int J Geriatr Psychiatry 26:687–694, 2011

Alexopoulos GS, Streim J, Carpenter D, et al: Using antipsychotic agents in older patients. Expert Consensus Panel for Using Antipsychotic Drugs in Older Patients. J Clin Psychiatry 65 (suppl 2):5–99, 2004

Al-Samarrai S, Dunn J, Newmark T, et al: Quetiapine for treatment-resistant delirium. Psychosomatics 44:350–351, 2003

American Psychiatric Association: Diagnostic and Statistical Manual: Mental Disorders. Washington, DC, American Psychiatric Association, 1952

American Psychiatric Association: Diagnostic and Statistical Manual of Mental Disorders, 2nd Edition. Washington, DC, American Psychiatric Association, 1968

American Psychiatric Association: Diagnostic and Statistical Manual of Mental Disorders, 3rd Edition. Washington, DC, American Psychiatric Association, 1980

American Psychiatric Association: Diagnostic and Statistical Manual of Mental Disorders, 3rd Edition, Revised. Washington, DC, American Psychiatric Association, 1987

American Psychiatric Association: Diagnostic and Statistical Manual of Mental Disorders, 4th Edition. Washington, DC, American Psychiatric Association, 1994

American Psychiatric Association: Practice guideline for the treatment of patients with delirium. Am J Psychiatry 156(5 suppl):1–20, 1999

American Psychiatric Association: Diagnostic and Statistical Manual of Mental Disorders, 4th Edition, Text Revision. Washington, DC, American Psychiatric Association, 2000

Anderson SD: Treatment of elderly patients with delirium. CMAJ 152:323–324, 1995

Armstrong DH, Dasts JF, Reilly TE, et al: Effect of haloperidol on dopamine-induced increase in renal blood flow. Drug Intell Clin Pharm 20:543–546, 1986

Armstrong SC, Cozza KL, Watanabe KS: The misdiagnosis of delirium. Psychosomatics 38:433–439, 1997

Bartlett EJ, Brodie JD, Simkowitz P, et al: Effects of haloperidol challenge on regional cerebral glucose utilization in normal human subjects. Am J Psychiatry 151:681–686, 1994

Bayindir O, Akpinar B, Can E, et al: The use of the 5-HT3-receptor antagonist ondansetron for the treatment of postcardiotomy delirium. J Cardiothorac Vasc Anesth 14:288–292, 2000

Bedford PD: General medical aspects of confusional states in elderly people. Br Med J 2:185–188, 1959

Bogardus ST Jr, Desai MM, Williams CS, et al: The effects of a targeted multicomponent delirium intervention on postdischarge outcomes for hospitalized older adults. Am J Med 114:383–390, 2003

Bostwick JM, Masterson BJ: Psychopharmacological treatment of delirium to restore mental capacity. Psychosomatics 39:112–117, 1998

Bourdel-Marchasson I, Vincent S, Germain C, et al: Delirium symptoms and low dietary intake in older inpatients are independent predictors of institutionalization: a 1-year prospective population-based study. J Gerontol A Biol Sci Med Sci 59:350–354, 2004

Bourgeois JA, Koike AK, Simmons JE, et al: Adjunctive valproic acid for delirium and/or agitation on a consultation-liaison service: a report of six cases. J Neuropsychiatry Clin Neurosci 17:232–238, 2005

Bourne RS, Tahir TA, Borthwick M, et al: Drug treatment of delirium: past, present and future. J Psychosom Res 65:273–282, 2008

Breitbart W, Marotta R, Platt MM, et al: A double-blind trial of haloperidol, chlorpromazine, and lorazepam in the treatment of delirium in hospitalized AIDS patients. Am J Psychiatry 153:231–237, 1996

Breitbart W, Rosenfeld B, Roth A, et al: The Memorial Delirium Assessment Scale. J Pain Symptom Manage 13:128–137, 1997

Breitbart W, Gibson C, Tremblay A: The delirium experience: delirium recall and delirium-related distress in hospitalized patients with cancer, their spouses/caregivers, and their nurses. Psychosomatics 43:183–194, 2002a

Breitbart W, Tremblay A, Gibson C: An open trial of olanzapine for the treatment of delirium in hospitalized cancer patients. Psychosomatics 43:175–182, 2002b

Brown RL, Henke A, Greenhalgh DG, et al: The use of haloperidol in the agitated, critically ill pediatric patient with burns. J Burn Care Rehabil 17:34–38, 1996

Burke WJ, Roccaforte WH, Wengel SP: Treating visual hallucinations with donepezil. Am J Psychiatry 156:1117–1118, 1999

Burns MJ, Linden CH, Graudins A, et al: A comparison of physostigmine and benzodiazepines for the treatment of anticholinergic poisoning. Ann Emerg Med 35:374–381, 2000

Caeiro L, Ferro JM, Albuquerque R, et al: Delirium in the first days of acute stroke. J Neurol 251:171–178, 2004

Camus V, Gonthier R, Dubos G, et al: Etiologic and outcome profiles in hypoactive and hyperactive subtypes of delirium. J Geriatr Psychiatry Neurol 13:38–42, 2000

Caplan GA, Coconis J, Board N, et al: Does home treatment affect delirium? A randomised controlled trial of rehabilitation of elderly and care at home or usual treatment (the REACH-OUT trial). Age Ageing 35:53–60, 2005

Carnes M, Howell T, Rosenberg M, et al: Physicians vary in approaches to the clinical assessment of delirium. J Am Geriatr Soc 51:234–239, 2003

Charlton BG, Kavanau JL: Delirium and psychotic symptoms: an integrative model. Med Hypotheses 58:24–27, 2002

Chatham MA: The effect of family involvement on patients' manifestations of postcardiotomy psychosis. Heart Lung 7:995–999, 1978

Chedru F, Geschwind N: Writing disturbances in acute confusional states. Neuropsychologia 10:343–353, 1972

Chen B, Cardasis W: Delirium induced by lithium and risperidone combination. Am J Psychiatry 153:1233–1234, 1996

Cole MG, McCusker J, Dendukuri N, et al: Symptoms of delirium among elderly medical inpatients with or without dementia. J Neuropsychiatry Clin Neurosci 14:167–175, 2002

Cole M, McCusker J, Dendukuri N, et al: The prognostic significance of subsyndromal delirium in elderly medical inpatients. J Am Geriatr Soc 51:754–760, 2003

Cutting J: The phenomenology of acute organic psychosis: comparison with acute schizophrenia. Br J Psychiatry 151:324–332, 1987

Dautzenberg PL, Mulder LJ, Olde Rikkert MG, et al: Delirium in elderly hospitalized patients: protective effects of chronic rivastigmine usage. Int J Geriatr Psychiatry 19:641–644, 2004

de Jonghe JF, Kalisvaart KJ, Eikelenboom P, et al: Early symptoms in the prodromal phase of delirium in elderly hip-surgery patients (abstract). Int Psychogeriatr 17 (suppl 2):148, 2005

Devlin JW, Roberts RJ, Fong JJ, et al: Efficacy and safety of quetiapine in critically ill patients with delirium: a prospective, multicenter, randomized, double-blind, placebo-controlled pilot study. Crit Care Med 38:419–427, 2010

Díaz V, Rodríguez J, Barrientos P, et al: [Use of procholinergics in the prevention of postoperative delirium in hip fracture surgery in the elderly: a randomized controlled trial.] (in Spanish) Rev Neurol 33:716–719, 2001

Drake ME, Coffey CE: Complex partial status epilepticus simulating psychogenic unresponsiveness. Am J Psychiatry 140:800–801, 1983

Dudley DL, Rowlett DB, Loebel PJ: Emergency use of intravenous haloperidol. Gen Hosp Psychiatry 1:240–246, 1979

Duppils GS, Wikblad K: Delirium: behavioural changes before and during the prodromal phase. J Clin Nurs 13:609–616, 2004

Easton C, MacKenzie F: Sensory-perceptual alterations: delirium in the intensive care unit. Heart Lung 17:229–237, 1988

Elie M, Boss K, Cole MG, et al: A retrospective, exploratory, secondary analysis of the association between antipsychotic use and mortality in elderly patients with delirium. Int Psychogeriatr 21:588–592, 2009

Ely EW, Dittus RS: Pharmacological treatment of delirium in the intensive care unit (letter). JAMA 292:168, 2004

Ely EW, Margolin R, Francis J, et al: Evaluation of delirium in critically ill patients: validation of the Confusion Assessment Method for the Intensive Care Unit (CAM-ICU). Crit Care Med 29:1370–1379, 2001

Ely EW, Stephens RK, Jackson JC, et al: Current opinions regarding the importance, diagnosis, and management of delirium in the intensive care unit: a survey of 912 healthcare professionals. Crit Care Med 32:106–112, 2004

Engel GL, Romano J: Delirium, II: reversibility of the electroencephalogram with experimental procedures. Arch Neurol Psychiatry 51:378–392, 1944

Engel GL, Romano J: Delirium, a syndrome of cerebral insufficiency. J Chronic Dis 9:260–277, 1959

Ewert J, Levin HS, Watson MG, et al: Procedural memory during posttraumatic amnesia in survivors of severe closed head injury: implications for rehabilitation. Arch Neurol 46:911–916, 1985

Fann JR, Alfano CM, Burington BE, et al: Clinical presentation of delirium in patients undergoing hematopoietic stem cell transplantation. Cancer 103:810–820, 2005

Farrell KR, Ganzini L: Misdiagnosing delirium as depression in medically ill elderly patients. Arch Intern Med 155:2459–2464, 1995

Fernandez F, Holmes VF, Adams F, et al: Treatment of severe, refractory agitation with a haloperidol drip. J Clin Psychiatry 49:239–241, 1988

Fernandez F, Levy JK, Mansell PWA: Management of delirium in terminally ill AIDS patients. Int J Psychiatry Med 19:165–172, 1989

Ferro JM, Caeiro L, Verdelho A: Delirium in acute stroke. Curr Opin Neurol 15:51–55, 2002

Flaherty JH, Tariq SH, Raghavan S, et al: A model for managing delirious older inpatients. J Am Geriatr Soc 51:1031–1035, 2003

Foley CM, Polinsky MS, Gruskin AB, et al: Encephalopathy in infants and children with chronic renal disease. Arch Neurol 38:656–658, 1981

Francis J: Sensory and environmental factors in delirium. Paper presented at Delirium: Current Advancements in Diagnosis, Treatment and Research, Geriatric Research, Education, and Clinical Center (GRECC), Veterans Administration Medical Center, Minneapolis, MN, September 13–14, 1993

Franco JG, Valencia C, Bernal C, et al: Relationship between cognitive status at admission and incident delirium in older medical inpatients. J Neuropsychiatry Clin Neurosci 22:329–337, 2010

Gagnon B, Low G, Schreier G: Methylphenidate hydrochloride improves cognitive function in patients with advanced cancer and hypoactive delirium: a prospective clinical study. J Psychiatry Neurosci 30:100–107, 2005

Gagnon P, Charbonneau C, Allard P, et al: Delirium in advanced cancer: a psychoeducational intervention for family caregivers. J Palliat Care 18:253–261, 2002

Gelfand SB, Indelicato J, Benjamin J: Using intravenous haloperidol to control delirium (abstract). Hosp Community Psychiatry 43:215, 1992

Girard TD, Pandharipande PP, Carson SS, et al; for MIND Trial Investigators: Feasibility, efficacy, and safety of antipsychotics for intensive care unit delirium: the MIND randomized, placebo-controlled trial. Crit Care Med 38:428–437, 2010

Hally O, Cooney C: Delirium in the hospitalised elderly: an audit of NCHD prescribing practice. Ir J Psychol Med 22:133–136, 2005

Han CS, Kim YK: A double-blind trial of risperidone and haloperidol for the treatment of delirium. Psychosomatics 45:297–301, 2004

Harrell R, Othmer E: Postcardiotomy confusion and sleep loss. J Clin Psychiatry 48:445–446, 1987

Hart RP, Levenson JL, Sessler CN, et al: Validation of a cognitive test for delirium in medical ICU patients. Psychosomatics 37:533–546, 1996

Hatta K, Takahashi T, Nakamura H, et al: The association between intravenous haloperidol and prolonged QT interval. J Clin Psychopharmacol 21:257–261, 2001

Heinrich TW, Biblo LA, Schneider J: Torsades de pointes associated with ziprasidone. Psychosomatics 47:264–268, 2006

Herrmann N, Mamdani M, Lanctôt KL: Atypical antipsychotics and risk of cerebrovascular accidents. Am J Psychiatry 161:1113–1115, 2004

Hill EH, Blumenfield M, Orlowski B: A modification of the Trzepacz Delirium Rating Scale—Revised-98 for use on the Palm Pilot, and a presentation of data of symptom monitoring using haloperidol, olanzapine, and risperidone in the treatment of delirious hospitalized patients (abstract). Psychosomatics 43:158, 2002

Horikawa N, Yamazaki T, Miyamoto K, et al: Treatment for delirium with risperidone: results of a prospective open trial with 10 patients. Gen Hosp Psychiatry 25:289–292, 2003

Hua H, Wei D, Hui Y, et al: Olanzapine and haloperidol for senile delirium: a randomized controlled observation. Chinese Journal of Clinical Rehabilitation 10:188–190, 2006

Hudetz JA, Iqbal Z, Gandhi SD, et al: Ketamine attenuates post-operative cognitive dysfunction after cardiac surgery. Acta Anaesthesiol Scand 53:864–872, 2009

Hustey FM, Meldon SW, Smith MD, et al: The effect of mental status screening on the care of elderly emergency department patients. Ann Emerg Med 41:678–684, 2003

Huyse F: Haloperidol and cardiac arrest. Lancet 2:568–569, 1988

Inouye SK, van Dyke CH, Alessi CA, et al: Clarifying confusion: the Confusion Assessment Method. Ann Intern Med 113:941–948, 1990

Inouye SK, Bogardus ST Jr, Charpentier PA, et al: A multicomponent intervention to prevent delirium in hospitalized older patients. N Engl J Med 340:669–676, 1999

Inouye SK, Foreman MD, Mion LC, et al: Nurses' recognition of delirium and its symptoms: comparison of nurse and researcher ratings. Arch Intern Med 161:2467–2473, 2001

Inouye SK, Bogardus ST Jr, Williams CS, et al: The role of adherence on the effectiveness of nonpharmacologic interventions: evidence from the delirium prevention trial. Arch Intern Med 163:958–964, 2003

Insau P, Lawley D: CSM guidance on antipsychotic use: care of the elderly in psychosis. Geriatric Medicine 14(suppl):6–7, 2004

Jacobson S, Jerrier H: EEG in delirium. Semin Clin Neuropsychiatry 5:86–92, 2000

Jacobson SA, Leuchter AF, Walter DO: Conventional and quantitative EEG diagnosis of delirium among the elderly. J Neurol Neurosurg Psychiatry 56:153–158, 1993a

Jacobson SA, Leuchter AF, Walter DO, et al: Serial quantitative EEG among elderly subjects with delirium. Biol Psychiatry 34:135–140, 1993b

Johnson JC, Kerse NM, Gottlieb G, et al: Prospective versus retrospective methods of identifying patients with delirium. J Am Geriatr Soc 40:316–319, 1992

Kain ZN, MacLaren JE, Herrmann L, et al: Preoperative melatonin and its effects on induction and emergence in children undergoing anesthesia and surgery. Anesthesiology 111:44–49, 2009

Kakuma R, du Fort GG, Arsenault L, et al: Delirium in older emergency department patients discharged home: effect on survival. J Am Geriatr Soc 51:443–450, 2003

Kalisvaart CJ, Boelaarts L, de Jonghe JF, et al: Successful treatment of three elderly patients suffering from prolonged delirium using the cholinesterase inhibitor rivastigmine [in Dutch]. Ned Tijdschr Geneeskd 148:1501–1504, 2004

Kalisvaart KJ, de Jonghe JF, Bogaards MJ, et al: Haloperidol prophylaxis for elderly hip-surgery patients at risk for delirium: a randomized placebo-controlled study. J Am Geriatr Soc 53:1658–1666, 2005

Kaneko T, Cai J, Ishikura T, et al: Prophylactic consecutive administration of haloperidol can reduce the occurrence of postoperative delirium in gastrointestinal surgery. Yonago Acta Med 42:179–184, 1999

Kapur S, Seeman P: Does fast dissociation from the dopamine D2 receptor explain the action of atypical antipsychotics? A new hypothesis. Am J Psychiatry 158:360–369, 2001

Karki SD, Masood GR: Combination risperidone and SSRI-induced serotonin syndrome. Ann Pharmacother 37:388–391, 2003

Kasahara H, Karasawa A, Ariyasu T, et al: Alcohol dementia and alcohol delirium in aged alcoholics. Psychiatry Clin Neurosci 50:115–123, 1996

Katz JA, Mahoney DH, Fernbach DJ: Human leukocyte alpha-interferon induced transient neurotoxicity in children. Invest New Drugs 6:115–120, 1988

Katznelson R, Djaiani GN, Borger MA, et al: Preoperative use of statins is associated with reduced early delirium rates after cardiac surgery. Anesthesiology 110:67–73, 2009

Kiely DK, Bergmann MA, Jones RN, et al: Characteristics associated with delirium persistence among newly admitted post-acute facility patients. J Gerontol A Biol Sci Med Sci 59:344–349, 2004

Kim JY, Jung IK, Han C, et al: Antipsychotics and dopamine transporter gene polymorphisms in delirium patients. Psychiatry Clin Neurosci 59:183–188, 2005

Kim KS, Pae CU, Chae JH, et al: An open pilot trial of olanzapine for delirium in the Korean population. Psychiatry Clin Neurosci 55:515–519, 2001

Kim KY, Bader GM, Kotlyar V, et al: Treatment of delirium in older adults with quetiapine. J Geriatr Psychiatry Neurol 16:29–31, 2003

Klijn IA, van der Mast RC: Pharmacotherapy of alcohol withdrawal delirium in patients admitted to a general hospital (comment). Arch Intern Med 165:346, 2005

Kolbeinsson H, Jonsson A: Delirium and dementia in acute medical admissions of elderly patients in Iceland. Acta Psychiatr Scand 87:123–127, 1993

Koponen H, Partanen J, Paakkonen A, et al: EEG spectral analysis in delirium. J Neurol Neurosurg Psychiatry 52:980–985, 1989

Koponen H, Sirvio J, Lepola U, et al: A long-term follow-up study of cerebrospinal fluid acetylcholinesterase in delirium. Eur Arch Psychiatry Clin Neurosci 243:347–351, 1994

Kriwisky M, Perry GY, Tarchitsky D, et al: Haloperidol-induced torsades de pointes. Chest 98:482–484, 1990

Kullmann F, Hollerbach S, Holstege A, et al: Subclinical hepatic encephalopathy: the diagnostic value of evoked potentials. J Hepatol 22:101–110, 1995

Larsen KA, Kelly SE, Stern TA, et al: Administration of olanzapine to prevent postoperative delirium in elderly joint-replacement patients: a randomized, controlled trial. Psychosomatics 51:409–418, 2010

Laurila JV, Pitkala KH, Strandberg TE, et al: Delirium among patients with and without dementia: does the diagnosis according to the DSM-IV differ from the previous classifications? Int J Geriatr Psychiatry 19:271–277, 2004

Lee KU, Won WY, Lee HK, et al: Amisulpride versus quetiapine for the treatment of delirium: a randomized, open prospective study. Int Clin Psychopharmacol 20:311–314, 2005

Lemey L, Vranken C, Simoens K, et al: The "flying delirium room": towards an adequate approach to acute delirium in a general hospital (abstract). Int Psychogeriatr 17 (suppl 2):260, 2005

Leso L, Schwartz TL: Ziprasidone treatment of delirium. Psychosomatics 43:61–62, 2002

Leung JM, Sands LP, Rico M, et al: Pilot clinical trial of gabapentin to decrease postoperative delirium in older patients. Neurology 67:1251–1253, 2006

Levenson JA: Should psychostimulants be used to treat delirious patients with depressed mood? (letter). J Clin Psychiatry 53:69, 1992

Levenson JL: High-dose intravenous haloperidol for agitated delirium following lung transplantation. Psychosomatics 36:66–68, 1995

Levkoff SE, Evans DA, Liptzin B, et al: Delirium: the occurrence and persistence of symptoms among elderly hospitalized patients. Arch Intern Med 152:334–340, 1992

Liptzin B, Levkoff SE, Gottlieb GL, et al: Delirium: background papers for DSM-IV. J Neuropsychiatry Clin Neurosci 5:154–160, 1993

Liptzin B, Laki A, Garb JL, et al: Donepezil in the prevention and treatment of postsurgical delirium. Am J Geriatr Psychiatry 13:1100–1106, 2005

Lundstrom M, Edlund A, Karlsson S, et al: A multifactorial intervention program reduces the duration of delirium, length of hospitalization, and mortality in delirious patients. J Am Geriatr Soc 53:622–628, 2005

Maldonado JR, Wysong A, van der Starre PJ, et al: Dexmedetomidine and the reduction of postoperative delirium after cardiac surgery. Psychosomatics 50:206–217, 2009

Marcantonio ER, Flacker JM, Wright RJ, et al: Reducing delirium after hip fracture: a randomized trial. J Am Geriatr Soc 49:516–522, 2001

Marcantonio E, Ta T, Duthie E, et al: Delirium severity and psychomotor types: their relationship with outcomes after hip fracture repair. J Am Geriatr Soc 50:850–857, 2002

Marcantonio ER, Simon SE, Bergmann MA, et al: Delirium symptoms in post-acute care: prevalent, persistent, and associated with poor functional recovery. J Am Geriatr Soc 51:4–9, 2003

Marcantonio ER, Kiely DK, Simon SE, et al: Outcomes of older people admitted to postacute facilities with delirium. J Am Geriatr Soc 53:963–969, 2005

Matsushima E, Nakajima K, Moriya H, et al: A psychophysiological study of the development of delirium in coronary care units. Biol Psychiatry 41:1211–1217, 1997

Mayo-Smith MF, Beecher LH, Fischer TL, et al; Working Group on the Management of Alcohol Withdrawal Delirium, Practice Guidelines Committee, American Society of Addiction Medicine: Management of alcohol withdrawal delirium: an evidence-based practice guideline. Arch Intern Med 164:1405–1412, 2004

McCaffrey R, Locsin R: The effect of music listening on acute confusion and delirium in elders undergoing elective hip and knee surgery. J Clin Nurs 13:91–96, 2004

McCusker J, Cole M, Abrahamowicz M, et al: Environmental risk factors for delirium in hospitalized older people. J Am Geriatr Soc 49:1327–1334, 2001

McCusker J, Cole MG, Dendukuri N, et al: The course of delirium in older medical inpatients: a prospective study. J Gen Intern Med 18:696–704, 2003

McKeith I, Fairbairn A, Perry R, et al: Neuroleptic sensitivity in patients with senile dementia of Lewy body type. BMJ 305:673–678, 1992

McNicoll L, Pisani MA, Zhang Y, et al: Delirium in the intensive care unit: occurrence and clinical course in older patients. J Am Geriatr Soc 51:591–598, 2003

Meagher D: Delirium episode as a sign of undetected dementia among community dwelling elderly subjects (letter). J Neurol Neurosurg Psychiatry 70:821, 2001a

Meagher D: Delirium: optimising management. BMJ 322(7279):144–149, 2001b

Meagher D: Clearing the confusion: psychopathology, cognition, and motoric profile in 100 consecutive cases of delirium. Int Psychogeriatr 17 (suppl 2):120–121, 2005

Meagher DJ, Trzepacz PT: Delirium phenomenology illuminates pathophysiology, management and course. J Geriatr Psychiatry Neurol 11:150–157, 1998

Meagher DJ, Trzepacz PT: Motoric subtypes of delirium. Semin Clin Neuropsychiatry 5:76–86, 2000

Meagher DJ, O'Hanlon D, O'Mahony E, et al: Use of environmental strategies and psychotropic medication in the management of delirium. Br J Psychiatry 168:512–515, 1996

Meagher DJ, Moran M, Raju B, et al: Phenomenology of 100 consecutive adult cases of delirium. Br J Psychiatry 190:135–141, 2007

Meagher DJ, Leonard M, Donnelly S, et al: A comparison of neuropsychiatric and cognitive profiles in delirium, dementia, comorbid delirium-dementia and cognitively intact controls. J Neurol Neurosurg Psychiatry 81:876–881, 2010

Mendelson G: Pheniramine aminosalicylate overdosage: reversal of delirium and choreiform movements with tacrine treatment. Arch Neurol 34:313, 1977

Metzger E, Friedman R: Prolongation of the corrected QT and torsades de pointes cardiac arrhythmia associated with intravenous haloperidol in the medically ill. J Clin Psychopharmacol 13:128–132, 1993

Milbrandt EB, Kersten A, Kong L, et al: Haloperidol use is associated with lower hospital mortality in mechanically ventilated patients. Crit Care Med 33:226–229, 2005

Milisen K, Foreman MD, Abraham IL, et al: A nurse-led interdisciplinary intervention program for delirium in elderly hip-fracture patients. J Am Geriatr Soc 49:523–532, 2001

Mittal D, Jimerson NA, Neely EP, et al: Risperidone in the treatment of delirium: results from a prospective open-label trial. J Clin Psychiatry 65:662–667, 2004

Montgomery EA, Fenton GW, McClelland RJ, et al: Psychobiology of minor head injury. Psychosom Med 21:375–384, 1991

Moretti R, Torre P, Antonello RM, et al: Cholinesterase inhibition as a possible therapy for delirium in vascular dementia: a controlled, open 24-month study of 246 patients. Am J Alzheimers Dis Other Demen 19:333–339, 2004

Morita T, Otani H, Tsunoda J, et al: Successful palliation of hypoactive delirium due to multi-organ failure by oral methylphenidate. Support Care Cancer 8:134–137, 2000

Morita T, Hirai K, Sakaguchi Y, et al: Family perceived distress about delirium-related symptoms of terminally ill cancer patients. Psychosomatics 45:107–113, 2004

Moulaert P: Treatment of acute nonspecific delirium with IV haloperidol in surgical intensive care patients. Acta Anaesthesiol Belg 40:183–186, 1989

Nagley SJ: Predicting and preventing confusion in your patients. J Gerontol Nurs 12:27–31, 1986

Nakamura J, Uchimura N, Yamada S, et al: [Effects of mianserin hydrochloride on delirium: comparison with the effects of oxypertine and haloperidol] (in Japanese). Nihon Shinkei Seishin Yakurigaku Zasshi 14:269–277, 1994

Nakamura J, Uchimura N, Yamada S, et al: The effect of mianserin hydrochloride on delirium. Hum Psychopharmacol 10:289–297, 1995

Nakamura J, Uchimura N, Yamada S, et al: Does plasma free-3-methoxy-4-hydroxy-phenyl(ethylene)glycol increase in the delirious state? A comparison of the effects of mianserin and haloperidol on delirium. Int Clin Psychopharmacol 12:147–152, 1997a

Nakamura J, Uchimura N, Yamada S, et al: Mianserin suppositories in the treatment of post-operative delirium. Hum Psychopharmacol 12:595–599, 1997b

Nicholas LM, Lindsey BA: Delirium presenting with symptoms of depression. Psychosomatics 36:471–479, 1995

O'Brien JM, Rockwood RP, Suh KI: Haloperidol-induced torsades de pointes. Ann Pharmacother 33:1046–1050, 1999

O'Keeffe ST: Rating the severity of delirium: the Delirium Assessment Scale. Int J Geriatr Psychiatry 9:551–556, 1994

O'Keeffe S: The experience of delirium in older people (abstract). Int Psychogeriatr 17 (suppl 2):120, 2005

O'Keeffe ST, Gosney MA: Assessing attentiveness in older hospitalized patients: global assessment vs. test of attention. J Am Geriatr Soc 45:470–473, 1997

O'Keeffe ST, Tormey WP, Glasgow R, et al: Thiamine deficiency in hospitalized elderly patients. Gerontology 40:18–24, 1994

O'Keeffe ST, Mulkerrin EC, Nayeem K, et al: Use of serial Mini-Mental State Examinations to diagnose and monitor delirium in elderly hospital patients. J Am Geriatr Soc 53:867–870, 2005

Okumura A, Nakano T, Fukumoto Y, et al: Delirious behavior in children with influenza: its clinical features and EEG findings. Brain Dev 27:271–274, 2005

Onofrj M, Curatola L, Malatesta G, et al: Reduction of P3 latency during outcome from post-traumatic amnesia. Acta Neurol Scand 83:273–279, 1991

Ovchinsky N, Pitchumoni S, Skotzko CE: Use of olanzapine for the treatment of delirium following traumatic brain injury. Psychosomatics 43:147–148, 2002

Owens JF, Hutelmyer CM: The effect of preoperative intervention on delirium in cardiac surgical patients. Nurs Res 31:60–62, 1982

Pae CU, Lee SJ, Lee CU, et al: A pilot trial of quetiapine for the treatment of patients with delirium. Hum Psychopharmacol 19:125–127, 2004

Pandharipande P, Shintani A, Peterson J, et al: Lorazepam is an independent risk factor for transitioning to delirium in intensive care unit patients. Anesthesiology 104:21–26, 2006

Pandharipande PP, Pun BT, Herr DL, et al: Effect of sedation with dexmedetomidine vs. lorazepam on acute brain dysfunction in mechanically ventilated patients: the MENDS randomized controlled trial. JAMA 298:2644–2653, 2007

Parellada E, Baeza I, de Pablo J, et al: Risperidone in the treatment of patients with delirium. J Clin Psychiatry 65:348–353, 2004

Passik SD, Cooper M: Complicated delirium in a cancer patient successfully treated with olanzapine. J Pain Symptom Manage 17:219–223, 1999

Patten SB, Lamarre CJ: Dysgraphia (letter). Can J Psychiatry 34:746, 1989

Perrault LP, Denault AY, Carrier M, et al: Torsades de pointes secondary to intravenous haloperidol after coronary bypass grafting surgery. Can J Anaesth 47:251–254, 2000

Platt MM, Breitbart W, Smith M, et al: Efficacy of neuroleptics for hypoactive delirium. J Neuropsychiatry Clin Neurosci 6:66–67, 1994a

Platt MM, Trautman P, Frager G, et al: Pediatric delirium: research update. Paper presented at the annual meeting of the Academy of Psychosomatic Medicine, Phoenix, AZ, November 1994b

Prakanrattana U, Prapaitrakool S: Efficacy of risperidone for prevention of postoperative delirium in cardiac surgery. Anaesth Intensive Care 35:714–719, 2007

Prugh DG, Wagonfeld S, Metcalf D, et al: A clinical study of delirium in children and adolescents. Psychosom Med 42:177–195, 1980

Rahkonen T, Luukkainen-Markkula R, Paanila S, et al: Delirium as a sign of undetected dementia among community dwelling elderly subjects: a 2 year follow up study. J Neurol Neurosurg Psychiatry 69:519–521, 2000

Ravona-Springer R, Dohlberg OT, Hirschman S, et al: Delirium in elderly patients treated with risperidone: a report of three cases. J Clin Psychopharmacol 18:171–172, 1998

Riker RR, Fraser GL, Cox PM: Continuous infusion of haloperidol controls agitation in critically ill patients. Crit Care Med 22:433–440, 1994

Riker RR, Fraser GL, Richen P: Movement disorders associated with withdrawal from high-dose intravenous haloperidol therapy in delirious ICU patients. Chest 111:1778–1781, 1997

Riker RR, Shehabi Y, Bokesch PM, et al: Dexmedetomidine vs. midazolam for sedation of critically ill patients: a randomized trial. JAMA 301:489–499, 2009

Robinson MJ: Probable Lewy body dementia presenting as "delirium." Psychosomatics 43:84–86, 2002

Rockwood K: The occurrence and duration of symptoms in elderly patients with delirium. J Gerontol 48:M162–M166, 1993

Rockwood K, Cosway S, Stolee P, et al: Increasing the recognition of delirium in elderly patients. J Am Geriatr Soc 42:252–256, 1994

Rockwood K, Cosway S, Carver D, et al: The risk of dementia and death after delirium. Age Ageing 28:551–556, 1999

Romano J, Engel GL: Delirium, I: electroencephalographic data. Arch Neurol Psychiatry 51:356–377, 1944

Rosenberg PB, Ahmed I, Hurwitz S: Methylphenidate in depressed medically ill patients. J Clin Psychiatry 52:263–267, 1991

Rubino AS, Onorati F, Caroleo S, et al: Impact of clonidine administration on delirium and related respiratory weaning after surgical correction of acute type-A aortic dissection: results of a pilot study. Interact Cardiovasc Thorac Surg 10:58–62, 2010 [Epub 2009 Oct 23]

Rudberg MA, Pompei P, Foreman MD, et al: The natural history of delirium in older hospitalized patients: a syndrome of heterogeneity. Age Ageing 26:169–174, 1997

Ruijs MB, Keyser A, Gabreels FJ, et al: Somatosensory evoked potentials and cognitive sequelae in children with closed head injury. Neuropediatrics 24:307–312, 1993

Ruijs MB, Gabreels FJ, Thijssen HM: The utility of electroencephalography and cerebral CT in children with mild and moderately severe closed head injuries. Neuropediatrics 25:73–77, 1994

Sampson EL, Raven PR, Ndhlovu PN, et al: A randomized, double-blind, placebo-controlled trial of donepezil hydrochloride (Aricept) for reducing the incidence of postoperative delirium after elective total hip replacement. Int J Geriatr Psychiatry 22:343–349, 2006

Samuels S, Fang M: Olanzapine may cause delirium in geriatric patients. J Clin Psychiatry 65:582–583, 2004

Sanders KM, Stern TA: Management of delirium associated with use of the intra-aortic balloon pump. Am J Crit Care 2:371–377, 1993

Sasaki Y, Matsuyama T, Inoue S, et al: A prospective, open-label, flexible-dose study of quetiapine in the treatment of delirium. J Clin Psychiatry 64:1316–1321, 2003

Schindler BA, Shook J, Schwartz GM: Beneficial effects of psychiatric intervention on recovery after coronary artery bypass graft surgery. Gen Hosp Psychiatry 11:358–364, 1989

Schneider A: Use of intravenous valproate (Depacon) in the treatment of delirium: a case series. Neurobiol Aging 25 (suppl 2):S302–S303, 2005

Schneider LS, Dagerman KS, Insel P: Risk of death with atypical antipsychotic drug treatment for dementia: meta-analysis of randomized placebo-controlled trials. JAMA 294:1934–1943, 2005

Schneir AB, Offerman SR, Ly BT, et al: Complications of diagnostic physostigmine administration to emergency department patients. Ann Emerg Med 42:14–19, 2003

Schofield I: A small exploratory study of the reaction of older people to an episode of delirium. J Adv Nurs 25:942–952, 1997

Sherer M, Nakas-Thompson R, Yablon SA, et al: Multidimensional assessment of acute confusion after traumatic brain injury. Arch Phys Med Rehabil 86:896–904, 2005

Shigeta H, Yasui A, Nimura Y, et al: Postoperative delirium and melatonin levels in elderly patients. Am J Surg 182:449–454, 2001

Sim FH, Brunet DG, Conacher GN: Quetiapine associated with acute mental status changes (letter). Can J Psychiatry 3:299, 2000

Sipahimalani A, Masand PS: Olanzapine in the treatment of delirium. Psychosomatics 39:422–430, 1998

Skrobik YK, Bergeron N, Dumont M, et al: Olanzapine vs. haloperidol: treating delirium in a critical care setting. Intensive Care Med 30:444–449, 2004

Stern TA: Continuous infusion of physostigmine in anticholinergic delirium: a case report. J Clin Psychiatry 44:463–464, 1983

Stern TA: Continuous infusion of haloperidol in agitated critically ill patients. Crit Care Med 22:378–379, 1994

Sternberg SA, Wolfson C, Baumgarten M: Undetected dementia in community-dwelling older people: the Canadian Study of Health and Aging. J Am Geriatr Soc 48:1430–1434, 2000

Straker DA, Shapiro PA, Muskin PR: Aripiprazole in the treatment of delirium. Psychosomatics 47:385–391, 2006

Sundaram M, Dostrow V: Epilepsy in the elderly. Neurologist 1:232–239, 1995

Swenson JR, Erman M, Labelle J, et al: Extrapyramidal reactions: neuropsychiatric mimics in patients with AIDS. Gen Hosp Psychiatry 11:248–253, 1989

Tahir TA, Eeles E, Karapareddy V, et al: A randomized controlled trial of quetiapine versus placebo in the treatment of delirium. J Psychosom Res 69:485–490, 2010

Takeuchi T, Furuta K, Hirasawa T, et al: Perospirone in the treatment of patients with delirium. Psychiatry Clin Neurosci 61:67–70, 2007

Teicher MH, Glod CA: Neuroleptic drugs: indications and guidelines for their rational use in children and adolescents. J Child Adolesc Psychopharmacol 1:33–56, 1990

Tesar GE, Murray GB, Cassem NH: Use of high-dose intravenous haloperidol in the treatment of agitated cardiac patients. J Clin Psychopharmacol 5:344–347, 1985

Toda H, Kusumi I, Sasaki Y, et al: Relationship between plasma concentration levels of risperidone and clinical effects in the treatment of delirium. Int Clin Psychopharmacol 20:331–333, 2005

Trzepacz PT: Neuropathogenesis of delirium: a need to focus our research. Psychosomatics 35:374–391, 1994

Trzepacz PT: Update on the neuropathogenesis of delirium. Dement Geriatr Cogn Disord 10:330–334, 1999

Trzepacz PT: Is there a final common neural pathway in delirium? Focus on acetylcholine and dopamine. Semin Clin Neuropsychiatry 5:132–148, 2000

Trzepacz PT, Dew MA: Further analyses of the Delirium Rating Scale. Gen Hosp Psychiatry 17:75–79, 1995

Trzepacz PT, Teague GB, Lipowski ZJ: Delirium and other organic mental disorders in a general hospital. Gen Hosp Psychiatry 7:101–106, 1985

Trzepacz PT, Baker RW, Greenhouse J: A symptom rating scale for delirium. Psychiatry Res 23:89–97, 1988

Trzepacz PT, Sclabassi R, Van Thiel D: Delirium: a subcortical mechanism? J Neuropsychiatry Clin Neurosci 1:283–290, 1989

Trzepacz PT, Mulsant BH, Dew MA, et al: Is delirium different when it occurs in dementia? A study using the Delirium Rating Scale. J Neuropsychiatry Clin Neurosci 10:199–204, 1998

Trzepacz PT, Mittal D, Torres R, et al: Validation of the Delirium Rating Scale-Revised-98: comparison to the Delirium Rating Scale and Cognitive Test for Delirium. J Neuropsychiatry Clin Neurosci 13:229–242, 2001

Trzepacz PT, Mittal D, Torres R, et al: Delirium vs. dementia symptoms: Delirium Rating Scale—Revised (DRS-R-98) and Cognitive Test for Delirium (CTD) item comparisons. Psychosomatics 43:156–157, 2002

Turkel SB, Braslow K, Tavare CJ, et al: The Delirium Rating Scale in children and adolescents. Psychosomatics 44:126–129, 2003

Turkel SB, Trzepacz PT, Tavare CJ: Comparison of delirium in adults and children. Psychosomatics 47:320–324, 2006

Uchiyama M, Tanaka K, Isse K, et al: Efficacy of mianserin on symptoms of delirium in the aged: an open trial study. Prog Neuropsychopharmacol Biol Psychiatry 20:651–656, 1996

Voyer P, Cole MG, McCusker J, et al: Prevalence and symptoms of delirium superimposed on dementia. Clin Nurs Res 15:46–66, 2006

Wahlund LA, Bjorlin GA: Delirium in clinical practice: experiences from a specialized delirium ward. Dement Geriatr Cogn Disord 10:389–392, 1999

Wanich CK, Sullivan-Marx EM, Gottlieb GL, et al: Functional status outcomes of a nursing intervention in hospitalized elderly. Image J Nurs Sch 24:201–207, 1992

Webster R, Holroyd S: Prevalence of psychotic symptoms in delirium. Psychosomatics 41:519–522, 2000

Wengel SP, Roccaforte WH, Burke WJ: Donepezil improves symptoms of delirium in dementia: implications for future research. J Geriatr Psychiatry Neurol 11:159–161, 1998

Wengel SP, Burke WJ, Roccaforte WH: Donepezil for postoperative delirium associated with Alzheimer's disease. J Am Geriatr Soc 47:379–380, 1999

Williams MA, Campbell EB, Raynor WJ, et al: Reducing acute confusional states in elderly patients with hip fractures. Res Nurs Health 8:329–337, 1985

Wilson LM: Intensive care delirium: the effect of outside deprivation in a windowless unit. Arch Intern Med 130:225–226, 1972

Wilt JL, Minnema AM, Johnson RF, et al: Torsades de pointes associated with the use of intravenous haloperidol. Ann Intern Med 119:391–394, 1993

Wolff HG, Curran D: Nature of delirium and allied states: the dysergastic reaction. Arch Neurol Psychiatry 33:1175–1215, 1935

World Health Organization: International Statistical Classification of Diseases and Related Health Problems, 10th Revision. Geneva, World Health Organization, 1992

Young LJ, George J: Do guidelines improve the process and outcomes of care in delirium? Age Ageing 32:525–528, 2003

Zee-Cheng CS, Mueller CE, Siefert CF, et al: Haloperidol and torsades de pointes (letter). Ann Intern Med 102:418, 1985

4

Traumatic Brain Injury

Jonathan M. Silver, M.D.

Robert E. Hales, M.D., M.B.A.

Stuart C. Yudofsky, M.D.

Each year in the United States, more than 2 million people sustain a traumatic brain injury (TBI); 300,000 of these persons require hospitalization, and more than 80,000 of the survivors are afflicted with the chronic sequelae of such injuries (Kraus and Sorenson 1994). In this population, psychosocial and psychological deficits are commonly the major source of disability for the victims and of stress for their families. The psychiatrist, neurologist, and neuropsychologist are often called on by other medical specialists or the families to treat these patients. In this chapter, we review the role these professionals play in the prevention, diagnosis, and treatment of the cognitive, behavioral, and emotional aspects of TBI.

Neuroanatomy

The patient who sustains brain injury from trauma may incur damage through several mechanisms. Contusions affect specific areas of the brain and usually occur as the result of low-velocity injuries, such as falls. Courville (1945) examined the neuroanatomical sites of contusions and found that most injuries were in the basal and polar portions of the temporal and frontal lobes. Most of these lesions were the result of the location of bony prominences that surround the orbital, frontal, and temporal areas along the base of the skull. Coup injuries occur at the site of impact due to local tissue strain. Contrecoup injuries occur away from the site of impact during sudden deceleration and translational and angular movements of the head. Impact is not required for contrecoup injuries to occur, and they usually occur in frontal and temporal areas (Gennarelli and Graham 1998).

Diffuse axonal injury refers to mechanical or chemical damage to the axons in cerebral white matter that commonly occurs with lateral angular or rotational acceleration. The axon is vulnerable to injury during high-velocity accidents when there is twisting and turning of the brain around the brain stem (as can occur in whiplash during car accidents). Axons are stretched, causing delayed (hours) disruption of the cytoskeleton and impaired axoplasm transport. This results in axoplasmic swelling and detachment, changes in membrane structure, disruption in neurofilaments, and wallerian degeneration of the distal stump of the axon (Gennarelli and Graham 2005). The disruption of axons can occur as late as 2 weeks after the injury (Gennarelli and Graham 1998). Chemically, metabolic changes occur, leading to axonal damage. The sites in the brain that are most vulnerable to axonal injury are the reticular formation, superior cerebellar peduncles, regions of the basal ganglia, hypothalamus, limbic fornices, and corpus callosum (Cassidy 1994).

Subdural hematomas (acute, subacute, and chronic) and intracerebral hematomas have effects that are specific to their locations and degree of neuronal damage. In general, subdural hematomas affect arousal and cognition.

Neuropsychiatric Assessment

History Taking

Although brain injuries subsequent to serious automobile, occupational, or sports accidents may not result in diagnostic enigmas for the psychiatrist, less severe trauma may first manifest as relatively subtle behavioral or affective change. Patients may fail to associate the traumatic event with subsequent symptoms.

Prototypic examples include the alcoholic man who is amnestic for a fall that occurred while he was inebriated, the 10-year-old boy who falls from his bicycle and hits his head but fails to inform his parents, and the wife who was beaten by her husband but who is either fearful or ashamed to report the injury to her family physician. Confusion, intellectual changes, affective lability, or psychosis may occur directly after the trauma or as late as many years afterward. Individuals who present for emergency treatment for blunt trauma may not be adequately screened for TBI (Chambers et al. 1996). Even individuals who identified themselves as "nondisabled" but who had experienced a blow to the head that left them at a minimum dazed and confused had symptoms and emotional distress similar to a group of individuals with known mild TBI (Gordon et al. 1998). Mild TBI, as defined by the Mild Traumatic Brain Injury Committee (1993, pp 86–87), is a "traumatically induced physiological disruption of brain function" with one or more of the following:

1. Any period of loss of consciousness;
2. Any loss of memory for events immediately before or after the accident;
3. Any alteration in mental state at the time of the accident (e.g., feeling dazed, disoriented, or confused);
4. Focal neurological deficit(s) that may or may not be transient; but where the severity of the injury does not exceed the following: loss of consciousness of approximately 30 minutes or less; after 30 minutes, an initial Glasgow Coma Scale (GCS) score of 13–15; and posttraumatic amnesia (PTA) not greater than 24 hours.

For every psychiatric patient, the clinician must specifically inquire whether the patient has been involved in situations that are associated with head trauma. The practitioner should ask about automobile, bicycle, and motorcycle accidents; falls; assaults; playground accidents; and participation in sports that are frequently associated with brain injury (e.g., football, soccer, rugby, boxing). Patients must be asked whether they experienced any alteration in consciousness after they were injured, including dazed or confused feelings, loss of consciousness (LOC), and a period of amnesia. The clinician should inquire whether the patients were hospitalized and whether they had posttraumatic symptoms, such as headache, dizziness, irritability, problems with concentration, and sensitivity to noise or light. Most patients will not volunteer this information without direct inquiry. Patients are usually unaware of the phenomenon of posttraumatic amnesia and may confuse posttraumatic amnesia with LOC. They assume that if they are unable to recall events, they must have been unconscious. Therefore, the clinician must document the source of this observation (e.g., whether there were observers who witnessed the period of unconsciousness).

Because many patients are unaware of, minimize, or deny the severity of behavioral changes that occur after TBI, family members also must be asked about the effects of the injury on their relative's behavior. For example, in evaluating the social adjustment of patients years after severe brain injury, Oddy et al. (1985) compared symptoms reported by both patients and their relatives. Forty percent of relatives of 28 patients with TBI reported that their relative behaved childishly; however, this symptom was not reported by the patients themselves. Although 28% of the patients complained of problems with their vision after the injury, this difficulty was not reported by relatives. Patients overestimate their level of functioning compared with the reporting of relatives, and they report more physical than nonphysical impairment (Sherer et al. 1998).

Family members also are more aware of emotional changes than are the victims of brain injury. Whereas individuals with TBI tend to view the cognitive difficulties as being more severe than the emotional changes (Hendryx 1989), mood disorders and frustration intolerance are viewed by family members as being more disabling than cognitive disabilities (Rappaport et al. 1989).

Laboratory Evaluation

Imaging Techniques

Brain imaging techniques are frequently used to demonstrate the location and extent of brain lesions (Belanger et al. 2007). Computed tomography (CT) is used for the acute assessment of the patient with head trauma to document hemorrhage, edema, midline shifts, herniation, fractures, and contusions. Imaging as soon as possible after the trauma is important for establishing a baseline injury scan, because lesions that cannot be seen during the acute phase may be visualized months after the injury (Bigler 2005). Thus, for a significant number of patients with severe brain injury, initial CT evaluations may not detect lesions that are observable on CT scans performed 1 and 3 months after the injury (Cope et al. 1988).

Magnetic resonance imaging (MRI) has been shown to detect clinically meaningful lesions in patients with severe brain injury when CT scans have not demonstrated anatomical bases for the degree of coma (Levin et al. 1987a; Wilberger et al. 1987). MRI is especially sensitive in detecting lesions in the frontal and temporal lobes that are not visualized by CT, and these loci are frequently related to the neuropsychiatric consequences of the injury (Levin et al. 1987a). MRI has been found to be more sensitive for the detection of contusions, shearing injury, and subdural and epidural hematomas (Orrison et al. 1994), and it has been able to document evidence of diffuse axonal injury in patients who have a normal CT scan after experiencing mild TBI (Mittl et al. 1994). When MRI is used, fluid-attenuated inversion recovery (FLAIR) is superior to the T2-weighted spin-echo technique, especially in visualizing central diffuse axonal injury of the fornix and corpus callosum (Ashikaga et al. 1997). MRI in the chronic stage is better correlated with neuropsychiatric symptoms (Bigler 2005). Quantitative analyses of individuals with TBI have revealed multiple affected brain structures, including the frontal and temporal lobes, thalamus, hippocampus, and basal ganglia (Bigler 2005).

Functional techniques in brain imaging, such as regional cerebral blood flow and positron emission tomography (PET), can be used to detect areas of abnormal function when CT and MRI scans fail to show any abnormalities of structure (Anderson et al. 2005). Single-photon emission computed tomography (SPECT) also shows promise in documenting brain damage after TBI. Abnormalities are visualized in patients who have experienced mild TBI (Gross et al. 1996; Masdeu et al. 1994; Nedd et al. 1993) or who have chronic TBI (Nagamachi et al. 1995), even in the presence of normally appearing areas on CT scans. Abnormalities on SPECT appear to correlate with the severity of trauma (Jacobs et al. 1994). These imaging techniques were used in examining a group of individuals with late whiplash syndrome (Bicik et al. 1998). Significant frontopolar hypometabolism was found, and it correlated significantly with scores on the Beck Depression Inventory (Beck et al. 1961). In individual cases, however, the reliability of the depiction of hypometabolism was low. A "normal" SPECT scan does not imply normal pathology; in addition, SPECT abnormalities after TBI have not been shown to correlate with cognitive deficits or behavioral symptoms (Anderson et al. 2005). SPECT abnormalities can also be seen in many of the concurrent problems experienced with TBI, including depression and substance use. Although some studies have found correlations between neuropsychological deficits and abnormalities on PET scans, other studies have found no relation between lesion location and deficits (Anderson et al. 2005).

Proton magnetic resonance spectroscopy, which provides information on intracellular function, has been investigated for the detection of abnormalities in TBI. *N*-acetylaspartate (NAA) is associated with neuronal or axonal loss. Cecil et al. (1998) examined 35 patients with TBI and found that a majority of those with mild TBI as well as those with severe TBI showed abnormal levels of NAA in the splenium, consistent with diffuse axonal injury. Early changes in NAA concentrations in gray matter were predictive of outcome in a group of 14 patients after TBI (Friedman et al. 1999). Ariza et al. (2004) found a correlation between performance on neuropsychological tests and NAA concentrations. Even in mild TBI, abnormalities may be found in areas that are frequent sites of diffuse axonal injury (Inglese et al. 2005).

McAllister et al. (1999, 2001) used functional MRI to assess patterns of regional brain activation in response to working memory loads in a group of individuals 1 month after they had sustained mild TBI. During a high-load task, this group demonstrated significantly increased activation, particularly in the right parietal and right dorsolateral frontal regions; however, no differences were found between the mild TBI group and the control group in terms of task performance. Findings from this study appear to correlate with the complaints of patients who state that they have to "work harder" to recall things but in whom no deficits are found on objective testing. Other studies suggest that individuals with TBI have impairment in brain structures required for appropriate responding to stimuli (Christodoulou et al. 2001; Easdon et al. 2004).

Caution must be observed in applying the findings in this literature to a clinical population. Physicians are unable to determine the presence of abnormalities before an accident. Abnormalities on SPECT or PET have been demonstrated in individuals with no history of brain injury who have psychiatric disorders, including posttraumatic stress disorder (PTSD) (Rauch et al. 1996), somatization disorder (Lazarus and Cotterell 1989), major depression (Dolan et al. 1992), and chronic alcoholism (Kuruoglu et al. 1996). After reviewing the evidence available in 1996, the American Academy of Neurology concluded that the evidence was insufficient to support the use of SPECT to diagnose TBI, and that the use of SPECT for this purpose should be considered investigational (Therapeutics and Technology Assessment Subcommittee 1996). Functional imaging results should be used only as part of an overall evaluation to confirm findings documented elsewhere (Silver and McAllister 1997).

Electrophysiological Techniques

Electrophysiological assessment of the patient after TBI may also assist in the evaluation. Electroencephalography can detect the presence of seizures or abnormal areas of functioning. For enhanced sensitivity of this technique, the electroencephalogram (EEG) should be obtained after sleep deprivation, with photic stimulation and hyperventilation and with anterotemporal and/or nasopharyngeal leads (Goodin et al. 1990).

Computerized interpretation of the EEG and brain electrical activity mapping may be useful in detecting areas of dysfunction not shown in the routine EEG (Watson et al. 1995). There is controversy regarding the usefulness of these techniques. The American Academy of Neurology and the American Clinical Neurophysiology Society have concluded that "the evidence of clinical usefulness or consistency of results [is] not considered sufficient for us to support [the] use [of quantitative electroencephalography] in diagnosis of patients with postconcussion syndrome, or minor or moderate head injury" (Nuwer 1997, p. 287). However, the EEG and Clinical Neuroscience Society addressed significant concerns regarding the interpretation of this report (Thatcher et al. 1999). Their opinion is that there is significant scientific literature on the use and interpretation of quantitative electroencephalography and that several findings have been consistent: reduced amplitude of high-frequency electroencephalography, especially in the frontal lobes; a shift toward lower increased electroencephalographic frequencies; and changes in electroencephalographic coherence (Thatcher et al. 1999). A detailed discussion of electrophysiological techniques can be found elsewhere (Arciniegas et al. 2005).

Neuropsychological Testing

Neuropsychological assessment of the patient with TBI is essential to document cognitive and intellectual deficits and strengths. Tests are administered to assess the patient's attention, concentration, memory, verbal capacity, and executive functioning. The latter capacity, which includes problem-solving skills, abstract thinking, planning, and reasoning abilities, is the most difficult to assess. A valid interpretation of these tests includes assessment of the patient's preinjury intelligence and other higher levels of functioning. Because multiple factors affect the results of neuropsychological tests, these tests must be performed and interpreted by a clinician with skill and experience.

Patients' complaints may not be easily or accurately categorized as either functional (i.e., primarily due to a psychiatric disorder) or neurological (i.e., primarily caused by the brain injury). Nonetheless, outside agencies—for example, insurance companies and lawyers—may request a neuropsychiatric evaluation to assist with this "differential." In reality, most symptoms result from the interaction of many factors, including neurological, social, emotional, educational, and vocational. Because important insurance and other reimbursement decisions may hinge on whether or not disabilities stem from brain injury, the clinician should take care that his or her impressions are based on data and are not misapplied to deprive the patient of deserved benefits. For example, mood disorders and cognitive sequelae of brain injury are often miscategorized as "mental illnesses" that are not covered by some insurance policies.

Clinical Features

Neuropsychiatric sequelae of TBI include problems with attention and arousal, concentration, and executive functioning; intellectual changes; memory impairment; personality changes; affective disorders; anxiety disorders; psychosis; posttraumatic epilepsy; sleep disorders; aggression; and irritability. Physical problems such as headache, chronic pain, vision impairment, and dizziness complicate recovery. The severity of the neuropsychiatric sequelae of the brain injury is determined by multiple factors existing before, during, and after the injury (Dikmen and Machamer 1995). In general, prognosis is associated with the severity of the injury.

Although duration of posttraumatic amnesia correlates with subsequent cognitive recovery (Levin et al. 1982), in an analysis of 1,142 patients assessed after hospitalization for TBI, the simple presence or absence of LOC was not significantly related to performance on neuropsychological tests (Smith-Seemiller et al. 1996). In patients with mild brain injury, a correlation between the occurrence of LOC and neuropsychological test results is lacking (Lovell et al. 1999). In addition, the symptoms of injury are correlated with the type of damage sustained. For example, those with diffuse axonal injury often experience arousal problems, attention problems, and slow cognitive processing. The presence of total anosmia in a group of patients with closed head injury predicted major vocational problems at least 2 years after these patients had been given medical clearance to return to work (Varney 1988). Posttraumatic anosmia may occur as a result of damage to the olfactory nerve, which is located adjacent to the orbitofrontal cortex, although involvement of the peripheral nerve also may result in anosmia. Impairment in olfactory naming and recognition frequently occurs in patients with moderate or severe brain injury and is related to frontal and temporal lobe damage (Levin et al. 1985).

In a review by Corrigan (1995), victims of TBI who were intoxicated with alcohol at the time of injury had longer periods of hospitalization, more complications during hospitalization, and a lower level of functioning at the time of discharge from the hospital than did patients with TBI who had no detectable blood alcohol level at the time of hospitalization. One factor complicating the interpretation of these data is that intoxication may produce decreased responsiveness even without TBI, which can result in a Glasgow Coma Scale (GCS) score that indicates greater severity of injury than is actually present. Furthermore, even a history of substance abuse is associated with increased morbidity and mortality rates.

Morbidity and mortality rates after brain injury increase with age. Elderly persons who experience TBI have longer periods of agitation and greater cognitive impairment and are more likely to develop mass lesions and permanent disability than are younger victims (Kim 2005). Individuals who have had a previous brain injury do not recover as well from subsequent injuries (Carlsson et al. 1987).

The interaction between brain injury and psychosocial factors cannot be underestimated. Demographic factors have been found to predict cognitive dysfunction after TBI (Smith-Seemiller et al. 1996). Preexisting emotional and behavioral problems are exacerbated after injury. Also, having a preexisting psychiatric disorder appears to increase the risk of TBI (Fann et al. 2002). Social conditions and support networks that existed before the injury affect the symptoms and course of recovery. In general, individuals with greater preinjury intelligence recover better after injury (Brown et al. 1981). Factors such as level of education, level of income, and socioeconomic status affect the ability to return to work after minor head injury (Rimel et al. 1981).

Personality Changes

Unlike many primary psychiatric illnesses that have a gradual onset, TBI often occurs suddenly and devastatingly. Although some patients recognize that they no longer have the same abilities and potential that they had before the injury, many others with significant disabilities deny any changes. Prominent behavioral traits such as disorderliness, suspiciousness, argumentativeness, isolativeness, disruptiveness, social inappropriateness, and anxiousness often become more pronounced after brain injury.

In a study of children with head injury, Brown et al. (1981) found that disinhibition, social inappropriateness, restlessness, and stealing were associated with injuries in which LOC extended for more than 7 days. In a survey of the relatives of victims of severe TBI, McKinlay et al. (1981) found that 49% of 55 patients had developed personality changes 3 months after the injury. After 5 years, 74% of these patients were reported to have changes in personality (Brooks et al. 1986). More than one-third of these patients had problems of "childishness" and "talking too much" (Brooks et al. 1986; McKinlay et al. 1981).

Thomsen (1984) found that 80% of 40 patients with severe TBI had personality changes that persisted for 2–5 years, and 65% had changes lasting 10–15 years after the injury. These changes included childishness (60% and 25%, respectively), emotional lability (40% and 35%, respectively), and restlessness (25% and 38%, respectively). Approximately two-thirds of patients had less social contact, and one-half had loss of spontaneity and poverty of interests after 10–15 years.

Because of the vulnerability of the prefrontal and frontal regions of the cortex to contusions, injury to these regions is common and gives rise to changes in personality known as the frontal lobe syndrome. For the prototypical patient with frontal lobe syndrome, the cognitive functions are preserved while personality changes abound. Psychiatric disturbances associated with frontal lobe injury commonly include impaired social judgment, labile affect, uncharacteristic lewdness, inability to appreciate the effects of one's behavior or remarks on others, loss of social graces (e.g., eating manners), diminution of attention to personal appearance and hygiene, and boisterousness. Impaired judgment may take the form of diminished concern for the future, increased risk taking, unrestrained drinking of alcohol, and indiscriminate selection of food. Patients may appear shallow, indifferent, or apathetic, with a global lack of concern for the consequences of their behavior.

Certain behavioral syndromes have been related to damage to specific areas of the frontal lobe (Auerbach 1986). The orbitofrontal syndrome is associated with behavioral excesses, such as impulsivity, disinhibition, hyperactivity, distractibility, and mood lability. Injury to the dorsolateral frontal cortex may result in slowness, apathy, and perseveration. This condition may be considered similar to the negative (deficit) symptoms associated with schizophrenia, wherein the patient may exhibit blunted affect, emotional withdrawal, social withdrawal, passivity, and lack of spontaneity (Kay et al. 1987). As with TBI, deficit symptoms in patients with schizophrenia are thought to result from disordered functioning of the dorsolateral frontal cortex (Berman et al. 1988). Outbursts of rage and violent behavior occur after damage to the inferior orbital surface of the frontal lobe and anterior temporal lobes.

Patients also develop changes in sexual behavior after brain injury, most commonly decreased sex drive, erectile function, and frequency of intercourse (Zasler 1994). Kleine-Levin syndrome—characterized by periodic hypersomnolence, hyperphagia, and behavioral disturbances that include hypersexuality—has also been reported to occur subsequent to brain injury (Will et al. 1988).

Although there have been studies examining personality changes after TBI, few studies have focused on Axis II psychopathology in individuals with TBI. Using a structured clinical interview to diagnose personality disorders in 100 individuals with TBI, Hibbard et al. (2000) found that several personality disorders developed after TBI that were reflective of persistent challenges and compensatory coping strategies facing these individuals. Whereas 24% of the sample population had personality disorders before TBI, 66% of the sample met criteria for personality disorders after TBI. The most common personality disorders were borderline, avoidant, paranoid, obsessive-compulsive, and narcissistic personality disorders. Koponen et al. (2002), in a 30-year follow-up study of 60 patients with TBI, found that the most frequent personality disorders were paranoid, schizoid, avoidant, and organic personality disorders.

In DSM-IV-TR (American Psychiatric Association 2000), these personality changes would be diagnosed as personality change due to TBI. Specific subtypes are provided for the most significant clinical problems.

Intellectual Changes

Problems with intellectual functioning may be among the most subtle manifestations of brain injury. Changes can occur in the ability to attend, concentrate, remember, abstract, calculate, reason, plan, and process information (McCullagh and Feinstein 2005). Problems with arousal can take the form of inattentiveness, distractibility, and difficulty switching and dividing attention (Ponsford and Kinsella 1992). Mental sluggishness, poor concentration, and memory problems are common complaints of both patients and relatives (Brooks et al. 1986; McKinlay et al. 1981; Thomsen 1984). High-level cognitive functions, termed *executive functions,* are frequently impaired after TBI (Table 4–1), although such impairments are difficult to detect and diagnose with cursory cognitive testing (McCullagh and Feinstein 2005). Only specific tests that mimic real-life decision-making situations may objectively demonstrate the problems that patients encounter in daily life (Bechara et al. 1994).

Children who survive head trauma often return to school with behavioral and learning problems (Mahoney et al. 1983). Children with behavioral disorders are much more likely to have a history of prior head injury (Michaud et al. 1993). In addition, children who sustained injury at or before age 2 years had significantly lower IQ scores in one study (Michaud et al. 1993). The risk factors for the sequelae of TBI in children are controversial (Max 2005). In a study of 43 children and adolescents who had sustained TBI, Max et al. (1998b) found that preinjury family functioning was a significant predictor of psychiatric disorders after 1 year. Whereas some investigators have demonstrated neuropsychological sequelae after mild TBI when careful testing is done (Gulbrandsen 1984), others have shown that mild TBI produces virtually no clinically significant long-term deficits (Fay et al. 1993). In patients who survive moderate to severe brain injury, the degree of memory impairment often exceeds the level of intellectual dysfunction (Levin et al. 1988). The following case example illustrates a typical presentation of an adolescent with TBI presenting with behavioral and academic problems.

Case Example

Ms. G, a 17-year-old girl, was referred by her father for neuropsychiatric evaluation because of many changes observed in her personality during the past 2 years. Whereas she had been an A student and had been involved in many ex-

Table 4–1. Aspects of executive functions potentially impaired after traumatic brain injury

Goal establishment, planning, and anticipation of consequences

Initiation, sequencing, and inhibition of behavioral responses

Generation of multiple response alternatives (in contrast to perseverative or stereotyped responses)

Conceptual/inferential reasoning, problem solving

Mental flexibility/ease of mental and behavioral switching

Transcending the immediately salient aspects of a situation (in contrast to "stimulus-bound behavior" or "environmental dependency")

Executive attentional processes

Executive memory processes

Self-monitoring and self-regulation, including emotional responses

Social adaptive functioning: sensitivity to others, using social feedback, engaging in contextually appropriate social behavior

Source. Reprinted from McCullagh S, Feinstein A: "Cognitive Changes," in *Textbook of Traumatic Brain Injury.* Edited by Silver JM, McAllister TW, Yudofsky SC. Washington, DC, American Psychiatric Publishing, 2005, pp. 321–335. Used with permission. Copyright © 2005 American Psychiatric Association.

tracurricular activities during her sophomore year in high school, substantial changes in her behavior had occurred during the past 2 years. She was barely able to maintain a C average, was "hanging around with the bad kids," and was frequently using marijuana and alcohol. A careful history revealed that 2 years earlier, her older brother had hit her in the forehead with a rake, which stunned her, but she did not lose consciousness. Although Ms. G had a headache after the accident, no psychiatric or neurological follow-up was pursued.

Neuropsychological testing at the time of evaluation revealed a significant decline in Ms. G's intellectual functioning from her "preinjury" state. Testing revealed poor concentration, attention, memory, and reasoning abilities. Academically, she was unable to "keep up" with the friends she had before her injury, and she began to socialize with a group of students with little interest in academics and began to conceptualize herself as being a rebel. When neuropsychological testing results were explained, the patient and her family learned that she had experienced a brain injury and they were able to understand her "defensive" reaction to her changed social behavior.

Psychiatric Disorders

Studies that use standard psychiatric diagnostic criteria have found that several psychiatric disorders are common in individuals with TBI (Deb et al. 1999; Fann et al. 1995; Hibbard et al. 1998; Jorge et al. 1993; van Reekum et al. 2000). In a group of patients referred to a brain injury rehabilitation center, Fann et al. (1995) found that 26% had current major depression, 14% had current dysthymia, 24% had current generalized anxiety disorder (GAD), and 8% had current substance abuse. Twelve percent reported pre-TBI depression. Deb et al. (1999) performed a psychiatric evaluation of 196 individuals who were hospitalized after TBI. They found that a psychiatric disorder was present in 21.7%, compared with 16.4% of a control population of individuals hospitalized for other reasons. Compared with the control group, the individuals with TBI had a higher rate of depression (13.9% vs. 2.1%) and panic disorder (9.0% vs. 0.8%). Factors associated with these psychiatric disorders included a history of psychiatric illness, preinjury alcohol use, unfavorable outcome, lower Mini-Mental State Examination scores, and fewer years of education. Hibbard et al. (1998) administered a structured psychiatric interview to 100 individuals with TBI. Major depression (61%), substance use disorder (28%), and PTSD (19%) were the most common psychiatric diagnoses elicited. Jorge et al. (1993) found that 26% of individuals had major depression 1 month after injury; 11% had comorbid GAD.

Several studies suggest that individuals who experience TBI have a higher than expected rate of preinjury psychiatric disorders. Histories of prior psychiatric disorders in individuals with TBI have varied between 17% and 44%, and pre-TBI substance use figures have ranged from 22% to 30% (Jorge et al. 1994; van Reekum et al. 1996). Fann et al. (1995) found that 50% of individuals who had sustained TBI reported a history of psychiatric problems prior to the injury. The Research and Training Center on Community Integration of Individuals with TBI at Mount Sinai Medical Center in New York found that in a group of 100 individuals with TBI, 51% had pre-TBI psychiatric disorders, most commonly major depression or substance use disorders, and these occurred at rates more than twice those reported in community samples (Hibbard et al. 1998). Fann et al. (2002) analyzed a health maintenance organization's database of 450,000 members for the occurrence of a TBI and evidence of a psychiatric condition. They found that the relative risk for TBI was 1.3–4 times higher in individuals with a preceding psychiatric diagnosis than in those without (24.2% vs. 14.3%). Interestingly, this held true for all psychiatric disorders except attention-deficit/hyperactivity disorder.

Affective Changes

Depression occurs frequently after TBI. Several diagnostic issues must be considered in the evaluation of the patient who appears depressed after TBI. Sadness is a common reaction after TBI. Patients who experience deficits in intellectual functioning and motoric abilities often describe "mourning" the loss of their "former selves." Careful psychiatric evaluation is required to distinguish grief reactions, sadness, and demoralization from major depression.

The clinician must distinguish major depression from mood lability, which occurs commonly after brain injury. Lability of mood and affect may be caused by temporal limbic and basal forebrain lesions (Ross and Stewart 1987) and has been shown to be responsive to standard pharmacological interventions for depression. In addition, apathy (diminished motivation) secondary to brain injury (which includes decreased motivation, decreased pursuit of pleasurable activities, and schizoid behavior) and complaints of slowness in thought and cognitive processing may resemble depression (Marin and Chakravorty 2005).

The clinician should endeavor to determine whether a patient may have been having an episode of major depression before an accident. Traumatic injury may occur as a result of the depression and suicidal ideation. Alcohol use, which frequently occurs with and complicates depressive illness, is also a known risk factor for motor vehicle accidents. One common scenario is depression leading to poor concentration, to substance abuse, and to risk taking (or even overt suicidal behavior), which together contribute to the motor vehicle accident and brain injury.

Prevalence of Depression After TBI

The prevalence of depression after brain injury has been assessed through self-report questionnaires, rating scales, and relatives' reports. For mild TBI, estimates of depressive complaints range from 6% to 39%. In patients with depression after severe TBI, who often have concomitant cognitive impairments, reported rates of depression vary from 10% to 77%.

Robert Robinson and his colleagues have performed prospective studies of the occurrence of depression after brain injury (Federoff et al. 1992; Jorge et al. 1993). They evaluated 66 hospitalized patients who had sustained acute TBI and followed the course of their mood over 1 year. Diagnoses were made using structured interviews and DSM-III-R (American Psychiatric Association 1987) criteria. The patients were evaluated 1 month, 3 months, 6 months, and 1 year after injury. At each period, approximately 25% of patients fulfilled criteria for major depressive disorder. The mean duration of depression was 4.7 months, with a range of 1.5–12 months. Of the entire group of patients, 42% developed major depression during the first year after injury. The researchers also found that patients with GAD and comorbid major depression have longer-lasting mood problems than do those patients with depression and no anxiety (Jorge et al. 1993). More recently, this group extended their observations to another group of 91 patients (Jorge et al. 2004). During the first year after TBI, 33% developed depression, significantly more than the "other injury" control group. Those depressed individuals had high rates of comorbid anxiety (75%) and aggression (56%) and reduced executive and social functioning.

Studies consistently report increased risk of suicide subsequent to TBI (Tate et al. 1997). Data from a follow-up study (N. Brooks, personal communication, 1990) of 42 patients with severe TBI showed that 1 year after injury, 10% of those surveyed had spoken about suicide and 2% had made suicide attempts. Five years after the traumatic event, 15% of the patients had made suicide attempts. In addition, many other patients expressed hopelessness about their condition and a belief that life was not worth living. Silver et al. (2001) found that individuals with a history of brain injury reported a higher frequency of suicide attempts than did individuals without TBI (8.1% vs. 1.9%). This difference remained significant even after controlling for sociodemographic factors, quality-of-life variables, and presence of any coexisting psychiatric disorder. Mann et al. (1999) found an increased occurrence of TBI in individuals who had made suicide attempts. Simpson and Tate (2002) evaluated 172 outpatients with TBI who were in a brain injury rehabilitation unit. Hopelessness was found in 35%, suicidal ideation in 23%, and a suicide attempt in 18%. The relationship between suicidal behavior and TBI is complicated. Oquendo et al. (2004) evaluated the predictors of suicidal ideation in 340 patients with major depression. Subjects with TBI reported more aggressive behavior during childhood than did subjects without TBI. Twenty percent of suicide attempters with TBI made their first suicide attempt prior to their brain injury. In addition, subjects with TBI had higher levels of aggressive behavior that antedated the TBI. In this study, suicidal behavior and TBI appeared to share an antecedent risk factor: aggression. Results suggest that the high incidence of suicide attempts in this population is caused by the combination of several factors—namely, major depression with disinhibition secondary to frontal lobe injury and preexisting risk factors such as aggressive behavior. The medical team, family, and other caregivers must work closely together, on a regular and continuing basis, to gauge a patient's suicide risk.

Mania After TBI

Manic episodes and bipolar disorder have also been reported to occur after TBI (Burstein 1993), although the occurrence is less frequent than that of depression after brain injury (Bakchine et al. 1989; Bamrah and Johnson 1991; Bracken 1987; Clark and Davison 1987; Nizamie et al. 1988). In a New Haven Epidemiologic Catchment Area (ECA) sample, bipolar disorder occurred in 1.6% of those with brain injury, although the odds ratio was no longer significant when sociodemographic factors and quality of life were controlled for (Silver et al. 2001). Predisposing factors for the development of mania after brain injury include damage to the basal region of the right temporal lobe (Starkstein et al. 1990) and right orbitofrontal cortex (Starkstein et al. 1988) in patients who have family histories of bipolar disorder.

Delirium

When a psychiatrist is consulted during the period when a patient with a brain injury is emerging from coma, the usual clinical picture is one of delirium with restlessness, agitation, confusion, disorientation, delusions, and/or hallucinations. As Trzepacz and Kennedy (2005) observed, this period of recovery is often termed *posttraumatic amnesia* in the brain injury literature and is classified as Level IV or V of the Rancho Los Amigos Levels of Cognitive Functioning Scale. Although delirium in patients with TBI is most often the result of the effects of the injury on brain tissue chemistry, the psychiatrist should be aware of other possible causes for the delirium (e.g., side effects of medication, withdrawal, or intoxication from drugs ingested before the traumatic event) and environmental factors (e.g., sensory monotony). Table 4–2 lists common factors that can result in posttraumatic delirium.

Table 4–2. Causes of delirium in patients with traumatic brain injury

Mechanical effects (acceleration or deceleration, contusion, and others)

Cerebral edema

Hemorrhage

Infection

Subdural hematoma

Seizure

Hypoxia (cardiopulmonary or local ischemia)

Increased intracranial pressure

Alcohol intoxication or withdrawal, Wernicke's encephalopathy

Reduced hemoperfusion related to multiple trauma

Fat embolism

Change in pH

Electrolyte imbalance

Medications (barbiturates, steroids, opioids, and anticholinergics)

Source. Reprinted from Trzepacz PT, Kennedy RE: "Delirium and Posttraumatic Amnesia," in *Textbook of Traumatic Brain Injury.* Edited by Silver JM, McAllister TW, Yudofsky SC. Washington, DC, American Psychiatric Publishing, 2005, pp. 175–200. Used with permission. Copyright © 2005 American Psychiatric Association.

Psychotic Disorders

Psychosis can occur either immediately after brain injury or after a latency of many months of normal functioning (Corcoran et al. 2005). McAllister (1998) observed that psychotic symptoms may result from a number of different post-TBI disorders, including mania, depression, and epilepsy. The psychotic symptoms may persist despite improvement in the cognitive deficits caused by trauma (Nasrallah et al. 1981). Review of the literature published between 1917 and 1964 (Davison and Bagley 1969) revealed that 1%–15% of schizophrenic inpatients have histories of brain injury. Violon and De Mol (1987) found that of 530 patients with head injury, 3.4% developed psychosis 1–10 years after the injury. Wilcox and Nasrallah (1987) found that a group of patients diagnosed with schizophrenia had a significantly greater history of brain injury with LOC before age 10 than did patients who were diagnosed with mania or depression or patients who were hospitalized for surgery. Achté et al. (1991) reported on a sample of 2,907 war veterans in Finland who had sustained brain injury. They found that 26% of these veterans had psychotic disorders. In a detailed evaluation of 100 of these veterans, the authors found that 14% had paranoid schizophrenia. In a comparison of patients who developed symptoms of schizophrenia or schizoaffective disorder subsequent to TBI, left temporal lobe abnormalities were found only in the group that developed schizophrenia (Buckley et al. 1993). The rate of schizophrenia in the group of individuals with a history of TBI in the New Haven ECA sample was 3.4% (Silver et al. 2001); however, after the authors controlled for alcohol abuse and dependence, the risk for the occurrence of schizophrenia was of borderline significance.

Patients with schizophrenia may have had brain injury, and this injury may remain undetected unless the clinician actively elicits a history specific for the occurrence of brain trauma. One high-risk group is homeless individuals with mental illness. To examine the relationship of TBI to schizophrenia and homelessness, Silver et al. (1993) conducted a case-control study of 100 homeless and 100 never-homeless indigent men with schizophrenia, and a similar population of women. In the group of men, 55 patients had a prior TBI (36 homeless, 19 domiciled; $P<0.01$). In the group of women, 35 had previous TBI (16 homeless, 19 domiciled; P value not significant). We believe that the cognitive deficits subsequent to TBI in conjunction with psychosis increase the risk for becoming homeless. In addition, those who are homeless and living in a shelter are at greater risk for experiencing trauma (Kass and Silver 1990).

Posttraumatic Epilepsy

Varying percentages of patients, depending on the location and severity of injury, will have seizures during the acute period after TBI. Within 5 years of the injury, posttraumatic epilepsy, with repeated seizures and the requirement for anticonvulsant medication, occurs in approximately 12%, 2%, and 1% of patients with severe, moderate, and mild head injuries, respectively (Annegers et al. 1980). Risk factors for posttraumatic epilepsy include skull fractures and wounds that penetrate the brain, a history of chronic alcohol use, intracranial hemorrhage, and increased severity of injury (Yablon 1993).

In a study of 421 Vietnam veterans who had sustained brain-penetrating injuries, Salazar et al. (1985) found that 53% had posttraumatic epilepsy. In 18% of these patients, the first seizure occurred after 5 years; in 7%, the first seizure occurred after 10 years. In addition, 26% of the patients with epilepsy had an organic mental syndrome as defined in DSM-III (American Psychiatric Association 1980). In a study of World War II veterans, patients with brain-penetrating injuries who developed posttraumatic epilepsy had a decreased life expectancy compared with patients with brain-penetrating injuries without epilepsy and patients with peripheral nerve injuries (Corkin et al. 1984). Patients who develop posttraumatic epilepsy have also been shown to have more difficulties with physical and social functioning and to require more intensive rehabilitation efforts (Armstrong et al. 1990).

Posttraumatic epilepsy is associated with psychosis, especially when seizures arise from the temporal lobes. Brief episodic psychoses may occur with epilepsy; about 7% of patients with epilepsy have persistent psychoses (McKenna et al. 1985). These psychoses have a number of atypical features, including confusion and rapid fluctuations in mood. Psychiatric evaluation of 101 patients with epilepsy revealed that 8% had organic delusional disorder that, at times, was difficult to differentiate symptomatically from schizophrenia (Garyfallos et al. 1988). Phenytoin has more profound effects on cognition than does carbamazepine (Gallassi et al. 1988), and negative effects on cognition have been found in patients who received phenytoin after traumatic injury (Dikmen et al. 1991). Minimal impairment of cognition was found with both valproate and carbamazepine in a group of patients with epilepsy (Prevey et al. 1996). Dikmen et al. (2000) found no adverse cognitive effects of valproate when it was administered for 12 months after a TBI was sustained. In a comparison of the effects of phenytoin and carbamazepine in patients recovering from TBI, Smith et al. (1994) found that both phenytoin and carbamazepine had negative effects on cognitive performance tasks, especially those that involved motor and speed performance. Intellectual deterioration in children undergoing long-term treatment with phenytoin or phenobarbital also has been documented (Corbett et al. 1985). Treatment with more than one anticonvulsant (polytherapy) has been associated with increased adverse neuropsychiatric reactions (Reynolds and Trimble 1985). Of the newer anticonvulsant medications, topiramate, but not gabapentin or lamotrigine, demonstrated adverse cognitive effects in healthy young adults (Martin et al. 1999; Salinsky et al.

2005). Hoare (1984) found that the use of multiple anticonvulsant drugs to control seizures resulted in an increase in disturbed behavior in children. Any patient with TBI who is treated with anticonvulsant medication requires regular reevaluations to substantiate continued clinical necessity.

Anxiety Disorders

Several anxiety disorders may develop after TBI (Warden and Labatte 2005). Jorge et al. (1993) found that 11% of 66 patients with TBI developed GAD in addition to major depression. Fann et al. (1995) evaluated 50 outpatients with TBI and found that 24% had GAD. Deb et al. (1999) evaluated 196 individuals who were hospitalized after TBI; panic disorder developed in 9%. Salazar et al. (2000) evaluated 120 military members after moderate to severe TBI. One year after enrollment in the study of cognitive rehabilitation, 15% met criteria for GAD. Hibbard et al. (1998) found that 18% of subjects with TBI developed PTSD, 14% developed obsessive-compulsive disorder, 11% developed panic disorder, 8% developed GAD, and 6% developed phobic disorder. All of these disorders were more frequent after TBI than before TBI. In analysis of data from the New Haven portion of the ECA study, Silver et al. (2001) found that of individuals with a history of brain injury during their lifetime, the incidences of anxiety disorders were 4.7% for obsessive-compulsive disorder, 11.2% for phobic disorder, and 3.2% for panic disorder. Dissociative disorders, including depersonalization (Grigsby and Kaye 1993) and dissociative identity disorder (Sandel et al. 1990), may occur. It is our clinical observation that patients with histories of prior trauma are at higher risk for developing these disorders.

Because of the potentially life-threatening nature of many of the causes of TBI, including motor vehicle accidents and assaults, one would expect these patients to be at increased risk of developing PTSD. There is a 9.2% risk of developing PTSD after exposure to trauma; the risk is highest for assaultive violence (Breslau et al. 1998). PTSD and acute stress response, including symptoms of peritraumatic dissociation (Ursano et al. 1999b), are not uncommon after serious motor vehicle accidents (Koren et al. 1999; Ursano et al. 1999a).

PTSD has been found in individuals with TBI (Bryant 1996; McMillan 1996; Ohry et al. 1996; Parker and Rosenblum 1996; Rattok 1996; Silver et al. 1997). Using the Structured Clinical Interview for DSM-IV to evaluate

100 individuals with a history of TBI, Hibbard et al. (1998) found that 18% met the criteria for PTSD. Harvey and Bryant conducted a 2-year study of 79 motor vehicle accident survivors who sustained mild TBI. They found that acute stress disorder developed in 14% of these patients at 1 month. After 2 years, 73% of the group with acute stress disorder developed PTSD (Harvey and Bryant 2000). Six months after severe TBI, 26 of 96 individuals (27.1%) had developed PTSD (Bryant et al. 2000). Although few patients had intrusive memories (19.2%), 96.2% reported emotional reactivity. Max et al. (1998a) evaluated 50 children who were hospitalized after TBI. Although only 4% of these subjects developed PTSD, 68% had one PTSD symptom after 3 months, suggesting subsyndromal PTSD despite neurogenic amnesia.

Because of the overlap among symptoms of PTSD and mild TBI, it can be difficult to ascribe specific symptoms to the brain injury or to the circumstances of the accident. In studies of patients with PTSD, memory deficits consistent with temporal lobe injury have been demonstrated (Bremner et al. 1993). Imaging studies have shown smaller hippocampal volumes with PTSD (Bremner et al. 1995, 1997). Apparently, exposure to extreme stressors results in brain dysfunction that may be similar to that found after TBI.

Case Example

While Mr. A was working, a machine was activated accidentally, and his head was crushed. He had full recall of the sound of his skull cracking and the sensation of blood coming down his forehead. It was several hours before he was transported to a hospital, but he never lost consciousness. An EEG revealed irregular right cerebral activity, and an MRI was compatible with contusion and infarction of the right temporal parietal region.

After the accident, Mr. A developed the full syndrome of PTSD; he experienced flashbacks, mood lability, sensitivity to noise, decreased interest, distress when looking at pictures of the accident, and problems with concentration.

Sleep Disorders

Individuals with TBI commonly complain of disrupted sleep patterns, ranging from hypersomnia to difficulty maintaining sleep (Rao et al. 2005). Fichtenberg et al. (2000) assessed 91 individuals with TBI who had been admitted to an outpatient neurorehabilitation clinic. The presence of depression (as indicated by scores on the Beck Depression Inventory) and mild severity of the TBI were correlated with the occurrence of insomnia. Guilleminault et al. (2000) assessed 184 patients with head trauma and hypersomnia. Abnormalities were demonstrated on the Multiple Sleep Latency Test. Sleep-disordered breathing was common (occurring in 59 of 184 patients). Hypersomnia must be differentiated from lack of motivation and apathy. In addition, the contribution of pain to disruption of sleep must be considered. Although depression and sleep disorders can be related and have similarities in sleep endocrine changes (Frieboes et al. 1999), in our experience with depressed individuals after TBI, the sleep difficulties persist after successful treatment of the mood disorder. In addition, we have seen patients who have developed sleep apnea or nocturnal myoclonus subsequent to TBI.

Mild Traumatic Brain Injury and Postconcussion Syndrome

Patients with mild TBI may present with somatic, perceptual, cognitive, and emotional symptoms that have been characterized as the postconcussion syndrome (Table 4–3). By definition, mild TBI is associated with a brief duration of LOC (less than 20 minutes) or no LOC, and posttraumatic amnesia of less than 24 hours; the patient usually does not require hospitalization after the injury (see section "Neuropsychiatric Assessment" earlier in this chapter). For each patient hospitalized with mild TBI, probably four to five others sustain mild TBIs but receive treatment as outpatients or perhaps get no treatment at all. The psychiatrist is often called to assess the patient years after the injury, and the patient may not associate brain-related symptoms such as depression and cognitive dysfunction with the injury. The results of laboratory tests, such as structural brain imaging studies, often do not reveal significant abnormalities. However, as discussed previously, functional imaging studies such as SPECT (Masdeu et al. 1994; Nedd et al. 1993) and computerized electroencephalography and brain stem auditory evoked potential recordings have demonstrated abnormal findings (Watson et al. 1995). Diffuse axonal injury may occur with mild TBI, as demonstrated in the pathological examination of brains from patients who have died from systemic injuries (Oppenheimer 1968), as well as in nonhuman primates (Gennarelli et al. 1982). In addition, the balance between cellular energy demand and supply can be disrupted (McAllister 2005).

Table 4–3.   Postconcussion syndrome

Somatic symptoms	Perceptual symptoms
Headache	Tinnitus
Dizziness	Sensitivity to noise
Fatigue	Sensitivity to light
Insomnia	**Emotional symptoms**
	Depression
Cognitive symptoms	Anxiety
Memory difficulties	Irritability
Impaired concentration	

Source.   Adapted from Lishman 1988.

Most studies of cognitive function subsequent to mild TBI suggest that patients report trouble with memory, attention, concentration, and speed of information processing, and patients can in fact be shown to have deficits in these areas shortly after their injury (1 week to 1 month) (Brown et al. 1994; McAllister 2005; McMillan and Glucksman 1987). In an evaluation of neuropsychological deficits in 53 patients who were experiencing postconcussive problems from 1 to 22 months after injury, Leininger et al. (1990) detected significantly poorer performance ($P<0.05$) on tests of reasoning, information processing, and verbal learning than that found in a control population. Hugenholtz et al. (1988) reported that significant attentional and information processing impairment ($P<0.01$) occurred in a group of adults after mild concussion. Although there was improvement over time, the patient group continued to have abnormalities 3 months after the injury. Warden et al. (2001) found that even in previously high-functioning individuals who sustained mild concussion (West Point cadets), there was impairment in processing speed several days after the injury.

Individuals with mild TBI have an increased incidence of somatic complaints, including headache, dizziness, fatigue, sleep disturbance, and sensitivity to noise and light (Brown et al. 1994; Dikmen et al. 1986; Levin et al. 1987a, 1987b; Rimel et al. 1981). In the behavioral domain, the most common problems include irritability, anxiety, and depression (Dikmen et al. 1986; Fann et al. 1995; Hibbard et al. 1998a). McAllister (2005) has opined that it may be more accurate to discuss postconcussive symptoms rather than a syndrome.

The majority of individuals with mild TBI recover quickly, with significant and progressive reduction of complaints in all three domains (cognitive, somatic, and behavioral) at 1, 3, and certainly 6 months from the injury (Bernstein 1999). Unfortunately, good recovery is not universal. A significant number of patients continue to complain of persistent difficulties 6–12 months and even longer after their injury. For example, Keshavan et al. (1981) found that 40% of their patients had significant symptoms 3 months after injury. Levin et al. (1987b), in a multicenter study, found that 3 months postinjury, 47% complained of headache, 22% of decreased energy, and 22% of dizziness. In a review of this topic, Bohnen et al. (1992) found a range of 16%–49% of patients with persistent symptoms at 6 months and 1%–50% with persistent symptoms at 1 year. Those with persistent symptoms have been found to have impaired cognitive function (Leininger et al. 1990). Brown et al. (1994) suggest that if symptoms are present at 3–6 months subsequent to injury, they tend to persist. Alves et al. (1993) prospectively assessed 587 patients with uncomplicated mild TBI for 1 year. The most frequent symptoms were headache and dizziness. The researchers found that fewer than 6% of these subjects complained of multiple symptoms consistent with postconcussion syndrome.

Therefore, there may be two groups of mild TBI patients: those who recover by 3 months and those who have persistent symptoms. It is not known whether the persistent symptoms are part of a cohesive syndrome or simply represent a collection of loosely related symptoms resulting from the vagaries of an individual injury (Alves et al. 1986). However, it is increasingly recognized that "mild" TBI and concussions that occur in sports injuries result in clinically significant neuropsychological impairment (Freeman et al. 2005).

In an extensive review of the literature, Alexander (1995) highlighted several important aspects regarding patients who develop prolonged postconcussion syndrome: 1) they are more likely to have been under stress at the time of the accident, 2) they develop depression and/or anxiety soon after the accident, 3) they have extensive social disruption after the accident, and 4) they have problems with physical symptoms such as headache and dizziness.

The treatment of patients with mild TBI involves initiating several key interventions (Kay 1993). In the early phase of treatment, the major goal is prevention of the postconcussion syndrome. This involves providing information and education about understanding and predicting symptoms and their resolution and actively managing a gradual process of return to functioning. Education about the postconcussion syndrome and its natural history improves prognosis (Wade et al. 1998). It is important to involve the patient's family or significant other, so that they understand the disorder and predicted recovery. After the postconcussion syndrome has developed, the clinician must develop an alliance with the patient and validate his or her experience of cognitive and emotional difficulties while not prematurely confronting emotional factors as primary. A combined treatment strategy is required that addresses the emotional problems along with cognitive problems.

Aggression

Individuals who have TBI may experience irritability, agitation, and aggressive behavior (Silver et al. 2005). These episodes range in severity from irritability to outbursts that result in damage to property or assaults on others. In severe cases, affected individuals cannot remain in the community or with their families and often are referred to long-term psychiatric or neurobehavioral facilities. Increased isolation and separation from others often occur.

In the acute recovery period, 35%–96% of patients with TBI reportedly exhibit agitated behavior (Silver et al. 2005). After the acute recovery phase, irritability or bad temper is common. In only one prospective study has the occurrence of agitation and restlessness been monitored by an objective rating instrument, the Overt Aggression Scale (Brooke et al. 1992b). The authors found that of 100 patients with severe TBI (defined as GCS score<8, >1 hour of coma, and >1 week of hospitalization), only 11 patients exhibited agitated behavior. Only 3 patients manifested these behaviors for more than 1 week. However, 35 patients were observed to be restless but not agitated. In a prospective sample of 100 patients admitted to a brain injury rehabilitation unit, 42% exhibited agitated behavior during at least one nursing shift (Bogner and Corrigan 1995). In follow-up periods ranging from 1 to 15 years after injury, these behaviors occurred in 31%–71% of patients who had experienced severe TBI (Silver et al. 2005). Studies of mild TBI have evaluated patients for much briefer periods; 1-year estimates of agitated behavior from these studies range from 5% to 70% (Silver et al. 2005). Tateno et al. (2003), studying an inpatient TBI population, found that aggression was associated with the presence of major depression, frontal lobe lesions, poor premorbid social functioning, and a history of alcohol and substance abuse.

Carlsson et al. (1987) examined the relationship between the number of TBIs associated with LOC and various symptoms, and they demonstrated that irritability increases with subsequent injuries. Of the men who did not have head injuries with LOC, 21% reported irritability, whereas 31% of men with one injury with LOC and 33% of men with two or more injuries with LOC admitted to this symptom ($P<0.0001$).

Explosive and violent behaviors have long been associated with focal brain lesions as well as with diffuse damage to the central nervous system (Anderson and Silver 1999). The current diagnostic category in DSM-IV-TR is personality change due to a general medical condition. Patients with aggressive behavior would be specified as having the aggressive type, whereas those with mood lability are specified as having the labile type. Characteristic behavioral features occur in many individuals who exhibit aggressive behavior after brain injury (Yudofsky et al. 1990):

- *Reactive*—The violence is triggered by modest or trivial stimuli.
- *Nonreflective*—The violence does not involve premeditation or planning.
- *Nonpurposeful*—The aggression serves no obvious long-term aims or goals.
- *Periodic*—Brief outbursts of rage and aggression are interspersed between long periods of relatively calm behavior.
- *Ego-dystonic*—The individual is often upset or embarrassed after the episode.
- *Explosive*—The aggression occurs suddenly with no apparent buildup.

Therapeutic Strategies

Many useful therapeutic approaches are available for people who have brain injuries. Patients with brain injuries may develop neuropsychiatric symptoms based on the location of their injury, the emotional reaction to their injury, their preexisting strengths and difficulties, and their social expectations and supports. Comprehensive rehabilitation centers address many of these issues with therapeutic strategies that are developed specifically for this population (Ben-Yishay and Lakin 1989; Binder and Rattok 1989; Pollack 1989; Prigatano 1989).

Although these programs meet many of the needs of patients with TBI, comprehensive neuropsychiatric evaluation (including daily evaluation and treatment of the patient by a psychiatrist) is rarely available. Although we propose a multifactorial, multidisciplinary, collaborative approach to treatment, for purposes of exposition we have divided treatment into psychopharmacological, behavioral and cognitive, and psychological and social interventions.

Psychopharmacological Treatment

Several general guidelines should be followed in the pharmacological treatment of the psychiatric syndromes that occur after TBI: 1) start low, go slow; 2) conduct a therapeutic trial of all medications; 3) maintain continuous reassessment of the clinical condition; 4) monitor drug-drug interactions; 5) augment a partial response; and 6) discontinue or lower the dosage of the most recently prescribed medication if a worsening of the treated symptom occurs soon after the medication is initiated (or increased). In our experience, patients with brain injury of any type are far more sensitive to the side effects of medications than are patients who do not have brain injury. As we explain below, dosages of psychotropic medications must be raised and lowered in small increments over protracted periods of time, although patients ultimately may require the same dosages and serum levels that are therapeutically effective for patients without brain injury (Silver and Yudofsky 1987).

When medications are prescribed, it is important that they be given in a manner that enhances the probability of benefit and reduces the possibility of adverse reactions. Medications often should be initiated at dosages that are lower than those usually administered to patients without brain injury. However, dosages comparable to those used to treat primary psychiatric disorders may be necessary to treat TBI-related neuropsychiatric conditions effectively. Dosage increments should be made gradually, to minimize side effects and enable the clinician to observe adverse consequences. Medications must be given sufficient time to impart their full effects. Thus, when a clinician decides to administer a medication, the patient must receive an adequate therapeutic trial of that medication in terms of dosage and duration of treatment.

Because of frequent changes in the clinical status of patients after TBI, continuous reassessment is necessary to determine whether each prescribed medication is still required. For depression following TBI, the standard guidelines for the treatment of major depression by the American Psychiatric Association (2010) may offer a reasonable framework within which to develop a working treatment plan, including continuation of medication for a minimum of 16–20 weeks following complete remission of depressive symptoms. For this and all other neuropsychiatric sequelae of TBI, however, no formal treatment guidelines specific to this population are available. Although literature regarding the types and dosages of medications useful for the treatment of such problems is increasing, few if any studies have been published regarding the optimal duration of treatment or the issues pertaining to treatment discontinuation and relapse risk. In general, if a patient has responded favorably to initial medication treatment for one or another neuropsychiatric problem after TBI, the clinician must use sound judgment and apply risk-benefit determinations to each specific case in deciding whether and/or when to taper and attempt to discontinue the medication following TBI. Continuous reassessment is necessary because spontaneous remission of some symptoms may occur, in which case the medication can be permanently discontinued, or a carryover effect of the medication may occur (i.e., its effects may persist after the duration of treatment), in which case a reinstatement of the medication may not be required.

When a new medication is initiated in combination with medications previously prescribed, the clinician must be vigilant for the development of drug-drug interactions. These interactions may include alteration of pharmacokinetics that results in increased half-lives and serum levels of medications, as can occur with the use of multiple anticonvulsants. Additionally, alterations of pharmacodynamics may develop during the administration of medications with additive or synergistic clinical effects (e.g., increased sedative effects when several sedating medications are administered simultaneously).

If a patient does not respond favorably to the initial medication prescribed, several alternatives are available. If the patient has had no response, changing to a medication with a different mechanism of action is suggested, much as is done in the treatment of depressed patients without brain injury. If the patient has had a partial response to the initial medication, addition of another medication may be useful. The selection of a supplementary or augmenting medication should be based on consideration of the possible complementary or contrary mechanisms of action of such agents and on the individual and combined side-effect profiles of the initial and secondary agents and their potential pharmacokinetic and pharmacodynamic interactions.

Although individuals after TBI may experience multiple concurrent neuropsychiatric symptoms (e.g., depressed mood, irritability, poor attention, fatigue, sleep disturbances), which together suggest a single "psychiatric diagnosis" such as major depression, we have found that some of these symptoms often persist despite treatment of the apparent "diagnosis." In other words, diagnostic parsimony should be sought but may not always be the best or most accurate diagnostic approach for this population. Therefore, the neuropsychiatric approach of evaluating and monitoring individual symptoms is necessary and differs from the usual "syndromal" approach of the present conventional psychiatric paradigm. Several medications may be required to alleviate several distinct symptoms following TBI, although the prudent course of action is to initiate each treatment one at a time, to determine the efficacy and side effects of each prescribed drug.

Studies of the effects of psychotropic medications in patients with TBI are few, and rigorous double-blind placebo-controlled studies are rare (see Arciniegas et al. 2000). The recommendations contained in this chapter represent a synthesis of the available treatment literature on TBI, the extensions of the known uses of these medications in phenotypically similar psychiatric populations of patients with other types of brain injury (e.g., stroke, multiple sclerosis), and our personal opinions. We recognize that the pathophysiology of these symptoms may differ in patients with TBI; thus, generalization of response to treatment seen in the context of other forms of brain dysfunction (e.g., stroke, Alzheimer's disease) to TBI may not always be valid. If treatment studies in the TBI population are available to offer guidance regarding medication treatments, we note and reference these for further consideration by interested readers.

Aggression and Agitation

Although no medication has been approved by the U.S. Food and Drug Administration (FDA) specifically for the treatment of aggression, medications are widely used (and commonly misused) in the management of patients with acute or chronic aggression. After appropriate assessment for the possible etiologies of these behaviors, the clinician should base treatment on the occurrence of comorbid neuropsychiatric conditions (depression, psychosis, insomnia, anxiety, delirium) (see Figure 4–1), whether the treatment is in the acute (hours to days) or chronic (weeks to months) phase, and the severity of the behavior

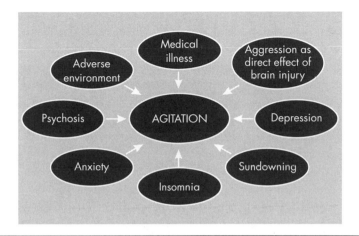

Figure 4–1. Factors associated with the psychopharmacological treatment of agitation in patients with traumatic brain injury.

Source. Reprinted from Silver JM, Hales RE, Yudofsky SC: "Neuropsychiatric Aspects of Traumatic Brain Injury," in *Essentials of Neuropsychiatry and Behavioral Neurosciences,* 2nd Edition. Edited by Yudofsky SC, Hales RE. Washington, DC, American Psychiatric Publishing, 2010, pp. 223–274. Used with permission. Copyright © 2010 American Psychiatric Association.

(mild to severe). The clinician must be aware that patients may not respond to just one medication but may require combination treatment, similar to the pharmacotherapeutic treatment for refractory depression.

Chronic aggression. If a patient continues to exhibit periods of agitation or aggression beyond several weeks, the use of specific antiaggressive medications should be initiated to prevent these episodes from occurring. Because no medication has been approved by the FDA for treatment of aggression, the clinician must use medications that may be antiaggressive but that have been approved for other uses (e.g., seizure disorders, depression, hypertension) (Silver and Yudofsky 1994; Yudofsky et al. 1998).

Antipsychotic medications. If, after thorough clinical evaluation, the clinician determines that the aggressive episodes result from psychosis, such as paranoid delusions or command hallucinations, then antipsychotic medications are the treatment of choice. Risperidone has had good results in treating agitation in elderly patients with dementia (Goldberg and Goldberg 1995). Olanzapine appears to be more sedating and quetiapine may have fewer extrapyramidal symptoms than risperidone. Clozapine may have greater antiaggressive effects than other antipsychotic medications (Michals et al. 1993; Ratey et al. 1993). The increased risk of seizures, however, must be carefully assessed.

Serotonin appears to be a key neurotransmitter in the modulation of aggressive behavior. In preliminary reports, buspirone, a serotonin type 1A agonist, has been reported to be effective in the management of aggression and agitation for patients with head injury, dementia, developmental disabilities, or autism (Silver and Yudofsky 1994; Yudofsky et al. 1998). In rare instances, some patients become more aggressive when treated with buspirone. Therefore, buspirone should be initiated at low dosages (i.e., 5 mg twice daily) and the dosage increased by 5 mg every 3–5 days. Dosages of 45–60 mg/day may be required before aggressive behavior improves, although we have noted dramatic improvement within 1 week.

Antianxiety medications.   Clonazepam may be effective in the long-term management of aggression, although controlled double-blind studies have not yet been conducted. We use clonazepam when pronounced aggression and anxiety occur together or when aggression occurs in association with neurologically induced tics and similarly disinhibited motor behaviors. The initial dosage should be 0.5 mg twice daily, and the dosage may be increased to as high as 2–4 mg twice daily, as tolerated. Sedation and ataxia are frequent side effects.

Anticonvulsive medications.   The anticonvulsant carbamazepine has been demonstrated to be effective for treatment of bipolar disorders and has also been advocated for control of aggression in both epileptic and nonepileptic populations. Reports indicate that the antiaggressive response of carbamazepine can be found in patients with and without electroencephalographic abnormalities (Silver and Yudofsky 1994; Yudofsky et al. 1998). Azouvi et al. (1999) found that 8 of 10 patients with aggressive behavior after TBI responded to carbamazepine.

In our experience and that of others, the anticonvulsant valproic acid may also be helpful to some patients with organically induced aggression (Geracioti

1994; Giakas et al. 1990; Horne and Lindley 1995; Mattes 1992; Wroblewski et al. 1997). For patients with aggression and epilepsy whose seizures are being treated with anticonvulsant drugs such as phenytoin and phenobarbital, switching to carbamazepine or to valproic acid may treat both conditions.

Gabapentin may be beneficial for the treatment of agitation in patients with dementia (Herrmann et al. 2000; Roane et al. 2000). Dosages have ranged from 200–2,400 mg/day. Childers and Holland (1997), however, reported an increase in anxiety and restlessness (i.e., agitation) in two cognitively impaired TBI patients for whom gabapentin was prescribed to reduce chronic pain.

Antimanic medications. Although lithium is known to be effective in controlling aggression related to manic excitement, many studies suggest that it may also have a role in the treatment of aggression in selected populations of patients without bipolar disorder (Yudofsky et al. 1998). Included are patients with TBI (Bellus et al. 1996; Glenn et al. 1989), as well as patients with mental retardation who exhibit self-injurious or aggressive behavior, children and adolescents with behavioral disorders, prison inmates, and patients with other organic brain syndromes.

Patients with brain injury have increased sensitivity to the neurotoxic effects of lithium (Hornstein and Seliger 1989; Moskowitz and Altshuler 1991). Because of lithium's potential for neurotoxicity and its relative lack of efficacy in many patients with aggression secondary to brain injury, we limit the use of lithium to patients whose aggression is related to manic effects or recurrent irritability related to cyclic mood disorders.

Antidepressants. The antidepressants that have been reported to control aggressive behavior are those that act preferentially (amitriptyline) or specifically (trazodone and fluoxetine) on serotonin. Fluoxetine has been reported to be effective in the treatment of aggressive behavior in patients who have sustained brain injury, as well as in patients with personality disorders and depression and in adolescents with mental retardation and self-injurious behavior (Silver and Yudofsky 1994; Yudofsky et al. 1998). We have used selective serotonin reuptake inhibitors with considerable success in aggressive patients with brain lesions. The dosages used are similar to those for the treatment of mood lability and depression.

We have evaluated and treated many patients with emotional lability that is characterized by frequent episodes of tearfulness and irritability and the full symptomatic picture of neuroaggressive syndrome (Silver and Yudofsky 1994). These patients—who would be diagnosed under DSM-IV-TR with personality change, labile type, due to TBI—have responded well to antidepressants.

Antihypertensive medications: β-blockers.   The first report of the use of β-adrenergic receptor blockers in the treatment of acute aggression appeared in 1977, and within the next 10 years more than 25 articles on this topic appeared in the neurological and psychiatric literature, reporting experience in using β-blockers with more than 200 patients with aggression (Yudofsky et al. 1987). Most of these patients had been unsuccessfully treated with antipsychotics, minor tranquilizers, lithium, and/or anticonvulsants before being treated with β-blockers. The β-blockers that have been investigated in controlled prospective studies include propranolol (a lipid-soluble, nonselective receptor antagonist), nadolol (a water-soluble, nonselective receptor antagonist), and pindolol (a lipid-soluble, nonselective β receptor antagonist with partial sympathomimetic activity). Evidence suggests that β-adrenergic receptor blockers are effective agents for the treatment of aggressive and violent behaviors, particularly those related to organic brain syndrome.

The effectiveness of propranolol in reducing agitation has been demonstrated during initial hospitalization after TBI (Brooke et al. 1992a). Guidelines for the use of propranolol are listed in Table 4–4. When a patient requires the use of a once-daily medication because of compliance difficulties, long-acting propranolol or nadolol can be used. When patients develop bradycardia that prevents them from taking therapeutic dosages of propranolol, the clinician can substitute pindolol, prescribing one-tenth the dosage of propranolol. The intrinsic sympathomimetic activity of pindolol stimulates the β receptor and restricts the development of bradycardia.

The major side effects of β-blockers when used to treat aggression are the lowering of blood pressure and of pulse rate. Because peripheral β receptors are fully blocked with dosages of 300–400 mg/day, further decreases in these vital signs usually do not occur even when dosages are increased to much higher levels. Despite reports of depression with the use of β-blockers, controlled trials and our experience indicate that it is a rare occurrence. Because the use of pro-

Table 4–4. Clinical use of propranolol

1. Conduct a thorough medical evaluation.

2. Exclude patients with the following disorders: bronchial asthma, chronic obstructive pulmonary disease, insulin-dependent diabetes mellitus, congestive heart failure, persistent angina, significant peripheral vascular disease, hyperthyroidism.

3. Avoid sudden discontinuation of propranolol (particularly in patients with hypertension).

4. Begin with a single test dose of 20 mg/day in patients for whom there are clinical concerns with hypotension or bradycardia. Increase dose of propranolol by 20 mg/day every 3 days.

5. Initiate propranolol on a 20-mg-three-times-daily schedule for patients without cardiovascular or cardiopulmonary disorder.

6. Increase the dosage of propranolol by 60 mg/day every 3 days.

7. Increase medication unless the pulse rate is reduced below 50 beats/minute or systolic blood pressure is less than 90 mm Hg.

8. Do not administer medication if severe dizziness, ataxia, or wheezing occurs. Reduce or discontinue propranolol if such symptoms persist.

9. Increase dose to 12 mg/kg of body weight or until aggressive behavior is under control.

10. Doses greater than 800 mg are not usually required to control aggressive behavior.

11. Maintain the patient on the highest dose of propranolol for at least 8 weeks before concluding that the patient is not responding to the medication. Some patients, however, may respond rapidly to propranolol.

12. Use concurrent medications with caution. Monitor plasma levels of all antipsychotic and anticonvulsive medications.

Source. Silver and Yudofsky 1987.

pranolol is associated with significant increases in plasma levels of thioridazine, which has an absolute dosage ceiling of 800 mg/day, the combination of these two medications should be avoided whenever possible.

Table 4–5 summarizes our recommendations for the use of various classes of medication in treatment of chronic aggressive disorders associated with TBI.

Table 4–5.   Pharmacotherapy of agitation and aggression

Acute agitation/severe aggression

Antipsychotic drugs

Benzodiazepines

Chronic agitation

Atypical antipsychotics

Anticonvulsants (valproic acid, carbamazepine, ?gabapentin)

Serotonergic antidepressants (SSRI, trazodone)

Buspirone

β-Blockers

Note.   SSRI=selective serotonin reuptake inhibitor.
Source.   Reprinted from Silver JM, Hales RE, Yudofsky SC: "Neuropsychiatric Aspects of Traumatic Brain Injury," in *Essentials of Neuropsychiatry and Behavioral Neurosciences,* 2nd Edition. Edited by Yudofsky SC, Hales RE. Washington, DC, American Psychiatric Publishing, 2010, pp. 223–274. Used with permission. Copyright © 2010 American Psychiatric Association.

Acute aggression may be treated by using the sedative properties of neuroleptics or benzodiazepines. In treating aggression, the clinician, when possible, should diagnose and treat underlying disorders and should use, when possible, antiaggressive agents specific for those disorders. When the patient has a partial response after a therapeutic trial with a specific medication, adjunctive treatment with a medication with a different mechanism of action should be instituted. For example, a patient who has a partial response to β-blockers can experience more improvement with the addition of an anticonvulsant.

Acute aggression and agitation.   In the treatment of agitation and of acute or severe episodes of aggressive behavior, medications that are sedating may be indicated. However, because these drugs are not specific in their ability to inhibit aggressive behavior, patients may experience detrimental effects on arousal and cognitive function. Therefore, the use of sedation-producing medications must be time limited, to avoid the emergence of seriously disabling side effects ranging from oversedation to tardive dyskinesia.

After the diagnosis and treatment of underlying causes of aggression and the evaluation and documentation of aggressive behaviors (such as with the Overt Aggression Scale), the clinician should consider the use of two categories of pharmacological interventions: 1) medications with sedating effects, as required in acute situations, so that the patient does not harm self or others; and 2) nonsedating antiaggressive medications for the treatment of chronic aggression (Silver and Yudofsky 1994; Yudofsky et al. 1995).

Antipsychotic drugs.   Antipsychotics are the most commonly used medications in the treatment of aggression. Although these agents are appropriate and effective when aggression is derivative of active psychosis, the use of neuroleptic agents to treat chronic aggression, especially that secondary to organic brain injury, is often ineffective and entails significant risks that the patient will develop serious complications. Usually, the sedative side effects rather than the antipsychotic properties of antipsychotics are used (i.e., misused) to "treat" (i.e., mask) the aggression. Often, patients develop tolerance to the sedative effects of the neuroleptics and therefore require increasing dosages. As a result, extrapyramidal and anticholinergic-related side effects occur. Paradoxically (and frequently), because of the development of akathisia, the patient may become more agitated and restless as the dosage of neuroleptic is increased, especially when a high-potency antipsychotic such as haloperidol is administered. The akathisia is often mistaken for increased irritability and agitation, and a vicious circle of increasing neuroleptics and worsening akathisia results.

In patients with brain injury and acute aggression, we recommend starting a neuroleptic such as risperidone at a low dose of 0.5 mg orally, with repeated administration every hour until control of aggression is achieved. If the patient's aggressive behavior does not improve after several administrations of risperidone, the hourly dose may be increased until the patient is so sedated that he or she no longer exhibits agitation or violence. Once the patient is not aggressive for 48 hours, the daily dosage should be decreased gradually (i.e., by 25% per day) to ascertain whether aggressive behavior reemerges. If the aggression reemerges, the clinician should then consider the next course of action: increasing the dosage of risperidone, initiating treatment with a more specific antiaggressive drug, or both.

Sedatives and hypnotics.   Inconsistent results have been reported in the literature on the effects of benzodiazepines in the treatment of aggression. The sedative properties of benzodiazepines are especially helpful in the management of acute agitation and aggression. Most likely, improvement is due to the effect of benzodiazepines on increasing the inhibitory neurotransmitter γ-aminobutyric acid (GABA). Paradoxically, several studies report increased hostility and aggression, as well as the induction of rage, in patients treated with benzodiazepines. However, these reports are balanced by the observation that this phenomenon is rare (Dietch and Jennings 1988). Benzodiazepines can produce amnesia, and preexisting memory dysfunction can be exacerbated by the use of benzodiazepines. Patients with brain injury may also experience increased problems with coordination and balance with benzodiazepine use.

For treatment of acute aggression, lorazepam 1–2 mg may be administered every hour by either oral or intramuscular route until sedation is achieved (Silver and Yudofsky 1994). Intramuscular lorazepam has been suggested as an effective medication in the emergency treatment of the violent patient (Bick and Hannah 1986). Intravenous lorazepam is also effective, although the onset of action is similar when the drug is administered intramuscularly. Caution must be taken with intravenous administration, and the drug should be injected in doses of less than 1 mg/minute to avoid laryngospasm. As with neuroleptics, gradual tapering of lorazepam may be attempted when the patient has been in control for 48 hours. If aggressive behavior recurs, medications for the treatment of chronic aggression may be initiated. Lorazepam in 1- or 2-mg doses, administered either orally or by injection, may be administered, if necessary, in combination with a neuroleptic medication (haloperidol 2–5 mg). Other sedating medications, such as paraldehyde, chloral hydrate, or diphenhydramine, may be preferable to sedative antipsychotic agents.

Behavioral and Cognitive Treatments

Behavioral treatments are important in the care of patients who have sustained TBI. Behavioral programs require careful design and execution by a staff well versed in these techniques. Behavioral methods can be used in response to aggressive outbursts and other maladaptive social behaviors (Corrigan and Bach 2005). One study (Eames and Wood 1985) found that behavior modification was 75% effective in dealing with disturbed behavior after severe brain injury.

After brain injury, patients may need specific cognitive strategies to assist with memory and concentration (Cicerone et al. 2005; Gordon and Hibbard 2005). As opposed to earlier beliefs that cognitive therapy should "exercise" the brain to develop skills that have been damaged, current therapies involve teaching the patient new strategies to compensate for lost or impaired functions. Salazar et al. (2000), for the Defense and Veterans Head Injury Program Study Group, compared an intensive 8-week in-hospital cognitive rehabilitation program and a limited home program. Both patient groups improved, and no significant difference was found between the two treatments. (For more information on cognitive treatments, see Chapter 12, "Cognitive Rehabilitation and Behavior Therapy for Patients With Neuropsychiatric Disorders.") We emphasize that for most patients, treatment strategies are synergistic. For example, the use of β-adrenergic receptor antagonists to treat agitation and aggression may enhance a patient's ability to benefit from behavioral and cognitive treatments.

Psychological and Social Interventions

In the broadest terms, patients who incur brain injury have psychological issues that revolve around four major themes: 1) psychopathology that preceded the injury, 2) psychological responses to the traumatic event, 3) psychological reactions to deficits brought about by brain injury, and 4) psychological issues related to potential recurrence of brain injury.

Preexisting psychiatric illnesses are most frequently intensified with brain injury. Therefore, the angry, obsessive patient or the patient with chronic depression will exhibit a worsening of these symptoms after brain injury. Specific coping mechanisms that were used before the injury may no longer be possible because of the cognitive deficits caused by the neurological disease. Therefore, patients need to learn new methods of adaptation to stress. In addition, as mentioned earlier in the subsection "Neuropsychological Testing," the patient's response to the injury is influenced by his or her social, economic, educational, and vocational status (and how each is affected by brain lesions).

The events surrounding brain injury often have far-reaching experiential and symbolic significance for the patient. Such issues as guilt, punishment, magical wishes, and fears crystallize about the nidus of a traumatic event. For example, a patient who sustains brain injury during a car accident may view his injury as punishment for long-standing violent impulses toward an aggressive father. In such cases, reassurance and homilies about his lack of responsibility for the accident are usually less productive than psychological exploration.

A patient's reactions to being disabled by brain damage have realistic as well as symbolic significance. When intense effort is required for a patient to form a word or to move a limb, frustration may be expressed as anger, depression, anxiety, or fear. Particularly in cases in which brain injury results in permanent impairment, a psychiatrist may experience countertransferential discomfort that results in failure to discuss directly with the patient and his or her family the implications of resultant disabilities and limitations. Gratuitous optimism, collaboration with the patient's denial, and facile solutions to complex problems are rarely effective and can erode the therapeutic alliance and ongoing treatment. Tyerman and Humphrey (1984) assessed 25 patients with severe brain injury for changes in self-concept. Patients viewed themselves as markedly changed after their injury but believed that they would regain preexisting capacities within a year. The authors concluded that these unrealistic expectations may hamper rehabilitation and adjustment of both the patient and his or her relatives. By gently and persistently directing the patient's attention to the reality of the disabilities, the psychiatrist may help the patient begin the process of acceptance and adjustment to the impairment. Clinical judgment will help the psychiatrist in deciding whether and when explorations of the symbolic significance of the patient's brain injury should be pursued.

Families of patients with neurological disorders are under severe stress. The relative with a brain injury may be unable to fulfill his or her previous role or function as parent or spouse, thus significantly affecting the other family members (Cavallo and Kay 2005). Oddy et al. (1978) evaluated 54 relatives of patients with brain injury within 1, 6, and 12 months of the traumatic event. Approximately 40% of the relatives showed depressive symptoms within 1 month of the event; 25% of the relatives showed significant physical or psychological illness within 6–12 months of the brain damage. Relatives also exhibit mood disturbances, especially anxiety, depression, and social role dysfunction, within this time (Kreutzer et al. 1994; Linn et al. 1994; Livingston et al. 1985a, 1985b). Family members may experience increased substance use, unemployment, and decreased financial status over time (Hall et al. 1994).

By treating relatives for their psychological responses to the brain injury, the clinician can foster a supportive and therapeutic atmosphere for the patient while significantly helping the relative. For both patients and their families, severe TBI results in multifaceted losses, including the loss of dreams about and expectations for the future. The psychiatrist may be of enormous benefit in treating the family and patient by providing support, insight, and other points of view. Educational and supportive treatment of families can be therapeutic when used together with appropriate social skills training. Patient advocacy groups, such as the National Brain Injury Foundation, can provide important peer support for families. Many patients require clear, almost concrete statements describing their behaviors because their insight and judgment may be impaired.

It is a distressing fact that brain injury can and often does recur. Repeated injury results in an increase in the incidence of neuropsychiatric and emotional symptoms (Carlsson et al. 1987). Patients' fears and anxieties about recurrence of injury are more than simply efforts at magical control over terrifying conditions. Therapeutic emphasis should be placed on actions and activities that will aid in preventing recurrence, including compliance with appropriate medications and abstinence from alcohol and other substances of abuse.

Prevention

Motor Vehicle Accidents

The proper use of seat belts with upper-torso restraints is 45% effective in preventing fatalities, 50% effective in preventing moderate to critical injuries, and 10% effective in preventing minor injuries among drivers and passengers (U.S. Department of Transportation 1984). This translates to 12,000–15,000 lives saved per year (National Safety Council 1986). Orsay et al. (1988) noted that victims of motor vehicle accidents who wore seat belts had a 60.1% reduction in injury severity. Without specific legislation, car restraints are used infrequently. Many brain injuries occur in side impacts, when the heads of occupants collide with the structural column between the windshield and the side window. More than 7,000 motor vehicle–related deaths are caused by side impacts, and nearly half of these deaths are due to brain trauma (Jagger 1992). In 2003, there were 44,800 motor vehicle accident–related fatalities (National Safety Council 2006). There were 2.2 million disabling injuries from motor vehicle accidents in 1998 (National Safety Council 1999).

The use of safety belts has prevented a significant number of deaths and injuries (Centers for Disease Control 1992; Kaplan and Cowley 1991). Driver and passenger air bags have decreased the number and severity of injuries, although they have not been as effective in controlling severe injuries of the lower extremities (Kuner et al. 1996).

Alcohol dependence is a highly prevalent and destructive illness. In addition, alcohol abuse is a common concomitant of affective and characterological disorders. Alcohol intoxication is frequently found in the patient who has suffered brain injury, whether from violence, falls, or motor vehicle accidents (Brismar et al. 1983). In the United States, the proportion of alcohol involvement in motor vehicle fatalities has been decreasing since 2002. Whereas during the week, 24% of fatally injured drivers have blood alcohol concentrations at or above 0.087%, on weekends, the proportion increases to 45% (Insurance Institute for Highway Safety 2005a). Alcohol-related deaths have been decreased by a combination of "zero tolerance" laws and laws lowering the allowable blood alcohol concentration for impaired driving from 0.10% to 0.08% (Insurance Institute for Highway Safety 2005a).

Drivers in fatal accidents more frequently have a history of alcohol use, previous accidents, moving traffic violations, psychopathology, stress, paranoid thinking, and depression. They often have less control of hostility and anger, a decreased tolerance for tension, and a history of increased risk taking (Tsuang et al. 1985). Therefore, we strongly advocate that all psychiatric and other medical histories include a detailed inquiry about alcohol use, seat belt use, and driving patterns. Questions about driving patterns, accident records, violations, driving while intoxicated, speeding patterns, car maintenance, the presence of distractions such as children and animals, and hazardous driving conditions should be included. The use of illicit substances and medications that may induce sedation, such as antihistamines, antihypertensive agents, anticonvulsants, minor tranquilizers, and antidepressants, should also be assessed and documented. Psychiatric patients are at greater risk for motor vehicle accidents because they often have several of these characteristics (Noyes 1985).

Significant preventive measures to reduce head trauma include counseling a patient about risk taking; the treatment of alcoholism and depression; the judicious prescription of medications and full explanations of sedation, cognitive impairment, and other potentially dangerous side effects; and public information activities on topics such as the proper use of seat belts, the dangers of drinking and driving, and automobile safety measures.

Clearly, motorcycle riding, with or without helmets, and using bicycles for commuting purposes are associated with head injuries, even when safety precautions are taken and when driving regulations are observed. In 2005, motorcyclist deaths totaled 4,439 (Insurance Institute for Highway Safety 2005d). It has been estimated that for every motorcycle-related death, another 37 injuries are reported and many more remain unreported to the police (Baker et al. 1987). Helmets can reduce the risk of on-highway motorcycle fatalities by about 37% and are 67% effective in preventing brain injuries (Insurance Institute for Highway Safety 2005d). Death rates from TBI are twice as high in states with weak or nonexistent helmet laws, compared with rates in states with helmet laws that apply to all riders (Sosin et al. 1989). Fewer than half of the states mandate that all riders wear helmets.

In 1988, the Centers for Disease Control reported that 1,300 bicyclists were killed annually in the United States. In 2005, 782 bicyclists were killed in crashes with motor vehicles, a number that has been decreasing over the years (Insurance Institute for Highway Safety 2005b). Virtually all of the riders who died were not wearing helmets (Insurance Institute for Highway Safety 2005b). The use of bicycle helmets can significantly decrease the morbidity and mortality resulting from bicycle-related head injuries (Thompson et al. 1989). However, only 16 states have mandatory helmet laws, and even these apply only to riders under age 18.

Brain Injury in Children

Beyond nurturance, children rely on their parents or guardians for guidance and protection. Each year in the United States, more than 1,500 children under age 13 die as motor vehicle passengers; more than 90% of these children were not using car seat restraints (Insurance Institute for Highway Safety 2005c). Child safety seats have been found to be 80%–90% effective in the prevention of injuries to children (National Safety Council 1985). In a sample of 494 children younger than age 4 years who had suffered motor vehicle accident trauma (Agran et al. 1985), 70% had been unrestrained, 12% were restrained with seat belts, and 22% were restrained in child safety seats. In general, restrained children tended to sustain less serious injuries than unrestrained children.

Children younger than 4 years who are not restrained in safety seats are 11 times more likely to be killed in motor vehicle accidents (National Safety Council 1985). A child should not sit on the lap of the parent, with or without restraints, because the adult's weight can crush the child during an accident. Young children traveling with drivers who themselves are not wearing seat belts are four times more likely to be left unrestrained (National Safety Council 1985). Legislation in Britain mandating the use of child safety seats has had a significant effect on decreasing fatal and serious injuries to children (Avery and Hayes 1985). In the United States, all 50 states and the District of Columbia have mandatory laws for child safety seats (National Safety Council 1985). Alcohol use by adults is frequently a factor in child injuries and fatalities (Li 2000). In the majority of drinking driver–related child passenger deaths, the child was an unrestrained passenger (Quinlan et al. 2000).

Children who ride in bicycle-mounted child seats are highly subject to injuries to the head and face and should wear bicycle helmets.

Children are often involved in sports that carry the risk of brain injury. Sports such as boxing, gymnastics, diving, soccer, football, basketball, and hockey are associated with considerable risk of TBI. In 1997, the Centers for Disease Control and Prevention estimated that 300,000 cases of TBI occurred annually during sports or recreation. For children ages 10–14 years, sports and recreational activities accounted for 43% of TBIs (Kraus and Nourjah 1988). Powell and Barber-Foss (1999) found that 3.9% of 17,815 high school athletes had sustained a mild TBI. Mild brain injury is not uncommon in football and can result in persistent symptoms and disabilities (Gerberich et al. 1983). According to Gerberich et al. (1983), an estimated 20% of high school football players sustained concussion during a single football season, with some reporting symptoms persisting as long as 6–9 months after the end of the season. Soccer, which may involve use of the head with sudden twists to strike the ball, may also result in neuropsychiatric abnormalities (Tysvaer et al. 1989).

The clinician must always be alert to the possibility that parents may be neglectful, may use poor judgment, and may even be directly violent in their treatment of children. Unfortunately, it is not uncommon for head trauma to result from overt child abuse on the part of parents, other adults, and peers. When these problems are discovered, clinicians must take direct actions to address them. We encourage direct counseling of parents who do not consistently use infant and child car seats for their children.

Conclusion

Invariably, brain injury leads to emotional damage in the patient and in the family. In this chapter, we have reviewed the most frequently occurring psychiatric symptoms that are associated with TBI. We have emphasized how the informed psychiatrist is not only effective but essential in both the prevention of brain injury and, when it occurs, the treatment of its sequelae. In addition to increased efforts devoted to the prevention of brain injury, we advocate a multidisciplinary and multidimensional approach to the assessment and treatment of neuropsychiatric aspects of brain injury.

Recommended Reading

Silver JM, McAllister TW, Yudofsky SC (eds): Textbook of Traumatic Brain Injury, 2nd Edition. Washington, DC, American Psychiatric Publishing, 2011

References

Achté K, Jarho L, Kyykka T, et al: Paranoid disorders following war brain damage: preliminary report. Psychopathology 24:309–315, 1991

Agran PF, Dunkie DE, Winn DG: Motor vehicle accident trauma and restraint usage patterns in children less than 4 years of age. Pediatrics 76:382–386, 1985

Alexander MP: Mild traumatic brain injury: pathophysiology, natural history, and clinical management. Neurology 45:1253–1260, 1995

Alves WM, Coloban ART, O'Leary TJ, et al: Understanding posttraumatic symptoms after minor head injury. J Head Trauma Rehabil 1:1–12, 1986

Alves W, Macciocchi SN, Barth JT: Postconcussive symptoms after uncomplicated mild head injury. J Head Trauma Rehabil 8:48–59, 1993

American Psychiatric Association: Diagnostic and Statistical Manual of Mental Disorders, 3rd Edition. Washington, DC, American Psychiatric Association, 1980

American Psychiatric Association: Diagnostic and Statistical Manual of Mental Disorders, 3rd Edition, Revised. Washington, DC, American Psychiatric Association, 1987

American Psychiatric Association: Diagnostic and Statistical Manual of Mental Disorders, 4th Edition, Text Revision. Washington, DC, American Psychiatric Association, 2000

American Psychiatric Association: Treatment of Patients With Major Depressive Disorder, 3rd Edition. Arlington, VA, American Psychiatric Association, November 2010. Available at: http://www.psychiatryonline.com/pracGuide/pracGuideTopic_7.aspx. Accessed September 8, 2010.

Anderson KE, Silver JM: Neurological and medical diseases and violence, in Medical Management of the Violent Patient: Clinical Assessment and Therapy. Edited by Tardiff K. New York, Marcel Dekker, 1999, pp 87–124

Anderson KE, Taber KH, Hurley RA: Functional imaging, in Textbook of Traumatic Brain Injury. Edited by Silver JM, McAllister TW, Yudofsky SC. Washington, DC, American Psychiatric Publishing, 2005, pp 107–134

Annegers JF, Grabow JD, Groover RV, et al: Seizures after head trauma: a population study. Neurology 30:683–689, 1980

Arciniegas DB, Topkoff J, Silver JM: Neuropsychiatric aspects of traumatic brain injury. Curr Treat Options Neurol 2:169–186, 2000

Arciniegas DB, Anderson CA, Rojas DC: Electrophysiological techniques, in Textbook of Traumatic Brain Injury. Edited by Silver JM, McAllister TW, Yudofsky SC. Washington, DC, American Psychiatric Publishing, 2005, pp 135–158

Ariza M, Junque C, Mataro M, et al: Neuropsychological correlates of basal ganglia and medial temporal lobe NAA/Cho reductions in traumatic brain injury. Arch Neurol 61:541–544, 2004

Armstrong KK, Sahgal V, Bloch R, et al: Rehabilitation outcomes in patients with posttraumatic epilepsy. Arch Phys Med Rehabil 71:156–160, 1990

Ashikaga R, Araki Y, Ishida O: MRI of head injury using FLAIR. Neuroradiology 39:239–242, 1997

Auerbach SH: Neuroanatomical correlates of attention and memory disorders in traumatic brain injury: an application of neurobehavioral subtypes. J Head Trauma Rehabil 1:1–12, 1986

Avery JG, Hayes HRM: Death and injury to children in cars in Britain. Br Med J (Clin Res Ed) 291:515, 1985

Azouvi P, Jokic C, Attal N, et al: Carbamazepine in agitation and aggressive behaviour following severe closed-head injury: results of an open trial. Brain Inj 13:797–804, 1999

Bakchine S, Lacomblez L, Benoit N, et al: Manic-like state after bilateral orbitofrontal and right temporoparietal injury: efficacy of clonidine. Neurology 39:777–781, 1989

Baker SP, Whitfield RA, O'Neill B: Geographic variations in mortality from motor vehicle crashes. N Engl J Med 316:1384–1387, 1987

Bamrah JS, Johnson J: Bipolar affective disorder following head injury. Br J Psychiatry 158:117–119, 1991

Bechara A, Damasio AR, Damasio H, et al: Insensitivity to future consequences following damage to human prefrontal cortex. Cognition 50:7–15, 1994

Beck AT, Ward CH, Mendelson M, et al: An inventory for measuring depression. Arch Gen Psychiatry 4:561–571, 1961

Belanger HG, Vanderploeg RD, Curtiss G, et al: Recent neuroimaging techniques in mild traumatic brain injury. J Neuropsychiatry Clin Neurosci 19:5–20, 2007

Bellus SB, Stewart D, Vergo JG, et al: The use of lithium in the treatment of aggressive behaviours with two brain-injured individuals in a state psychiatric hospital. Brain Inj 10:849–860, 1996

Ben-Yishay Y, Lakin P: Structured group treatment for brain-injury survivors, in Neuropsychological Treatment After Brain Injury. Edited by Ellis DW, Christensen A-L. Boston, MA, Kluwer Academic, 1989, pp 271–295

Berman KF, Illowsky BP, Weinberger DR: Physiological dysfunction of dorsolateral prefrontal cortex in schizophrenia, IV: further evidence for regional and behavioral specificity. Arch Gen Psychiatry 45:616–622, 1988

Bernstein DM: Recovery from head injury. Brain Inj 13:151–172, 1999

Bicik I, Radanov BP, Schäfer N, et al: PET with 18fluorodeoxyglucose and hexamethylpropylene amine oxime SPECT in late whiplash syndrome. Neurology 51:345–350, 1998

Bick PA, Hannah AL: Intramuscular lorazepam to restrain violent patients. Lancet 1:206–207, 1986

Bigler ED: Structural imaging, in Textbook of Traumatic Brain Injury. Edited by Silver JM, McAllister TW, Yudofsky SC. Washington, DC, American Psychiatric Publishing, 2005, pp 79–106

Binder LM, Rattok J: Assessment of the postconcussive syndrome after mild head trauma, in Assessment of the Behavioral Consequences of Head Trauma. Edited by Lezak MD. New York, Alan R Liss, 1989, pp 37–48

Bogner JA, Corrigan JD: Epidemiology of agitation following brain injury. NeuroRehabilitation 5:293–297, 1995

Bohnen N, Twijnstra A, Jolles J: Post-traumatic and emotional symptoms in different subgroups of patients with mild head injury. Brain Inj 6:481–487, 1992

Bracken P: Mania following head injury. Br J Psychiatry 150:690–692, 1987

Bremner JD, Scott TM, Delaney RC, et al: Deficits in short-term memory in posttraumatic stress disorder. Am J Psychiatry 150:1015–1019, 1993

Bremner JD, Randall P, Scott TM, et al: MRI-based measurement of hippocampal volume in patients with combat-related posttraumatic stress disorder. Am J Psychiatry 152:973–981, 1995

Bremner JD, Randall P, Vermetten E, et al: Magnetic resonance imaging–based measurement of hippocampal volume in posttraumatic stress disorder related to childhood physical and sexual abuse: a preliminary report. Biol Psychiatry 41:23–32, 1997

Breslau N, Kessler RC, Chilcoat HD, et al: Trauma and posttraumatic stress disorder in the community: the 1996 Detroit Area Survey of Trauma. Arch Gen Psychiatry 55:626–632, 1998

Brismar B, Engstrom A, Rydberg U: Head injury and intoxication: a diagnostic and therapeutic dilemma. Acta Chir Scand 149:11–14, 1983

Brooke MM, Patterson DR, Questad KA, et al: The treatment of agitation during initial hospitalization after traumatic brain injury. Arch Phys Med Rehabil 73:917–921, 1992a

Brooke MM, Questad KA, Patterson DR, et al: Agitation and restlessness after closed head injury: a prospective study of 100 consecutive admissions. Arch Phys Med Rehabil 73:320–323, 1992b

Brooks N, Campsie L, Symington C, et al: The five year outcome of severe blunt head injury: a relative's view. J Neurol Neurosurg Psychiatry 49:764–770, 1986

Brown G, Chadwick O, Shaffer D, et al: A prospective study of children with head injuries, III: psychiatric sequelae. Psychol Med 11:63–78, 1981

Brown SJ, Fann JR, Grant I: Postconcussional disorder: time to acknowledge a common source of neurobehavioral morbidity. J Neuropsychiatry Clin Neurosci 6:15–22, 1994

Bryant RA: Posttraumatic stress disorder, flashbacks, and pseudomemories in closed head injury. J Trauma Stress 9:621–629, 1996

Bryant RA, Marosszeky JE, Crooks J, et al: Posttraumatic stress disorder after severe traumatic brain injury. Am J Psychiatry 157:629–631, 2000

Buckley P, Stack JP, Madigan C, et al: Magnetic resonance imaging of schizophrenia-like psychoses associated with cerebral trauma: clinicopathological correlates. Am J Psychiatry 150:146–148, 1993

Burstein A: Bipolar and pure mania disorders precipitated by head trauma. Psychosomatics 34:194–195, 1993

Carlsson GS, Svardsudd K, Welin L: Long-term effects of head injuries sustained during life in three male populations. J Neurosurg 67:197–205, 1987

Cassidy JW: Neuropathology, in Neuropsychiatry of Traumatic Brain Injury. Edited by Silver JM, Yudofsky SC, Hales RE. Washington, DC, American Psychiatric Press, 1994, pp 43–80

Cavallo MM, Kay T: The family system, in Textbook of Traumatic Brain Injury. Edited by Silver JM, McAllister TW, Yudofsky SC. Washington, DC, American Psychiatric Publishing, 2005, pp 533–558

Cecil KM, Hills EC, Sandel ME, et al: Proton magnetic resonance spectroscopy for detection of axonal injury in the splenium of the corpus callosum of brain-injured patients. J Neurosurg 88:795–801, 1998

Centers for Disease Control: Bicycle-related injuries: data from the National Electronic Injury Surveillance System. MMWR Morb Mortal Wkly Rep 36:269–271, 1988

Centers for Disease Control: Increased safety-belt use: United States, 1991. MMWR Morb Mortal Wkly Rep 41:421–423, 1992

Centers for Disease Control and Prevention: Sports-related recurrent brain injuries— United States. MMWR Morb Mortal Wkly Rep 46:224–227, 1997

Chambers J, Cohen SS, Hemminger L, et al: Mild traumatic brain injuries in low-risk trauma patients. J Trauma 41:976–979, 1996

Childers MK, Holland D: Psychomotor agitation following gabapentin use in brain injury. Brain Inj 11:537–540, 1997

Christodoulou C, DeLuca J, Ricker JH, et al: Functional magnetic resonance imaging of working memory impairment after traumatic brain injury. J Neurol Neurosurg Psychiatry 71:161–168, 2001

Cicerone KD, Dahlberg C, Malec JF, et al: Evidence-based cognitive rehabilitation: updated review of the literature from 1998 through 2002. Arch Phys Med Rehabil 86:1681–1692, 2005

Clark AF, Davison K: Mania following head injury: a report of two cases and a review of the literature. Br J Psychiatry 150:841–844, 1987

Cope DN, Date ES, Mar EY: Serial computerized tomographic evaluations in traumatic head injury. Arch Phys Med Rehabil 69:483–486, 1988

Corbett JA, Trimble MR, Nichol TC: Behavioral and cognitive impairments in children with epilepsy: the long-term effects of anticonvulsant therapy. J Am Acad Child Psychiatry 24:17–23, 1985

Corcoran C, McAllister TW, Malaspina D: Psychotic disorders, in Textbook of Traumatic Brain Injury. Edited by Silver JM, McAllister TW, Yudofsky SC. Washington, DC, American Psychiatric Publishing, 2005, pp 213–229

Corkin S, Sullivan EV, Carr A: Prognostic factors for life expectancy after penetrating head injury. Arch Neurol 41:975–977, 1984

Corrigan JD: Substance abuse as a mediating factor in outcome from traumatic brain injury. Arch Phys Med Rehabil 76:302–309, 1995

Corrigan PW, Bach PA: Behavioral treatment, in Textbook of Traumatic Brain Injury. Edited by Silver JM, McAllister TW, Yudofsky SC. Washington, DC, American Psychiatric Publishing, 2005, pp 661–678

Courville CB: Pathology of the Nervous System, 2nd Edition. Mountain View, CA, Pacific Press Publications, 1945

Davison K, Bagley CR: Schizophrenic-like psychoses associated with organic disorders of the central nervous system: a review of the literature, in Current Problems in Neuropsychiatry: Schizophrenia, Epilepsy, the Temporal Lobe (British Journal of Psychiatry Special Publication No 4). Edited by Herrington RN. London, Headley Brothers, 1969, pp 113–184

Deb S, Lyons I, Koutzoukis C, et al: Rate of psychiatric illness 1 year after traumatic brain injury. Am J Psychiatry 156:374–378, 1999

Dietch JT, Jennings RK: Aggressive dyscontrol in patients treated with benzodiazepines. J Clin Psychiatry 49:184–189, 1988

Dikmen S, Machamer JE: Neurobehavioral outcomes and their determinants. J Head Trauma Rehabil 10:74–86, 1995

Dikmen S, McLean A, Temkin N: Neuropsychological and psychosocial consequences of minor head injury. J Neurol Neurosurg Psychiatry 49:1227–1232, 1986

Dikmen SS, Temkin NR, Miller B, et al: Neurobehavioral effects of phenytoin prophylaxis of posttraumatic seizures. JAMA 265:1271–1277, 1991

Dikmen SS, Machamer JE, Win HR, et al: Neuropsychological effects of valproate in traumatic brain injury: a randomized trial. Neurology 54:895–902, 2000

Dolan RJ, Bench CJ, Brown RG, et al: Regional cerebral blood flow abnormalities in depressed patients with cognitive impairment. J Neurol Neurosurg Psychiatry 55:768–773, 1992

Eames P, Wood R: Rehabilitation after severe brain injury: a follow-up study of a behavior modification approach. J Neurol Neurosurg Psychiatry 48:613–619, 1985

Easdon C, Levine B, O'Connor C, et al: Neural activity associated with response inhibition following traumatic brain injury: an event-related fMRI investigation. Brain Cogn 54:136–138, 2004

Fann JR, Katon WJ, Uomoto JM, et al: Psychiatric disorders and functional disability in outpatients with traumatic brain injuries. Am J Psychiatry 152:1493–1499, 1995

Fann JR, Leonetti A, Jaffe K, et al: Psychiatric illness and subsequent traumatic brain injury: a case control study. J Neurol Neurosurg Psychiatry 72:615–620, 2002

Fay GC, Jaffe KM, Polissar NL, et al: Mild pediatric brain injury: a cohort study. Arch Phys Med Rehabil 74:895–901, 1993

Federoff PJ, Starkstein SE, Forrester AW, et al: Depression in patients with acute traumatic brain injury. Am J Psychiatry 149:918–923, 1992

Fichtenberg NL, Millis SR, Mann NR, et al: Factors associated with insomnia among post-acute traumatic brain injury survivors. Brain Inj 14:659–667, 2000

Freeman JR, Barth JT, Broshek DK, et al: Sports injuries, in Textbook of Traumatic Brain Injury. Edited by Silver JM, McAllister, Yudofsky SC. Washington, DC, American Psychiatric Publishing, 2005, pp 453–476

Frieboes R-M, Muller U, Murck H, et al: Nocturnal hormone secretion and the sleep EEG in patients several months after traumatic brain injury. J Neuropsychiatry Clin Neurosci 11:354–360, 1999

Friedman SD, Brooks WM, Jung RE, et al: Quantitative proton MRS predicts outcome after traumatic brain injury. Neurology 52:1384–1391, 1999

Gallassi R, Morreale A, Lorusso S, et al: Carbamazepine and phenytoin: comparison of cognitive effects in epileptic patients during monotherapy and withdrawal. Arch Neurol 45:892–894, 1988

Garyfallos G, Manos N, Adamopoulou A: Psychopathology and personality characteristics of epileptic patients: epilepsy, psychopathology and personality. Acta Psychiatr Scand 78:87–95, 1988

Gennarelli TA, Graham DI: Neuropathology of the head injuries. Semin Clin Neuropsychiatry 3:160–175, 1998

Gennarelli TA, Thibault LE, Adams JH, et al: Diffuse axonal injury and traumatic coma in the primate. Ann Neurol 12:564–574, 1982

Gennarelli TA, Graham DI: Neuropathology, in Textbook of Traumatic Brain Injury. Edited by Silver JM, McAllister TW, Yudofsky SC. Washington, DC, American Psychiatric Publishing, 2005, pp 27–50

Geracioti TD: Valproic acid treatment of episodic explosiveness related to brain injury. J Clin Psychiatry 55:416–417, 1994

Gerberich SG, Priest JD, Boen JR, et al: Concussion incidences and severity in secondary school varsity football players. Am J Public Health 73:1370–1375, 1983

Giakas WJ, Seibyl JP, Mazure CM: Valproate in the treatment of temper outbursts (letter). J Clin Psychiatry 51:525, 1990

Glenn MB, Wroblewski B, Parziale J, et al: Lithium carbonate for aggressive behavior or affective instability in ten brain-injured patients. Am J Phys Med Rehabil 68:221–226, 1989

Goldberg RJ, Goldberg JS: Low-dose risperidone for dementia related disturbed behavior in nursing homes. Paper presented at the annual meeting of the American Psychiatric Association, Miami, FL, May 20–25, 1995

Goodin DS, Aminoff MJ, Laxer KD: Detection of epileptiform activity by different noninvasive EEG methods in complex partial epilepsy. Ann Neurol 27:330–334, 1990

Gordon WA, Hibbard MR: Cognitive rehabilitation, in Textbook of Traumatic Brain Injury. Edited by Silver JM, McAllister TW, Yudofsky SC. Washington, DC, American Psychiatric Publishing, 2005, pp 655–660

Gordon WA, Brown M, Sliwinski M, et al: The enigma of "hidden" traumatic brain injury. J Head Trauma Rehabil 13:1–18, 1998

Grigsby J, Kaye K: Incidence and correlates of depersonalization following head trauma. Brain Inj 7:507–513, 1993

Gross H, Kling A, Henry G, et al: Local cerebral glucose metabolism in patients with long-term behavioral and cognitive deficits following mild traumatic brain injury. J Neuropsychiatry Clin Neurosci 8:324–334, 1996

Guilleminault C, Yuen KM, Gulevich MG, et al: Hypersomnia after head-neck trauma: a medicolegal dilemma. Neurology 54:653–659, 2000

Gulbrandsen GB: Neuropsychological sequelae of light head injuries in older children 6 months after trauma. J Clin Neuropsychol 6:257–268, 1984

Hall KM, Karzmark P, Stevens M, et al: Family stressors in traumatic brain injury: a two-year follow-up. Arch Phys Med Rehabil 75:876–884, 1994

Harvey AG, Bryant RA: Two-year prospective evaluation of the relationship between acute stress disorder and posttraumatic stress disorder following mild traumatic brain injury. Am J Psychiatry 15:626–628, 2000

Hendryx PM: Psychosocial changes perceived by closed-head-injured adults and their families. Arch Phys Med Rehabil 70:526–530, 1989

Herrmann N, Lanctôt K, Myszak M: Effectiveness of gabapentin for the treatment of behavioral disorders in dementia. J Clin Psychopharmacol 20:90–93, 2000

Hibbard MR, Uysal S, Kepler K, et al: Axis I psychopathology in individuals with traumatic brain injury. J Head Trauma Rehabil 13:24–39, 1998

Hibbard MR, Bogdany J, Uysal S, et al: Axis II psychopathology in individuals with traumatic brain injury. Brain Inj 14:45–61, 2000

Hoare P: The development of psychiatric disorder among schoolchildren with epilepsy. Dev Med Child Neurol 26:3–13, 1984

Horne M, Lindley SE: Divalproex sodium in the treatment of aggressive behavior and dysphoria in patients with organic brain syndromes. J Clin Psychiatry 56:430–431, 1995

Hornstein A, Seliger G: Cognitive side effects of lithium in closed head injury (letter). J Neuropsychiatry Clin Neurosci 1:446–447, 1989

Hugenholtz H, Stuss DT, Stethem LL, et al: How long does it take to recover from a mild concussion? Neurosurgery 22:853–858, 1988

Inglese M, Makani S, Johnson G, et al: Diffuse axonal injury in mild traumatic brain injury. J Neurosurg 103:298–303, 2005

Insurance Institute for Highway Safety, Highway Loss Data Institute: Fatality facts 2005: alcohol. Washington, DC, Insurance Institute for Highway Safety, Highway Loss Data Institute, 2005a. Available at: http://www.iihs.org/research/fatality_facts_ 2005/alcohol.html. Accessed March 3, 2011.

Insurance Institute for Highway Safety, Highway Loss Data Institute: Fatality facts 2005: bicycles. Washington, DC, Insurance Institute for Highway Safety, Highway Loss Data Institute, 2005b. Available at: http://www.iihs.org/research/fatality_facts_2005/bicycles.html. Accessed March 3, 2011.

Insurance Institute for Highway Safety, Highway Loss Data Institute: Fatality facts 2005: children. Washington, DC, Insurance Institute for Highway Safety, Highway Loss Data Institute, 2005c. Available at: http://www.iihs.org/research/fatality_facts_2005/children.html. Accessed March 3, 2011.

Insurance Institute for Highway Safety, Highway Loss Data Institute: Fatality facts 2005: motorcycles. Washington, DC, Insurance Institute for Highway Safety, Highway Loss Data Institute, 2005d. Available at: http://www.iihs.org/research/fatality_facts_2005/motorcycles.html. Accessed January 10, 2007.

Jacobs A, Put E, Ingels M, et al: Prospective evaluation of technetium-99m-HMPAO SPECT in mild and moderate traumatic brain injury. J Nucl Med 35:942–947, 1994

Jagger J: Prevention of brain trauma by legislation, regulation, and improved technology: a focus on motor vehicles. J Neurotrauma 9(suppl):S313–S316, 1992

Jorge RE, Robinson RG, Starkstein SE, et al: Depression and anxiety following traumatic brain injury. J Neuropsychiatry Clin Neurosci 5:369–374, 1993

Jorge RE, Robinson RG, Starkstein SE, et al: Influence of major depression on 1-year outcome in patients with traumatic brain injury. J Neurosurg 81:726–733, 1994

Jorge RE, Robinson RG, Moser D, et al: Major depression following traumatic brain injury. Arch Gen Psychiatry 61:42–50, 2004

Kaplan BH, Cowley RA: Seatbelt effectiveness and cost of noncompliance among drivers admitted to a trauma center. Am J Emerg Med 9:4–10, 1991

Kass F, Silver JM: Neuropsychiatry and the homeless. J Neuropsychiatry Clin Neurosci 2:15–19, 1990

Kay SR, Fiszbein A, Opler LA: The Positive and Negative Syndrome Scale (PANSS) for schizophrenia. Schizophr Bull 13:261–276, 1987

Kay T: Neuropsychological treatment of mild traumatic brain injury. J Head Trauma Rehabil 8:74–85, 1993

Keshavan MS, Channabasavanna SM, Narahana Reddy GN: Post-traumatic psychiatric disturbances: patterns and predictors of outcome. Br J Psychiatry 138:157–160, 1981

Kim E: Elderly, in Textbook of Traumatic Brain Injury. Edited by Silver JM, McAllister TW, Yudofsky SC. Washington, DC, American Psychiatric Publishing, 2005, pp 495–508

Koponen S, Taiminen T, Portin R, et al: Axis I and II psychiatric disorders after traumatic brain injury: a 30 year follow-up study. Am J Psychiatry 159:1315–1321, 2002

Koren D, Arnon I, Klein E: Acute stress response and posttraumatic stress disorder in traffic victims: a one-year prospective, follow-up study. Am J Psychiatry 156:367–373, 1999

Kraus JF, Nourjah P: The epidemiology of mild, uncomplicated brain injury. J Trauma 28:1637–1643, 1988

Kraus JF, Sorenson SB: Epidemiology, in Neuropsychiatry of Traumatic Brain Injury. Edited by Silver JM, Yudofsky SC, Hales RE. Washington, DC, American Psychiatric Press, 1994, pp 3–41

Kreutzer JS, Gervasio AH, Camplair PS: Primary caregivers' psychological status and family functioning after traumatic brain injury. Brain Inj 8:197–210, 1994

Kuner EH, Schlickewei W, Oltmanns D: Injury reduction by the airbag in accidents. Injury 27:185–188, 1996

Kuruoglu AC, Arikan Z, Vural G, et al: Single photon emission computerised tomography in chronic alcoholism: antisocial personality disorder may be associated with decreased frontal perfusion. Br J Psychiatry 169:348–354, 1996

Lazarus A, Cotterell KP: SPECT scan reveals abnormality in somatization disorder patient. J Clin Psychiatry 50:475–476, 1989

Leininger BE, Gramling SE, Farrell AD, et al: Neuropsychological deficits in symptomatic minor head injury patients after concussion and mild concussion. J Neurol Neurosurg Psychiatry 53:293–296, 1990

Levin HS, Benton AL, Grossman RG: Neurobehavioral Consequences of Closed Head Injury. New York, Oxford University Press, 1982

Levin HS, High WM, Eisenberg HM: Impairment of olfactory recognition after closed head injury. Brain 108 (Pt 3):579–591, 1985

Levin HS, Amparo E, Eisenberg HM, et al: Magnetic resonance imaging and computerized tomography in relation to the neurobehavioral sequelae of mild and moderate head injuries. J Neurosurg 66:706–713, 1987a

Levin HS, Mattis S, Ruff RM, et al: Neurobehavioral outcome following minor head injury: a three-center study. J Neurosurg 66:234–243, 1987b

Levin HS, Goldstein FC, High WM Jr, et al: Disproportionately severe memory deficit in relation to normal intellectual functioning after closed head injury. J Neurol Neurosurg Psychiatry 51:1294–1301, 1988

Li G: Child injuries and fatalities from alcohol-related motor vehicle crashes: call for a zero-tolerance policy. JAMA 283:2291–2292, 2000

Linn RT, Allen K, Willer BS: Affective symptoms in the chronic stage of traumatic brain injury: a study of married couples. Brain Inj 8:135–147, 1994

Lishman WA: Physiogenesis and psychogenesis in the "post-concussional syndrome." Br J Psychiatry 153:460–469, 1988

Livingston MG, Brooks DN, Bond MR: Patient outcome in the year following severe head injury and relatives' psychiatric and social functioning. J Neurol Neurosurg Psychiatry 48:876–881, 1985a

Livingston MG, Brooks DN, Bond MR: Three months after severe head injury: psychiatric and social impact on relatives. J Neurol Neurosurg Psychiatry 48:870–875, 1985b

Lovell MR, Iverson GL, Collins MW, et al: Does loss of consciousness predict neuropsychological decrements after concussion? Clin J Sport Med 9:193–198, 1999

Mahoney WJ, D'Souza BJ, Haller JA, et al: Long-term outcome of children with severe head trauma and prolonged coma. Pediatrics 71:754–762, 1983

Mann JJ, Waternaux C, Haas GL, et al: Toward a clinical model of suicidal behavior in psychiatric patients. Am J Psychiatry 156:181–189, 1999

Marin RS, Chakravorty S: Disorders of diminished motivation, in Textbook of Traumatic Brain Injury. Edited by Silver JM, McAllister TW, Yudofsky SC. Washington, DC, American Psychiatric Publishing, 2005, pp 337–352

Martin R, Kuzniecky R, Ho S, et al: Cognitive effects of topiramate, gabapentin, and lamotrigine in healthy young adults. Neurology 52:321–327, 1999

Masdeu JC, Van Heertum RL, Kleiman A, et al: Early single-photon emission computed tomography in mild head trauma: a controlled study. J Neuroimaging 4:177–181, 1994

Mattes JA: Valproic acid for nonaffective aggression in the mentally retarded. J Nerv Ment Dis 180:601–602, 1992

Max JE: Children and adolescents, in Textbook of Traumatic Brain Injury. Edited by Silver JM, McAllister TW, Yudofsky SC. Washington, DC, American Psychiatric Publishing, 2005, pp 477–494

Max JE, Castillo CS, Robin DA, et al: Posttraumatic stress symptomatology after childhood traumatic brain injury. J Nerv Ment Dis 186:589–596, 1998a

Max JE, Robin DA, Lindgren SD, et al: Traumatic brain injury in children and adolescents: psychiatric disorders at one year. J Neuropsychiatry Clin Neurosci 10:290–297, 1998b

McAllister TW: Traumatic brain injury and psychosis: what is the connection? Semin Clin Neuropsychiatry 3:211–223, 1998

McAllister TW: Mild brain injury and the postconcussion syndrome, in Textbook of Traumatic Brain Injury. Edited by Silver JM, McAllister TW, Yudofsky SC. Washington, DC, American Psychiatric Publishing, 2005, pp 279–308

McAllister TW, Saykin AJ, Flashman LA, et al: Brain activation during working memory 1 month after mild traumatic brain injury: a functional MRI study. Neurology 53:1300–1308, 1999

McAllister TW, Sparling MB, Flashman LA, et al: Differential working memory load effects after mild traumatic brain injury. Neuroimage 14:1004–1012, 2001

McCullagh S, Feinstein A: Cognitive changes, in Textbook of Traumatic Brain Injury. Edited by Silver JM, McAllister TW, Yudofsky SC. Washington, DC, American Psychiatric Publishing, 2005, pp 321–335

McKenna PJ, Kane JM, Parrish K: Psychotic syndromes in epilepsy. Am J Psychiatry 142:895–904, 1985

McKinlay WW, Brooks DN, Bond MR, et al: The short-term outcome of severe blunt head injury as reported by the relatives of the injured person. J Neurol Neurosurg Psychiatry 44:527–533, 1981

McMillan TM: Post-traumatic stress disorder following minor and severe closed head injury: 10 single cases. Brain Inj 10:749–758, 1996

McMillan TM, Glucksman EE: The neuropsychology of moderate head injury. J Neurol Neurosurg Psychiatry 50:393–397, 1987

Michals ML, Crismon ML, Roberts S, et al: Clozapine response and adverse effects in nine brain-injured patients. J Clin Psychopharmacol 13:198–203, 1993

Michaud LJ, Rivara FP, Jaffe KM, et al: Traumatic brain injury as a risk factor for behavioral disorders in children. Arch Phys Med Rehabil 74:368–375, 1993

Mild Traumatic Brain Injury Committee, Head Injury Interdisciplinary Special Interest Group, American Congress of Rehabilitation Medicine: Definition of mild traumatic brain injury. J Head Trauma Rehabil 8:86–87, 1993

Mittl RL, Grossman RI, Hiehle JF, et al: Prevalence of MR evidence of diffuse axonal injury in patients with mild head injury and normal head CT findings. AJNR Am J Neuroradiol 15:1583–1589, 1994

Moskowitz AS, Altshuler L: Increased sensitivity to lithium-induced neurotoxicity after stroke: a case report. J Clin Psychopharmacol 11:272–273, 1991

Nagamachi S, Nichikawa T, Ono S, et al: A comparative study of 123I-IMP SPET and CT in the investigation of chronic-stage head trauma patients. Nucl Med Commun 16:17–25, 1995

Nasrallah HA, Fowler RC, Judd LL: Schizophrenia-like illness following head injury. Psychosomatics 22:359–361, 1981

National Safety Council: Accident Facts. Chicago, IL, National Safety Council, 1985

National Safety Council: Accident Facts. Chicago, IL, National Safety Council, 1986

National Safety Council: Accident Facts. Chicago, IL, National Safety Council, 1999

National Safety Council: Report on Injuries in America. 2006. Available at: http://www.nsc.org/library/report_injury_ usa.htm. Accessed January 15, 2007.

Nedd K, Sfakianakis G, Ganz W, et al: 99mTc-HMPAO SPECT of the brain in mild to moderate traumatic brain injury patients: compared with CT—a prospective study. Brain Inj 7:469–479, 1993

Nizamie SH, Nizamie A, Borde M, et al: Mania following head injury: case reports and neuropsychological findings. Acta Psychiatr Scand 77:637–639, 1988

Noyes R Jr: Motor vehicle accidents related to psychiatric impairment. Psychosomatics 26:569–580, 1985

Nuwer MR: Assessment of digital EEG, quantitative EEG and EEG brain mapping: report of the American Academy of Neurology and the American Clinical Neurophysiology Society. Neurology 49:277–292, 1997

Oddy M, Humphrey M, Uttley D: Stresses upon the relatives of head-injured patients. Br J Psychiatry 133:507–513, 1978

Oddy M, Coughlan T, Tyerman A, et al: Social adjustment after closed head injury: a further follow-up seven years after injury. J Neurol Neurosurg Psychiatry 48:564–568, 1985

Ohry A, Rattok J, Solomon Z: Post-traumatic stress disorder in brain injury patients. Brain Inj 10:687–695, 1996

Oppenheimer DR: Microscopic lesions in the brain following head injury. J Neurol Neurosurg Psychiatry 31:299–306, 1968

Oquendo MA, Friedman JH, Grunebaum MF, et al: Mild traumatic brain injury and suicidal behavior in major depression. J Nerv Ment Dis 192:430–434, 2004

Orrison WW, Gentry LR, Stimac GK, et al: Blinded comparison of cranial CT and MR in closed head injury evaluation. AJNR Am J Neuroradiol 15:351–356, 1994

Orsay EM, Turnbull TL, Dunne M, et al: Prospective study of the effect of safety belts on morbidity and health care costs in motor-vehicle accidents. JAMA 260:3598–3603, 1988

Parker RS, Rosenblum A: IQ loss and emotional dysfunctions after mild head injury in a motor vehicle accident. J Clin Psychol 52:32–43, 1996

Pollack IW: Traumatic brain injury and the rehabilitation process: a psychiatric perspective, in Neuropsychological Treatment After Brain Injury. Edited by Ellis D, Christensen A-L. Boston, MA, Kluwer Academic, 1989, pp 105–127

Ponsford J, Kinsella G: Attention deficits following closed head injury. J Clin Exp Neuropsychol 14:822–838, 1992

Powell JW, Barber-Foss KD: Traumatic brain injury in high school athletes. JAMA 282:958–963, 1999

Prevey ML, Delaney RC, Cramer JA, et al: Effect of valproate on cognitive functioning: comparison with carbamazepine. Arch Neurol 53:1008–1016, 1996

Prigatano GP: Work, love, and play after brain injury. Bull Menninger Clin 53:414–431, 1989

Quinlan KP, Brewer RD, Sleet DA, et al: Characteristics of child passenger deaths and injuries involving drinking drivers. JAMA 283:2249–2252, 2000

Rao V, Rollings P, Spiro J: Fatigue and sleep problems, in Textbook of Traumatic Brain Injury. Edited by Silver JM, McAllister TW, Yudofsky SC. Washington, DC, American Psychiatric Publishing, 2005, pp 369–384

Rappaport M, Herrero-Backe C, Rappaport ML, et al: Head injury outcome up to ten years later. Arch Phys Med Rehabil 70:885–892, 1989

Ratey JJ, Leveroni C, Kilmer D, et al: The effects of clozapine on severely aggressive psychiatric inpatients in a state hospital. J Clin Psychiatry 54:219–223, 1993

Rattok J: Do patients with mild brain injuries have posttraumatic stress disorder, too? J Head Trauma Rehabil 11:95–97, 1996

Rauch SL, van der Kolk BA, Fisler RE, et al: A symptom provocation study of posttraumatic stress disorder using positron emission tomography and script-driven imagery. Arch Gen Psychiatry 53:380–387, 1996

Reynolds EH, Trimble MR: Adverse neuropsychiatric effects of anticonvulsant drugs. Drugs 29:570–581, 1985

Rimel RW, Giordani B, Barht JT, et al: Disability caused by minor head injury. Neurosurgery 9:221–228, 1981

Roane DM, Feinberg TE, Meckler L, et al: Treatment of dementia-associated agitation with gabapentin. J Neuropsychiatry Clin Neurosci 12:40–43, 2000

Ross ED, Stewart RS: Pathological display of affect in patients with depression and right frontal brain damage. An alternative mechanism. J Nerv Ment Dis 176:165–172, 1987

Salazar AM, Jabbari B, Vance SC, et al: Epilepsy after penetrating head injury, I: clinical correlates: a report of the Vietnam Head Injury Study. Neurology 35:1406–1414, 1985

Salazar AM, Warden DL, Schwab K, et al: Cognitive rehabilitation for traumatic brain injury: a randomized trial. Defense and Veterans Head Injury Program (DVHIP) Study Group. JAMA 283:3075–3081, 2000

Salinsky MC, Storzbach D, Spencer DC, et al: Effects of topiramate and gabapentin on cognitive abilities in healthy volunteers. Neurology 64:792–798, 2005

Sandel ME, Weiss B, Ivker B: Multiple personality disorder: diagnosis after a traumatic brain injury. Arch Phys Med Rehabil 71:523–535, 1990

Sherer M, Boake C, Levin E, et al: Characteristics of impaired awareness after traumatic brain injury. J Int Neuropsychol Soc 4:380–387, 1998

Silver JM, McAllister TW: Forensic issues in the neuropsychiatric evaluation of the patient with mild traumatic brain injury. J Neuropsychiatry Clin Neurosci 9:102–113, 1997

Silver JM, Yudofsky SC: Pharmacologic treatment of aggression. Psychiatr Ann 17:397–407, 1987

Silver JM, Yudofsky SC: Aggressive disorders, in Neuropsychiatry of Traumatic Brain Injury. Edited by Silver JM, Yudofsky SC, Hales RE. Washington, DC, American Psychiatric Press, 1994, pp 313–356

Silver JM, Caton CM, Shrout PE, et al: Traumatic brain injury and schizophrenia. Paper presented at the annual meeting of the American Psychiatric Association, San Francisco, CA, May 22–27, 1993

Silver JM, Rattok J, Anderson K: Post-traumatic stress disorder and traumatic brain injury. Neurocase 3:151–157, 1997

Silver JM, Weissman M, Kramer R, et al: The association between severe head injuries and psychiatric disorders: findings from the New Haven NIMH Epidemiologic Catchment Area Study. Brain Inj 15:935–945, 2001

Silver JM, Yudofsky SC, Anderson KE: Aggressive disorders, in Textbook of Traumatic Brain Injury. Edited by Silver JM, McAllister TW, Yudofsky SC. Washington, DC, American Psychiatric Publishing, 2005, pp 259–278

Simpson G, Tate R: Suicidality after traumatic brain injury: demographic, injury and clinical correlates. Psychol Med 32:687–697, 2002

Smith KR, Goulding PM, Wilderman D, et al: Neurobehavioral effects of phenytoin and carbamazepine in patients recovering from brain trauma: a comparative study. Arch Neurol 51:653–660, 1994

Smith-Seemiller L, Lovell MR, Smith SS: Cognitive dysfunction after closed head injury: contributions of demographics, injury severity and other factors. Appl Neuropsychol 3:41–47, 1996

Sosin DM, Sacks JJ, Smith SM: Head injury–associated deaths in the United States from 1979 to 1986. JAMA 262:2251–2255, 1989

Starkstein SE, Boston JD, Robinson RG: Mechanisms of mania after brain injury: 12 case reports and review of the literature. J Nerv Ment Dis 176:87–100, 1988

Starkstein SE, Mayberg HS, Berthier ML, et al: Mania after brain injury: neuroradiological and metabolic findings. Ann Neurol 27:652–659, 1990

Tate R, Simpson G, Flanagan S, et al: Completed suicide after traumatic brain injury. J Head Trauma Rehabil 12:16–20, 1997

Tateno A, Jorge RE, Robinson RG: Clinical correlates of aggressive behavior after traumatic brain injury. J Neuropsychiatry Clin Neurosci 15:155–160, 2003

Thatcher RW, Moore N, John ER, et al: QEEG and traumatic brain injury: rebuttal of the American Academy of Neurology 1997 report by the EEG and Clinical Neuroscience Society. Clin Electroencephalogr 30:94–98, 1999

Therapeutics and Technology Assessment Subcommittee of the American Academy of Neurology: Assessment of brain SPECT. Neurology 46:278–285, 1996

Thompson RS, Rivara FP, Thompson DC: A case-control study of the effectiveness of bicycle safety helmets. N Engl J Med 320:1361–1367, 1989

Thomsen IV: Late outcome of very severe blunt head trauma: a 10–15 year second follow-up. J Neurol Neurosurg Psychiatry 47:260–268, 1984

Trzepacz PT, Kennedy RE: Delirium and posttraumatic amnesia, in Textbook of Traumatic Brain Injury. Edited by Silver JM, McAllister TW, Yudofsky SC. Washington, DC, American Psychiatric Publishing, 2005, pp 175–200

Tsuang MT, Boor M, Fleming JA: Psychiatric aspects of traffic accidents. Am J Psychiatry 142:538–546, 1985

Tyerman A, Humphrey M: Changes in self-concept following severe head injury. Int J Rehabil Res 7:11–23, 1984

Tysvaer AT, Storli O, Bachen NI: Soccer injuries to the brain. Acta Neurol Scand 80:151–156, 1989

Ursano RJ, Fullerton CS, Epstein RS, et al: Acute and chronic posttraumatic stress disorder in motor vehicle accident victims. Am J Psychiatry 156:589–595, 1999a

Ursano RJ, Fullerton CS, Epstein RS, et al: Peritraumatic dissociation and posttraumatic stress disorder following motor vehicle accidents. Am J Psychiatry 156:1808–1810, 1999b

U.S. Department of Transportation: Final regulatory impact analysis—amendment to Federal Motor Vehicle Safety Standard 208, Passenger Car Front Seat Occupant Protection (DOT Publ No HS-806-572). Washington, DC, U.S. Department of Transportation, 1984

van Reekum R, Bolago I, Finlayson MA, et al: Psychiatric disorders after traumatic brain injury. Brain Inj 10:319–327, 1996

van Reekum R, Cohen T, Wong J: Can traumatic brain injury cause psychiatric disorders? J Neuropsychiatry Clin Neurosci 12:316–327, 2000

Varney NR: Prognostic significance of anosmia in patients with closed-head trauma. J Clin Exp Neuropsychol 10:250–254, 1988

Violon A, De Mol J: Psychological sequelae after head trauma in adults. Acta Neurochir (Wien) 85:96–102, 1987

Wade DT, King NS, Crawford S, et al: Routine follow up after head injury: a second randomised clinical trial. J Neurol Neurosurg Psychiatry 65:177–183, 1998

Warden DL, Labbate LA: Posttraumatic stress disorder and other anxiety disorders, in Textbook of Traumatic Brain Injury. Edited by Silver JM, McAllister TW, Yudofsky SC. Washington, DC, American Psychiatric Publishing, 2005, pp 231–243

Warden D, Bleiberg J, Cameron KL, et al: Persistent prolongation of simple reaction time in sports concussion. Neurology 57:524–526, 2001

Watson MR, Fenton GW, McClelland RJ, et al: The post-concussional state: neurophysiological aspects. Br J Psychiatry 167:514–521, 1995

Wilberger JE, Deeb A, Rothfus W: Magnetic resonance imaging in cases of severe head injury. Neurosurgery 20:571–576, 1987

Wilcox JA, Nasrallah HA: Childhood head trauma and psychosis. Psychiatry Res 21:303–306, 1987

Will RG, Young JPR, Thomas DJ: Klein-Levin syndrome: report of two cases with onset of symptoms precipitated by head trauma. Br J Psychiatry 152:410–412, 1988

Wroblewski BA, Joseph AB, Kupfer J, et al: Effectiveness of valproic acid on destructive and aggressive behaviours in patients with acquired brain injury. Brain Inj 11:37–47, 1997

Yablon SA: Posttraumatic seizures. Arch Phys Med Rehabil 74:983–1001, 1993

Yudofsky SC, Silver JM, Schneider SE: Pharmacologic treatment of aggression. Psychiatr Ann 17:397–407, 1987

Yudofsky SC, Silver JM, Hales RE: Pharmacologic management of aggression in the elderly. J Clin Psychiatry 51 (suppl 10):22–28, 1990

Yudofsky SC, Silver JM, Hales RE: Psychopharmacology of aggression, in The American Psychiatric Press Textbook of Psychopharmacology. Edited by Schatzberg AF, Nemeroff CB. Washington, DC, American Psychiatric Press, 1995, pp 735–751

Yudofsky SC, Silver JM, Hales RE: Treatment of agitation and aggression, in The American Psychiatric Press Textbook of Psychopharmacology, 2nd Edition. Edited by Schatzberg AF, Nemeroff CB. Washington, DC, American Psychiatric Press, 1998, pp 881–900

Zasler N: Sexual dysfunction, in Neuropsychiatry of Traumatic Brain Injury. Edited by Silver JM, Yudofsky SC, Hales RE. Washington, DC, American Psychiatric Press, 1994, pp 443–470

5

Seizure Disorders

H. Florence Kim, M.D., M.S.

Frank Y. Chen, M.D.

Stuart C. Yudofsky, M.D.

Robert E. Hales, M.D., M.B.A.

Gary J. Tucker, M.D.

$\mathbf{B}$efore the development of the electroencephalogram (EEG) by Dr. Hans Berger in the 1930s, all seizure disorders were classified with mental disorders (Berger 1929–1938). Indeed, a strong link between epilepsy and psychiatry has been known for more than a century. Epilepsy is an important natural model of behavioral disturbance because of its ability to cause behavioral symptoms without overt classical seizures. Epilepsy can cause both chronic and episodic behavior disorders. Unfortunately, the cause of the epilepsy itself is often unclear, because laboratory diagnostic evidence may not be present on EEGs or imaging modalities.

Seizure Disorders

Seizures and Epilepsy

Epilepsy is a term applied to a broad group of disorders, with a vast variety of clinical manifestations. The defining feature of any of the epilepsies is the *epileptic seizure*. The definition of both terms has evolved and changed dramatically since 1970. Past attempts to the epileptic seizure have focused on clinical symptoms, nature of onsent and termination, cause, or diagnosis. The current consensus definition of an epileptic seizure is a "transient occurrence of signs and/or symptoms due to abnormal excessive or synchronous neuronal activity in the brain" (Fisher et al. 2005). Seizures can manifest in multiple ways, as they can affect behavior and emotions, cognition, and consciousness, as well as motor, sensory, and autonomic function.

The diagnosis of epilepsy is made when a person has had at least one epileptic seizure and demonstrates an enduring alteration or disturbance of the brain that may cause a predisposition to future seizures. The definition of epilepsy also includes neurobiological, psychological, cognitive, and social changes or disturbances that are associated with the epileptic seizure (Fisher et al. 2005).

Classification of Seizures

The classification of seizures and epilepsy is also constantly evolving. It has shifted away from terms such as *generalized* and *focal* as defining classifications, to focus instead on characterizing seizures on the basis of brain networks. Hence, a *focal seizure* is defined as an epileptic seizure that begins unilaterally in one hemisphere of the brain networks. A *generalized seizure,* on the other hand, will rapidly engage bilateral networks of the brain. In the past, distinction was made between different types of focal (or partial) seizures, such as *simple partial* or *complex partial seizures* or *secondary generalization,* but more recently this distinction has been eliminated (Berg et al. 2010).

Past classification schemas have also focused on the etiology of seizures as a means of categorizing and grouping epilepsy syndromes, dividing them into idiopathic, symptomatic, and cryptogenic (hidden) causes. Although it is still useful to consider the etiology in the classification of epileptic seizures, these categories have changed to encompass the following three groups: 1) genetic etiology, in which the seizures are considered a direct result of a genetic defect (known or presumed); 2) structural/metabolic cause, in which the seizures are associated with a known structural or metabolic disease; and 3) unknown etiology (Berg et al. 2010).

The terms in the next subsection are presented as long-standing descriptors of epileptic seizures but are no longer used in classification or grouping of epilepsy syndromes.

Seizure Descriptors

Generalized Seizures

Generalized seizures (generalized attacks) manifest immediately and spread bilaterally through the brain networks. No preceding motor or perceptual experiences occur, and there is almost invariably total loss of consciousness.

Focal (Partial) Seizures

Focal seizures (partial or localization-related) result in epileptic firing in a specific focus in the brain (usually the cerebral cortex). *Simple partial seizures* (previously called *elementary partial seizures*) involve no alteration in consciousness. *Complex partial seizures* (CPSs) involve a defect in consciousness (i.e., confusion, dizziness). Some authors further subdivide CPSs into type 1 (temporal lobe) and type 2 (extratemporal). Forty percent of all patients with epilepsy will have CPSs (International League Against Epilepsy 1985). The terms *simple* and *complex partial seizures* are no longer recommended for use in classification of specific seizure types but may still be used as descriptive terms.

Tonic-Clonic Seizures

Tonic-clonic seizures (grand mal seizures) are the most common form of generalized seizure, with a total loss of consciousness and a tetanic muscular phase lasting usually several seconds (tonic), followed by a phase of repetitive jerking lasting usually 1–2 minutes (clonic). These seizures may be generalized, or they may begin as partial seizures and secondarily generalize.

Partial seizures secondarily generalized start as partial seizures and then spread bilaterally throughout the cerebral cortex, producing secondary generalization. These seizures are distinct from a previous classification of secondary generalized epilepsy, which referred to a kind of epilepsy generalized from the start, with features of a diffuse cerebral pathology.

Absence Seizures

Typical *absence seizures* (*petit mal* seizures) occur primarily in children. These start generalized, with loss of consciousness for a few seconds without any motor phase. Typical electroencephalographic findings are bilateral and synchronous and have spike waves of 3–4 Hz.

Status Epilepticus

Status epilepticus, a continuous seizure state that involves two or more seizures superimposed on each other without total recovery of consciousness, is a true medical emergency. Generalized status epilepticus can be convulsive (tonic-clonic seizures) or nonconvulsive (behavioral or cognitive changes from baseline such as confusion, stupor, or coma, accompanied by continuous or near continuous seizure activity on EEGs). Several other forms of status epilepticus exist, including absence status epilepticus and focal status epilepticus types, when consciousness may be preserved, and the diagnosis is often made by electroencephalography (Novak et al. 1971).

Causes of Epilepsy

The genetic or unknown epilepsies, in which no central nervous system (CNS) pathology is evident, are usually childhood syndromes. In patients older than 30 years, the onset of epilepsy or recurrent seizures is usually associated with CNS pathology. These syndromes are usually described as symptomatic or secondary seizure disorders, or epilepsy. Conditions such as head injury, encephalitis, birth trauma, or hyperpyrexia represent rather static and permanent lesions that can cause epilepsy or seizures. Conditions that are progressive (change over time) include medication overdose or withdrawal, tumor, infections, metabolic disease (e.g., hypoglycemia and uremia), and endocrine diseases. Alzheimer's disease and other dementias, multiple sclerosis, cerebral arteriopathy, and other degenerative or infiltrative conditions can all lead to a progressive and changing picture of seizures.

Seizures can also be a reaction to various medical or physiological stresses. This fact is particularly evident at both ends of the age spectrum. For example, febrile conditions are more likely to cause seizures in young people and older people.

Table 5–1. Behavioral symptoms often associated with seizures, particularly temporal lobe epilepsy

Hallucinations: all sensory modalities

Illusions

Déjà vu

Jamais vu

Depersonalization

Repetitive thoughts and nightmares

Flashbacks and visual distortions

Epigastric sensations

Automatisms

Affective and mood changes

Catatonia

Cataplexy

Amnestic episodes

Source. Reprinted from Kim HF, Chen FY, Yudofsky SC, et al.: "Neuropsychiatric Aspects of Seizure Disorders," in *Essentials of Neuropsychiatry and Behavioral Neurosciences,* 2nd Edition. Edited by Yudofsky SC, Hales RE. Washington, DC, American Psychiatric Publishing, 2010, pp. 275–298. Used with permission. Copyright © 2010 American Psychiatric Association.

Temporal Lobe Epilepsy

Temporal lobe epilepsy is no longer recognized by the ILAE, but we use the term in the descriptive sense, implying both complex and simple partial seizures, including psychomotor automatisms and tonic-clonic seizures that may originate from the temporal lobe. Many such phenomena interpreted as having originated in the temporal lobe may, in fact, be extratemporal.

Although the term *temporal lobe epilepsy* has formally been superseded, in practice it is still commonly used in the absence of an adequate alternative. The phenomena of temporal lobe epilepsy are *not* synonymous with those of its proposed nonanatomical replacement, CPSs, because CPSs are restricted to patients who have focal firing with defects of consciousness.

Table 5–1 describes some of the symptoms that have often been associated with temporal lobe disturbances.

Epidemiology

Obtaining a clear idea of the epidemiology of epilepsy is often difficult. Prevalence is 5–40 per 1,000 people. The incidence is 40–70 per 100,000 people per year in industrialized countries and more than twice that high in developing countries. Worldwide, 50 million people are affected by epilepsy, with 2.4 million new cases occurring every year (GCAE Secretariat 2003). The incidence of epilepsy is highest in young children, decreases in adults, and peaks again in elderly people (Dekker 2002).

Diagnosis

Diagnosis of epilepsy is clinical, similar to that of schizophrenia or other psychiatric disorders. Although an EEG can be confirmatory, 20% of patients with epilepsy have a normal EEG, and 2% of patients without epilepsy have spike and wave formations (Engel 1992). The best diagnostic test for seizures is the observation of a seizure or the report of someone who has observed the seizure. Thus, history is crucial. Important information includes age at onset of seizures, history of illness or trauma to the nervous system, a family history, and some idea of whether the condition is progressive or static. Attempts should be made to determine whether the seizures are idiopathic or secondary. Certainly, these descriptions are most helpful in the diagnosis of major motor or generalized seizures. They are also useful in determining the relation between the seizures and various behavioral disturbances. Because the seizure focus can reside in any location in the brain, the number of behavioral symptoms associated with seizures is considerable (see Table 5–1).

Laboratory

An elevated prolactin level is the only major laboratory value used in the diagnostic workup of seizure disorders. Serum prolactin is released by epileptic activity spreading from the temporal lobe to the hypothalamic-pituitary axis (Bauer 1996). A threefold to fourfold rise in prolactin levels occurs within 15–20 minutes of a generalized tonic-clonic seizure. Because prolactin level normalizes within 60 minutes, blood should be drawn 15–20 minutes after the seizure. In a study of 200 consecutive patients seen in the emergency department setting with a diagnosis of seizure followed by syncope, the sensitivity of serum prolactin level was 42%, specificity was 82%, positive predictive value was 74%, negative predictive value was 54%, and overall diagnostic accuracy was 60% (Vukmir 2004). Furthermore, elevated prolactin levels have not been helpful in differentiating true seizures from nonepileptic seizures (Shukla et al. 2004; Willert et al. 2004). Some data indicate that repeated seizures and shorter seizure-free periods decrease the prolactin response (Malkowicz et al. 1995). Prolactin levels also may be elevated by neuroleptic use. Thus, elevated serum prolactin levels may be helpful as a confirmatory test for suspected seizure but not as a singular diagnostic test.

Imaging

Structural imaging techniques such as magnetic resonance imaging and computed tomography scans are crucial for the evaluation of symptomatic epilepsies. Both structural and functional imaging modalities are also useful for localization of seizure foci to evaluate candidates for surgical intervention. Functional imaging such as single-photon emission computed tomography (SPECT) and positron emission tomography (PET) has been valuable in evaluating ictal events and blood flow to focal lesions during a seizure. Postictal and interictal evaluations are much less informative. SPECT studies are very reliable for localizing ictal events, whereas PET is better in the detection of interictal temporal lobe hypermetabolism (Ho et al. 1995). As these instruments become more sensitive, their use will increase in the clinical evaluation of seizure disorders.

Electroencephalography

The EEG is one of the most important tests in the evaluation of seizures, suspected seizures, or episodic behavioral disturbances. Paroxysmal interictal EEGs with spikes and wave complexes can confirm the clinical diagnosis of a seizure disorder. The EEG can, when positive, differentiate between seizure types (e.g., absence seizures from generalized seizures) and indicate the possibility of a structural lesion when there are focal findings in the EEG. A normal electroencephalographic result does not eliminate the possibility of the presence of a seizure disorder. The EEG is a reflection of surface activity in the cortex and may not reflect seizure activity deep in the brain. Most clinicians, when confronted with a behavior disorder that does not fit the usual clinical picture of a schizophrenic psychosis (particularly if the disorder is episodic), will obtain an EEG. A negative electroencephalographic result may deter further seizure workup. The diagnosis of epilepsy (as with schizophrenia) is a clinical one, and although the EEG can confirm the diagnosis, it cannot exclude it. Even with elaborate recordings (24-hour EEGs) and concomitant videotaping, a seizure disorder cannot always be diagnosed.

Special techniques, such as use of nasopharyngeal electrodes (Bickford 1979), sphenoidal electrodes (Ebersole and Leroy 1983), buccal skin electrodes (Sadler and Goodwin 1986), or cerebral cortical placements (Heath 1982), may assist with diagnosis by electroencephalography.

Medications that should be avoided in all patients who are to undergo electroencephalography include benzodiazepines, which may have, by virtue of their strong antiepileptic effects, profound effects in normalizing the EEG. Because effects on receptor activity may last weeks, even with the short-acting benzodiazepines, demonstration of abnormal activity after administration of benzodiazepines may decrease substantially. L-Tryptophan should also be avoided. Adamec and Stark (1983) found that L-tryptophan has some effect in raising the seizure threshold during electroconvulsive therapy (ECT). Some psychotropic medications, such as neuroleptics, tricyclic and heterocyclic antidepressants, and benzodiazepines (Pincus and Tucker 1985), also may increase synchronization of the EEG (leading to a seizurelike pattern). One report (Ryback and Gardner 1991) described a small series in which procaine activation of the EEG was useful in identifying patients with episodic behavior disorders who were responsive to anticonvulsants.

Recent advances in electroencephalographic technology may ultimately change the whole perspective of its use in psychiatry. Evoked potentials and quantitative electroencephalography are promising research tools that have yet to show specific clinical utility in the diagnosis and treatment of neuropsychiatric disorders.

Differential Diagnosis of Behavioral Symptoms Associated With Epilepsy

Medical conditions that must be distinguished from seizures include panic disorder, hyperventilation, hypoglycemia, various transient cerebral ischemias, migraine, narcolepsy, malingering, and conversion reactions.

Characteristics of temporal lobe epilepsy are subjective experiences or feelings, automatisms, and, more rarely, catatonia or cataplexy. Because the symptoms are usually related to a focal electrical discharge in the brain, they are generally consistent and few in number. Although the list of possible symptoms may be quite large (see Table 5–1), each patient will have a limited number of specific symptoms—for example, auditory hallucinations (usually voices), repetitive sounds, or visual hallucinations and misperceptions of a consistent type that includes a visual disturbance. The automatisms are simple (e.g., chewing, swallowing, pursing of the lips, looking around, smiling, grimacing, crying). Other types of automatisms are attempting to sit up, examining or fumbling with objects, and buttoning or unbuttoning clothes. Complex, goal-directed behavior is unusual during these episodes. Aggressive behavior is also rare. Typically, the patient will become aggressive only when an attempt is made to restrain or prevent ambulation (Rodin 1973). Typical attacks consist of a cessation of activity, followed by automatism and impairment of consciousness. The entire episode usually lasts from 10 seconds to as long as 30 minutes. Motor phenomena and postural changes, such as catatonia, are rarer (Fenton 1986; Kirubakaran et al. 1987).

The profile of patients who present primarily with behavioral symptoms is usually of episodic "brief" disturbances lasting for variable time periods (hours to days). These patients often state that such episodes have occurred once a month or once every 3 months. The patients seek psychiatric attention when the frequency of the episodes increases to daily or several per day, with resultant impairment of functioning.

Pseudoseizures (the terms *pseudoseizure, nonepileptic seizure,* and *conversion reaction* are used synonymously) can at times be extremely difficult to differentiate from true seizures (Table 5–2), a task that is often complicated by the fact that the person who is suspected of having "seizures," primarily related to psychological reasons, often has a history of true seizures. Devinsky and Gordon (1998) noted that nonepileptic seizures often can follow epileptic seizures. These authors postulated that the epileptic seizure, particularly a CPS, leads to possible loss of inhibition of impulses and emotions. Patients with nonepileptic seizures differ from patients with seizure disorder in that the former may have significantly more stress, more negative life events, and a history of child abuse, and more somatic symptoms and awareness of their bodies (Arnold and Privitera 1996; Tojek et al. 2000). Most patients with nonepileptic seizures have somatoform disorders, particularly conversion, rather than dissociative disorders. Interestingly, patients with nonepileptic seizures who do not fit the criteria for conversion have a high incidence of anxiety and psychotic disorders (Alper et al. 1995; Kuyk et al. 1999). A significant number of patients with non-

Table 5–2.   General features of nonepileptic seizures ("pseudoseizures")

Setting

Environmental gain (audience usually present)

Seldom sleep related

Often triggered (e.g., by stress)

Suggestive profile on Minnesota Multiphasic Personality Inventory

Attack

Atypical movements, often bizarre or purposeful

Seldom results in injury

Often starts and ends gradually

Out-of-phase movements of extremities

Side-to-side movements

Examination

Restraint accentuates the seizure

Inattention decreases over time

Plantar flexor reflexes

Reflexes intact (corneal, pupillary, and blink)

Consciousness preserved

Autonomic system uninvolved

Autonomically intact

After attack

No postictal features (lethargy, tiredness, abnormal electroencephalogram findings)

Prolactin normal (after 30 minutes)

No or little amnesia

Memory exists (hypnosis or amobarbital sodium)

Source.   Reprinted from Kim HF, Chen FY, Yudofsky SC, et al.: "Neuropsychiatric Aspects of Seizure Disorders," in *Essentials of Neuropsychiatry and Behavioral Neurosciences,* 2nd Edition. Edited by Yudofsky SC, Hales RE. Washington, DC, American Psychiatric Publishing, 2010, pp. 275–298. Used with permission. Copyright © 2010 American Psychiatric Association.

epileptic seizures also have concomitant mood and anxiety disorders. There-fore, combination treatment with individual psychotherapy and psychotropic medications, such as selective serotonin reuptake inhibitors (SSRIs), benzodi-azepines, or atypical antipsychotics, can be extremely helpful in decreasing the frequency and morbidity associated with nonepileptic seizures (Thomas and Jankovic 2004).

Frontal lobe epilepsy can also include bizarre behavioral symptoms and can be confused with nonepileptic seizures. Laskowitz et al. (1995) noted that the symptoms of frontal lobe epilepsy often appear as spells with an aura of panic symptoms, with weird vocalizations and with bilateral limb movements but no periods of postictal tiredness and no confusion; also, no oral or alimentary movements occur. These spells last about 60–70 seconds. Fortunately, most of these seizures are symptomatic of a CNS lesion, and usually the correct diag-nosis is made with the EEG or imaging studies. Thomas et al. (1999) described a form of nonconvulsive status epilepticus of frontal origin; patients often pre-sented with a mood disturbance similar to hypomania, subtle cognitive im-pairments, some disinhibition, and some indifference.

Etiological Links of Seizures to Psychopathology

The increased incidence of psychopathology and seizure disorders is clear and evident, but the exact etiology of this increased incidence is unclear. There have been two major theories historically. One is an affinity theory, best exemplified by the classic articles of Slater et al. (1963), who described a group of patients with epilepsy and psychosis. An opposing theory was first postulated by Von Meduna (1937), who observed (incorrectly) that the patients with schizophre-nia under his care had few epileptic conditions (Fink 1984). He then hypothe-sized that the induction of a seizure in a psychotic patient might be therapeutic. Landolt (1958) observed a group of patients whose electroencephalographic re-sults seemed to normalize during a psychotic episode. This has been called "forced normalization." This inverse relation between seizures and behavioral disturbances has been noted by many clinicians. For example, it is not uncom-mon for a patient with epilepsy to have a marked decrease in seizures for a pro-longed time and then later to have an increase in behavioral disturbances. After a seizure, the behavior seems to normalize again. Although these observations are clinically and statistically apparent (Schiffer 1987), their exact etiological importance to all patients with epilepsy and behavioral disturbance is unclear.

The relation between psychopathology and seizures is further complicated by whether the behavioral disturbance is a preictal event, an ictal event, or a postictal event. *Kindling*, a pathophysiological event, is the sequence whereby repetitive subthreshold electrical or chemical stimuli to specific brain areas eventually induce a seizure or a behavioral disturbance that persists, but it has never been demonstrated in humans (Adamec and Stark 1983). The kindling process has been hypothesized as one of the possible causes of psychopathology.

Comorbid Psychiatric Syndromes

The relation of psychopathology and seizure disorders is difficult to establish. Most of the studies rest at the level of case report, and even large-scale studies usually deal with populations that have come to psychiatric attention rather than community-based samples (Popkin and Tucker 1994). The following question constantly arises: Is the person's behavior associated with a seizure disorder, or is the behavior associated with another underlying disease of the CNS that can cause seizures? At the symptom level, the clinician is frequently dealing with general symptoms related to damage of the CNS that are not specific to any one condition or region of the brain. The symptoms can be episodic changes in mood, irritability or impulsiveness, psychosis, anxiety disorders, or confusional syndromes. The other major types of symptoms usually seen with CNS dysfunction are related to more insidious disorders, such as dementia, depression, various motor diseases, or distinctive personality changes such as those seen after head trauma (Popkin and Tucker 1994).

Because the temporal relation of mood or psychotic symptoms to seizure episodes is important, a patient's symptoms should be classified as peri-ictal, ictal, postictal, or interictal. The term *peri-ictal* (or premonitory) refers to psychiatric symptoms immediately before and after the seizure. These symptoms may last hours to days and may resolve when the seizure itself occurs. *Ictal* symptoms are affective or psychotic symptoms that occur during the seizure itself. *Postictal* psychiatric symptoms begin shortly after the cessation of seizure activity. *Interictal* refers to chronic psychiatric symptoms that appear during seizure-free periods. This classification is important in that each type appears to follow a differing constellation and severity of symptoms and thus may require different treatment approaches.

Psychosis

Clinical Features

All of the symptoms described in patients with schizophrenia can also occur in patients with seizure disorders (Toone et al. 1982). Seizure disorders and schizophrenia have many empirical similarities that also make the differential diagnosis difficult. The peak age at onset is similar. Both disorders may first appear in early to late adolescence, although epilepsy often presents in childhood and may occur at any age. The neurotransmitter dopamine appears to be related to both conditions: dopamine antagonists are antipsychotic and mildly epileptogenic, whereas dopamine agonists are psychotogenic and mildly antiepileptic (Trimble 1977). The family history can be of help in that the genetic frequencies are similar for both conditions, with 10%–13% of the offspring of parents with either schizophrenia or epilepsy having the same condition (Metrakos and Metrakos 1961). Most cases, however, have no family history of either condition.

Clinically, a psychiatrist typically sees three psychotic presentations with seizure disorders. One is an episodic course that is usually related to seizure activity, manifested by perceptual changes, alterations in consciousness, and poor memory for the events. Peri-ictal, ictal, and postictal psychoses often follow this episodic course. The second type is a chronic interictal psychotic condition in which the patient may have simple auditory hallucinations, paranoia, or other perceptual changes; this condition closely resembles schizophrenia. The third type is simply a variation in which the patient usually has some type of persistent experience of depersonalization or visual distortion that, for lack of a better name, is usually labeled as psychotic. This third type is probably a variant of the chronic psychotic state.

Although Slater et al. (1963) postulated a long period between the onset of seizures and subsequent psychosis, it is not uncommon for a clinician to treat a patient for "schizophrenia" and find that the patient is completely unresponsive to antipsychotic medications. During the course of this treatment, the patient has a grand mal seizure. An EEG is then obtained that confirms the diagnosis of epilepsy.[1] The patient is then given anticonvulsant medication, and a marked decrease in the "psychotic" symptoms occurs.

Many of these patients with psychosis seem quite intact when experiencing the symptoms, particularly between episodes. Their mental status examinations seem to show no evidence of other schizophrenic symptoms. During the episode, what is often seen is a confusional state and an alteration in consciousness rather than an inability to communicate. What the patients and their families describe is an abrupt change in personality, mood, or ability to function. The clinician needs to remain suspicious of altered perceptual experiences that do not completely meet DSM-IV-TR (American Psychiatric Association 2000) criteria for schizophrenia and to reevaluate patients whose symptoms do not respond to antipsychotic medication.

Treatment of Psychotic Conditions

The major treatment of the episodic psychotic conditions is usually the appropriate use of anticonvulsant medications. The treatment of chronic conditions involves both anticonvulsant and antipsychotic medications. In general, the use of medication in patients with seizures and psychosis is difficult in that very small dosages of any medication often cause an increase in symptoms that diminishes over time. Consequently, very small dosages and infrequent changes seem to be the major guidelines in treating these conditions. Although all of the neuroleptics can lower the seizure threshold, the rate of seizures with atypical antipsychotic agents is quite low, and their use is increasing in patients with seizures and psychosis, despite lack of controlled clinical trials as to their efficacy in treating seizure-related psychosis. Of the traditional neuroleptics, haloperidol, fluphenazine, molindone, pimozide, and trifluoperazine seem to lower the seizure threshold the least. The propensity for clozapine to lower the seizure threshold is quite well known, so it is only used in patients whose symptoms do not respond to all other antipsychotic medications. Furthermore, the concomitant use of clozapine and carbamazepine is contraindicated because of the risk of agranulocytosis.

---

[1]It is important to note that although neuroleptics may lower the seizure threshold, they do not usually cause seizures in patients who are not predisposed to them. Among inpatients taking psychotropic medication, seizures were infrequent, occurring in 0.03% of psychiatric inpatients (Popli et al. 1995).

Anxiety Disorders

Clinical Features

The correspondence between seizure disorders and anxiety disorders is a fascinating topic, and the substantial overlapping of symptoms often makes differentiation between these classes of disorders complex. Either type of syndrome can be confused with the other, and the same class of medications (benzodiazepines) helps to reduce the symptoms and subsequent impairment of both types. Panic disorder and CPSs are each included in the differential diagnosis of the other. Although many symptoms overlap, evidence of neurophysiological linkage between anxiety and seizure disorder remains tenuous, except that both involve underlying limbic dysfunction (see Fontaine et al. 1990).

Roth and Harper (1962) pointed out some of the similarities between epilepsy and anxiety disorders. Both are episodic disorders with sudden onset without a precipitating event; both sometimes include dissociative symptoms—depersonalization, derealization, and déjà vu; both often include abnormal perceptual and emotional disturbances, such as intense fear and terror; and both have associated physical symptoms. Significant clinical differences between panic disorder and CPSs help to differentiate the two: in panic disorders, consciousness is usually preserved, olfactory hallucinations are unusual, the patient has a positive family history, electroencephalographic results are usually normal, and many patients do not respond well to anticonvulsants (Handal et al. 1995).

Treatment of Comorbid Anxiety

Patients with seizure disorders and comorbid anxiety disorder should receive treatment for their anxiety. Clinical experience indicates that SSRIs (first-line treatments for primary anxiety disorders) are helpful in the treatment of anxiety disorders in patients with epilepsy. SSRIs have potential interactions with hepatically metabolized antiepileptic medications because they can inhibit various cytochrome P450 enzymes. Benzodiazepines such as clonazepam and alprazolam also can be helpful in the treatment of anxiety disorders in patients with epilepsy. Psychotherapeutic approaches such as cognitive-behavioral therapy, behavioral modification, short-term symptom-focused therapies, and psychoeducation may be helpful.

Mood Disorders

Clinical Features

CNS disorders and chronic medical illnesses, including epilepsy, are frequently associated with increased incidence of mood disorders (Silver et al. 1990). Suicide is of special concern because its prevalence is greater in patients with epilepsy than in the general population (Gehlert 1994; Nilsson et al. 2002). Suicide is the cause of death in 10% of all patients with epilepsy, compared with 1% in the general population (Jones et al. 2003).

Patients with uncontrolled seizures have a prevalence of depression up to 10 times greater than in the general population and up to 5 times greater than in patients with controlled seizures (Harden and Goldstein 2002; Hermann et al. 2000; Lambert and Robertson 1999). Depressed epilepsy patients had twice as many emergency department and nonpsychiatric office visits as did their nondepressed counterparts (Cramer et al. 2004). Little is known, however, about the prevalence of other mood disorders such as mania and dysthymia in patients with seizure disorders.

Several features of depression in patients with epilepsy require special consideration before one diagnoses a comorbid mood disorder. Peri-ictal depression or premonitory dysphoria may occur before or after the seizure, lasting hours to days. Depressive or dysphoric symptoms of this type may stop when the seizure occurs or may continue for days after the seizure. Ictal depressive symptoms occur during the seizure and are characterized by sudden onset of symptoms without precipitating factors and can even manifest as impulsive suicidality (Prueter and Norra 2005). Postictal depressive episodes occur after seizure activity resolves and may last for up to 2 weeks. The most common type of depression in epilepsy is interictal depression, which may manifest as major depressive or dysthymic episodes. Interictal depression does not fit DSM-IV-TR classification well because it tends to have a chronic course and atypical mood symptoms of pain, mixed phases of euphoria and dysphoria, and short intervals without affective symptoms (Kanner 2003).

In evaluating depression in a patient with epilepsy, the clinician needs to examine the medications the patient is taking. Anticonvulsants have been identified as causal agents of depression and cognitive impairments; phenobarbital, the anticonvulsant vigabatrin, and multiple combinations of anticonvulsants appear to contribute to mood disturbance (Bauer and Elger 1995; Brent et al.

1990; Levinson and Devinsky 1999; Mendez et al. 1993). Other anticonvulsants have minimal effect, and some, such as carbamazepine and lamotrigine, may have beneficial effects on mood.

Treatment of Comorbid Mood Disorders

Data on the treatment of depression in seizure patients are extremely limited. In general, preictal and ictal depressive symptoms may not require antidepressant treatment because these episodes are often self-limited and improved seizure control will reduce their occurrence (Lambert and Robertson 1999). However, postictal or interictal depression requires treatment with antidepressant medication.

When depression does occur, the clinician should determine whether the patient has had a recent change in antiepileptic medication regimen. If the patient is taking an antiepileptic medication with known depressogenic effects, it should be replaced, if possible, by one with mood-stabilizing effects, such as carbamazepine, valproate, or lamotrigine. For patients with a bipolar diathesis or suspected mood lability, monotherapy with carbamazepine, valproic acid, or lamotrigine may suffice to prevent episodes, decrease severity of symptoms, and minimize overall decompensation.

All antidepressants, including the SSRI antidepressants, are proconvulsive, although the incidence of seizures in healthy individuals is low (Alldredge 1999). Despite limited controlled clinical data on the efficacy of SSRI antidepressants in the treatment of mood disorders in patients with epilepsy, SSRIs are generally recommended as first-line treatments (Kanner and Nieto 1999). Citalopram and sertraline are often used because of their minimal interactions with antiepileptic medications. It is important to start any medication with smaller dosages than are conventionally given for primary psychiatric disorders, with gradual dosage increases over time. Regular monitoring of interval EEGs and antiepileptic medication levels is recommended. Of the older antidepressant medications, most of the tricyclic antidepressants are known to lower the seizure threshold. This is particularly true of amitriptyline, maprotiline, and clomipramine. Bupropion is also very likely to cause seizures. However, doxepin, trazodone, and the monoamine oxidase inhibitors have less of a tendency to lower the seizure threshold (Rosenstein et al. 1993). Most of the seizures reported with any of these medications are dose related; therefore, blood level monitoring in these patients can be quite useful.

In most cases, treating the depression often improves seizure control. In an open study evaluating the use of fluoxetine as an adjunctive medication in patients with CPSs, 6 of 17 patients showed a dramatic improvement, and the others had a 30% reduction in seizure frequency over 14 months (Favale et al. 1995). To date, no evidence shows that any one particular antidepressant is more effective than another, and the choice should be made on clinical grounds. Epileptic patients with refractory or severe depression and even mania should be considered for ECT because it is not contraindicated in people with epilepsy. ECT raises the seizure threshold by more than 50% (Sackeim 1999). However, controlled clinical trials with ECT are lacking in epilepsy patients (Zwil and Pelchat 1994).

Few empirical studies have evaluated psychotherapeutic approaches for treatment of depression in patients with seizures (Fenwick 1994; Mathers 1992; Regan et al. 1993). A study by Gillham (1990) reported that psychological intervention with education to improve coping skills could be helpful in reducing seizure frequency and psychological symptoms (as well as depressive symptoms) in patients with refractory seizures.

Vagus nerve stimulation is a well-tolerated, efficacious treatment for refractory epilepsy. This procedure's efficacy in the treatment of mood disorders is not conclusively established, although results from open, long-term studies of treatment-resistant depression are promising. Repetitive transcranial magnetic stimulation is currently being investigated as a treatment for epilepsy and mood disorders but is not recommended for clinical use at this time.

Behavioral and Personality Disturbances

The literature and clinical experience clearly point to an association between seizure disorders and behavioral disturbances (Blumer 1999; Blumer et al. 1995; Neppe and Tucker 1988). Most of the knowledge in this area comes from cross-sectional case-control studies, case reports, and tertiary centers that treat the most severe cases. Several factors, such as the stigma of seizure disorders, adverse social factors, level of social support, cultural acceptability, consequences of the illness on psychosocial adaptation, and interpersonal relationships, play important roles in shaping patterns of behavior and have a significant effect on the integrity of personality development. Factors that may assume a role in the pathogenesis of personality and behavioral disturbances are age at onset of the seizure disorder, type of seizure disorder, location and laterality, frequency of seizures, etiology, presence of a structural lesion, presence of another medical illness or behavioral dysfunction, and ongoing administration of anticonvulsants.

An increase in episodic and impulsive aggression also has been associated with seizure disorders, particularly CPSs (Blake et al. 1995; Mann 1995). Following the postictal period, uncooperative and aggressive behavior may occur when a confused patient is restrained or may occur in a patient who develops a postictal paranoid psychosis (Rodin 1973). Aggressive behavior during a seizure is very unusual, and aggressive activity is usually carried out in a disordered, uncoordinated, and nondirected way (Fenwick 1986). The prevalence of interictal aggression is increased in some seizure disorders, CPSs, and generalized seizure disorders, but such aggression may be an epiphenomenon of epilepsy and probably can be accounted for by other factors associated with violence and aggression: exposure to violence as a child, male sex, low IQ, low socioeconomic status, adverse social factors, focal or diffuse neurological lesions, refractory seizures, cognitive impairment, history of institutionalization, and drug use (Devinsky and Vazquez 1993).

Overall Guidelines for Treatment of Comorbid Psychiatric Syndromes

With any chronic illness, basic principles should be applied in developing a treatment plan. Seizure disorders are no exception, and guidelines for treatment are summarized in Table 5–3. A thorough assessment of premorbid functioning, past episodes, previous trials and responses, duration of the current episode, and level of impairment and psychosocial dysfunction facilitates proper intervention and guides subsequent management. Given that insults to the CNS produce only a limited amount of symptom expression, the mood, anxiety, psychotic, cognitive, and behavioral symptoms and signs associated with seizure disorders do not fit neatly into the DSM psychiatric categories (Tucker 1996). The neuropsychiatrist may elect to treat patients with a suspected seizure disorder empirically. These patients, including those with refractory psychiatric illness, may find benefit with an anticonvulsant (Post et al. 1985). In a few patients with concomitant psychiatric illness, anticonvulsant monotherapy for the seizure disorder may suffice (Neppe et al. 1988). Patients taking anticonvulsants should have serum blood levels checked at the first indication of incipient or worsening psychiatric symptoms or signs. An increase in the dosage of an anticonvulsant may be all that is necessary to diminish symptoms

Table 5–3.   Basic principles of treating patients with a seizure disorder and concomitant psychiatric symptoms

1.   Perform a thorough assessment of biopsychosocial factors that aggravate neuropsychiatric symptoms.

2.   Evaluate the need for adjustment of the anticonvulsant.

3.   Consider psychotherapeutic approaches (individual, group, family) that are specific for the syndrome or that target behaviors or stressors.

4.   Preferably—but not always—use anticonvulsant monotherapy.

5.   Optimize the addition of psychotropic medication by targeting specific psychiatric symptoms.

6.   Start with a smaller-than-usual dose and wait until symptoms stabilize (often weeks) before changing the dose.

7.   Anticipate interactions between anticonvulsant and psychotropic medications.

8.   Collaborate with other caregivers.

Source.   Reprinted from Kim HF, Chen FY, Yudofsky SC, et al.: "Neuropsychiatric Aspects of Seizure Disorders," in *Essentials of Neuropsychiatry and Behavioral Neurosciences,* 2nd Edition. Edited by Yudofsky SC, Hales RE. Washington, DC, American Psychiatric Publishing, 2010, pp. 275–298. Used with permission. Copyright © 2010 American Psychiatric Association.

and prevent decompensation. Conversely, patients with complex medication regimens may realize symptom improvement after dosage reduction (Trimble and Thompson 1983).

Most patients will require treatment of psychiatric syndromes. Individual, group, family, or couples therapy can provide specific syndrome-focused treatments. Psychotherapeutic approaches have many advantages. They avoid drug interactions, circumvent the tendency of psychotropic medications to alter seizure thresholds, and can teach patients behavior and coping skills that may have a positive effect on symptoms and dysfunction.

Many patients will require pharmacotherapy, either combined with psychotherapeutic approaches or alone. Patients with temporal lobe epilepsy have a wide variety of mood, anxiety, dissociative, psychotic, and behavioral disturbances that frequently resemble psychiatric disorders. Discriminating the symptoms of previous seizures from target psychiatric symptoms will ensure a greater likelihood of response to medication.

Although we recommend an aggressive approach for the treatment of co-morbid psychiatric syndromes, we are judicious with the dosing of psychotropics and prefer gradual increases. Clinical experience shows that many patients with seizure disorders seem to respond to smaller dosages. When a new drug is added, the clinician must be vigilant for potential drug interactions.

Many anticonvulsants will lower the serum drug level of psychotropics through enzyme induction (Perucca et al. 1985), and psychotropics may increase the levels of anticonvulsants secondary to increased cytochrome P450 hepatic enzyme competition (Cloyd et al. 1986). Monitoring of serum levels is recommended for patients receiving tricyclic antidepressants (Preskorn and Fast 1992). After the addition of a psychotropic, anticonvulsant blood levels should be monitored, weekly at first and then monthly. After a few months, serum levels can be checked less frequently. Thereafter, any changes in medication dosage require reexamination of serum blood levels.

The importance of coordinating care with other professionals and health care providers cannot be overemphasized. It behooves the psychiatrist to work with a neurologist (if available) to develop a long-term strategy. Often, psychiatrists will assume the role of supervising all treatment planning (Schoenenberger et al. 1995).

Specific Aspects of Anticonvulsant Use

Management

Often, when treating patients who have suspected seizure disorders, the psychiatrist will have to manage the anticonvulsants single-handedly. As valproic acid and carbamazepine have become more common in the treatment of bipolar illness, the basic principles have become known to most psychiatrists (McElroy et al. 1988; Neppe et al. 1988). Until the psychiatrist is comfortable with these medications, however, collaboration with a neurologist is helpful and serves as a good learning technique.

Pharmacokinetic Interactions

Anticonvulsant administration is particularly important and particularly difficult by virtue of enzyme induction and inhibition occurring in the liver. This enzyme induction tends to affect predominantly the cytochrome P450 enzyme system in the liver; this implies that both the metabolism of anticonvulsants (particularly carbamazepine) and the metabolism of other lipid-soluble compounds are accelerated (Alldredge 1999; Post et al. 1985). However, some of the newer anticonvulsants—oxcarbazepine, gabapentin, and vigabatrin— have few drug interactions (Dichter and Brodie 1996). Of the major anticonvulsants, phenobarbital, phenytoin, carbamazepine, lamotrigine, topiramate, and tiagabine have potent drug interactions.

Phenobarbital

Phenobarbital is the most potent of the enzyme inducers; when it is used in combination, it reduces levels of other anticonvulsants. In addition, phenobarbital may cause psychological depression and may lead to addiction, or to lethal overdose, which was a major cause of death in the 1950s. It also produces a cognitive impairment, which may explain the rigidity of personality observed in patients with seizure disorders who take phenobarbital.

Barbiturates have little role in the outpatient management of seizure disorders except in patients who are already taking and tolerating them. Side effects may include CNS depression, psychological depression, and cognitive impairments. It is extremely difficult to taper off barbiturates without inducing an epileptic seizure.

Phenytoin

Despite being an outstanding anticonvulsant in controlling generalized tonic-clonic and partial seizures, diphenylhydantoin sodium (or phenytoin) has limited use in treating the neuropsychiatric patient. The side-effect profile (see Pulliainen and Jokelainen 1994) includes mild cognitive impairment. Because phenytoin has a small therapeutic range, patients can easily become drug toxic and, ironically, may experience seizures or worsening of them. Gum hyperplasia is a classic finding (Trimble 1979, 1988).

Carbamazepine

The increasing use of carbamazepine rather than phenytoin is due to psychotropic properties, fewer side effects, and proven value in severe disorders and bipolar illness. Carbamazepine is as effective as phenytoin in both generalized tonic-clonic seizures and partial seizures and thus is the drug of choice for such conditions. It is ineffective in absence seizures, for which sodium valproate or ethosuximide is preferred.

Carbamazepine may be used in treating nonresponsive psychotic or atypical psychotic patients with any temporal lobe abnormalities on EEG, with episodic hostility, or with affective lability (Blumer et al. 1988; Cowdry and Gardner 1988; Neppe et al. 1991).

Carbamazepine and the other anticonvulsants involved in enzyme induction can cause many unanticipated side effects (Cloyd et al. 1986) (e.g., patients taking oral contraceptives may have their steroid levels lowered, patients may become vitamin D deficient, folic acid may be depleted). Elevation in hepatic enzyme levels (γ-glutamyltransferase) commonly occurs; this does not imply that the anticonvulsant drugs should be stopped.

Patients taking neuroleptics who are given carbamazepine may have more side effects as a consequence of raised levels from competition at enzyme system pathways.

In addition to the phenomenon of induction of hepatic enzymes, a second phenomenon of deinduction of hepatic enzyme systems occurs (Neppe and Kaplan 1988).

Valproate

Sodium valproate is useful in combined tonic-clonic and absence seizures. It also appears to be effective against CPSs. Valproate does not induce enzymes but metabolically competes; it raises levels of psychotropics and itself. It is safe, relatively nontoxic, and generally well tolerated. The major concern is potentially fatal but rare hepatotoxicity in young children, particularly when valproate is used with other anticonvulsants (McElroy et al. 1988).

Newer Antiepileptic Drugs

There are many newer antiepileptic drugs: gabapentin, felbamate, oxcarbazepine, tiagabine, topiramate, vigabatrin, levetiracetam, and lamotrigine. Most of these drugs for which the actions are known affect either the inhibitory γ-aminobutyric acid (GABA) system (gabapentin, tiagabine, vigabatrin) or the excitatory glutaminergic system (felbamate, lamotrigine). These drugs have been well studied, and all have various mild to serious side effects (Dichter and Brodie 1996; Ketter et al. 1999). Gabapentin, lamotrigine, and topiramate have been increasingly used in psychiatry for bipolar disorder and anxiety disorders and may have uses for similar disorders in seizure disorder patients (Ghaemi and Gaughan 2000; Ketter et al. 1999).

Conclusion

Psychopathology occurs in only a minority of persons with epilepsy. Medications used to treat seizure disorders often do not alleviate behavior changes, and at times agents such as neuroleptics and antidepressants help behavior change but not seizure disturbances. The exact etiology of these conditions remains to be determined. Clinical judgment in the individual case remains the essential standard of care in the absence of solid evidence for specific indications and protocols for the use of anticonvulsant-psychotropic combinations in specific populations.

Recommended Readings

Barry JJ, Ettinger AB, Friel P, et al: Consensus statement: the evaluation and treatment of people with epilepsy and affective disorders. Epilepsy Behav 13(suppl):S1–S29, 2008

Cavanna AE, Ali F, Rickards HE, et al: Behavioral and cognitive effects of anti-epileptic drugs. Discov Med 9:138–144, 2010

Marcangelo MJ, Ovsiew F: Psychiatric aspects of epilepsy. Psychiatr Clin North Am 30:781–802, 2007

Trimble M, Schmitz B (eds): The Neuropsychiatry of Epilepsy. Cambridge, UK, Cambridge University Press, 2002

References

Adamec RE, Stark AC: Limbic kindling and animal behavior: implications for human psychopathology associated with complex partial seizures. Biol Psychiatry 18:269–293, 1983

Alldredge BK: Seizure risk associated with psychotropic drugs: clinical and pharmacokinetic considerations. Neurology 53 (suppl 2):S68–S75, 1999

Alper K, Devinsky O, Perrine K, et al: Psychiatric classification of nonconversion nonepileptic seizures. Arch Neurol 52:199–201, 1995

American Psychiatric Association: Diagnostic and Statistical Manual of Mental Disorders, 4th Edition, Text Revision. Washington, DC, American Psychiatric Association, 2000

Arnold LM, Privitera MD: Psychopathology and trauma in epileptic and psychogenic seizure patients. Psychosomatics 37:438–443, 1996

Bauer J: Epilepsy and prolactin in adults: a clinical review. Epilepsy Res 24:1–7, 1996

Bauer J, Elger CE: Anticonvulsive drug therapy: historical and current aspects. Nervenarzt 66:403–411, 1995

Berg AT, Berkovic SF, Brodie MJ, et al: Revised terminology and concepts for organization of seizures and epilepsies: report of the ILAE Commission on Classification and Terminology, 2005–2009. Epilepsia 51:676–685, 2010

Berger H: Über das Elektrenkephalogramm des Menschen. Arch Psychiatr Nervenkr 1929–1938

Bickford RG: Activation procedures and special electrodes, in Current Practice of Unusual Electroencephalography. Edited by Kass D, Daly DD. New York, Raven, 1979, pp 269–306

Blake P, Pincus J, Buckner C: Neurologic abnormalities in murderers. Neurology 45:1641–1647, 1995

Blumer D: Evidence supporting the temporal lobe epilepsy personality syndrome. Neurology 53.S9–S12, 1999

Blumer D, Heilbronn M, Himmelhoch J: Indications for carbamazepine in mental illness: atypical psychiatric disorder or temporal lobe syndrome? Compr Psychiatry 29:108–122, 1988

Blumer D, Montouris G, Hermann B: Psychiatric morbidity in seizure patients on a neurodiagnostic monitoring unit. J Neuropsychiatry Clin Neurosci 7:445–456, 1995

Brent DA, Crumrine PK, Varma R, et al: Phenobarbital treatment and major depressive disorder in children with epilepsy: a naturalistic follow-up. Pediatrics 85:1086–1091, 1990

Cloyd JC, Levy RH, Wedlund RH: Relationship between carbamazepine concentration and extent of enzyme autoinduction (abstract). Epilepsia 27:592, 1986

Cowdry R, Gardner DL: Pharmacotherapy of borderline personality disorder. Arch Gen Psychiatry 45:111–119, 1988

Cramer JA, Blum D, Fanning K, et al: The impact of comorbid depression on health resource utilization in a community sample of people with epilepsy. Epilepsy Behav 5:337–342, 2004

Dekker PA: Epilepsy: A Manual for Medical and Clinical Officers in Africa. Geneva, World Health Organization, 2002

Devinsky O, Gordon E: Epileptic seizures progressing into nonepileptic conversion seizures. Neurology 51:1293–1296, 1998

Devinsky O, Vazquez B: Behavioral changes associated with epilepsy. Neurol Clin 11:127–149, 1993

Dichter M, Brodie M: New antiepileptic drugs. N Engl J Med 334:1583–1590, 1996

Ebersole JS, Leroy RJ: Evaluation of ambulatory EEG monitoring. Neurology 33:853–860, 1983

Engel J: The epilepsies, in Cecil Textbook of Medicine, 19th Edition. Edited by Wyngaarden JB, Smith LH Jr, Bennett JC. Philadelphia, PA, WB Saunders, 1992, pp 2202–2213

Favale E, Rubino P, Mainardi P, et al: Anticonvulsant effect of fluoxetine in humans. Neurology 45:1926–1927, 1995

Fenton GW: The EEG, epilepsy and psychiatry, in What Is Epilepsy? Edited by Trimble MR, Reynolds EH. Edinburgh, UK, Churchill Livingstone, 1986, pp 139–160

Fenwick P: Is dyscontrol epilepsy? in What Is Epilepsy? Edited by Trimble MR, Reynolds EH. Edinburgh, UK, Churchill Livingstone, 1986, pp 161–182

Fenwick P: The behavioral treatment of epilepsy generation and inhibition of seizures. Neurol Clin 12:175–202, 1994

Fink M: Meduna and the origins of convulsive therapy. Am J Psychiatry 141:1034–1041, 1984

Fisher RS, Boas WV, Blume W, et al: Epileptic seizures and epilepsy: definitions proposed by the International League Against Epilepsy (ILAE) and the International Bureau for Epilepsy (IBE). Epilepsia 46:470–472, 2005

Fontaine R, Breton G, Déry R, et al: Temporal lobe abnormalities in panic disorder: an MRI study. Biol Psychiatry 27:304–310, 1990

GCAE Secretariat: Epilepsy: Out of the Shadows. ILAE/IBE/WHO Global Campaign Against Epilepsy. Heemstede, The Netherlands, World Health Organization, 2003

Gehlert S: Perceptions of control in adults with epilepsy. Epilepsia 35:81–88, 1994

Ghaemi S, Gaughan S: Novel anticonvulsants: a new generation of mood stabilizers. Harv Rev Psychiatry 8:1–7, 2000

Gillham RA: Refractory epilepsy: an evaluation of psychological methods in outpatient management. Epilepsia 31:427–432, 1990

Handal N, Masand P, Weilburg J: Panic disorder and complex partial seizures: a truly complex relationship. Psychosomatics 36:498–502, 1995

Harden CL, Goldstein MA: Mood disorders in patients with epilepsy: epidemiology and management. CNS Drugs 16:291–302, 2002

Heath RG: Psychosis and epilepsy: similarities and differences in the anatomic-physiologic substrate. Advances in Biological Psychiatry 8:106–116, 1982

Hermann BP, Seidenberg M, Bell B: Psychiatric comorbidity in chronic epilepsy: identification, consequences, and treatment of major depression. Epilepsia 41 (suppl 2):S31–S41, 2000

Ho S, Berkovic S, Berlangieri S, et al: Comparison of ictal SPECT and interictal PET in the presurgical evaluation of TLE. Ann Neurol 37:738–745, 1995

International League Against Epilepsy, Commission on Classification and Terminology: Proposal for classification of epilepsies and epileptic syndromes. Epilepsia 26:268–278, 1985

Jones JE, Hermann BP, Barry JJ, et al: Rates and risk factors for suicide, suicidal ideation, and suicide attempts in chronic epilepsy. Epilepsy Behav 4 (suppl 3):S31–S38, 2003

Kanner AM: Depression in epilepsy: a frequently neglected multifaceted disorder. Epilepsy Behav 4 (suppl 4):S11–S19, 2003

Kanner AM, Nieto JC: Depressive disorders in epilepsy. Neurology 53 (5 suppl 2):S26–S32, 1999

Ketter T, Post R, Theodore W: Positive and negative psychiatric effects of antiepileptic drugs in patients with seizure disorders. Neurology 53 (suppl 2):S53–S67, 1999

Kirubakaran V, Sen S, Wilkinson C: Catatonic stupor: unusual manifestation of TLE. Psychiatr J Univ Ott 12:244–246, 1987

Kuyk J, Spinhoven P, Boas W, et al: Dissociation in temporal lobe epilepsy and pseudoepileptic seizure patients. J Nerv Ment Dis 187:713–720, 1999

Lambert MV, Robertson MM: Depression in epilepsy: etiology, phenomenology, and treatment. Epilepsia 40 (suppl 10):S21–S47, 1999

Landolt H: Serial encephalographic investigations during psychotic episodes in epileptic patients and during schizophrenic attacks, in Lectures on Epilepsy. Edited by Lorentz de Haas AM. London, Elsevier, 1958, pp 91–133

Laskowitz D, Sperling M, French J, et al: The syndrome of frontal lobe epilepsy. Neurology 45:780–787, 1995

Levinson D, Devinsky O: Psychiatric events during vigabatrin therapy. Neurology 53:1503–1511, 1999

Malkowicz D, Legido A, Jackel R, et al: Prolactin secretion following repetitive seizures. Neurology 45:448–452, 1995

Mann JJ: Violence and aggression, in Psychopharmacology: The Fourth Generation of Progress. Edited by Bloom FE, Kupfer DJ. New York, Raven, 1995, pp 1919–1928

Mathers CB: Group therapy in the management of epilepsy. Br J Med Psychol 65:279–287, 1992

McElroy SL, Keck P, Pope HG Jr, et al: Valproate in primary psychiatric disorders, in Use of Anticonvulsants in Psychiatry. Edited by McElroy SL, Pope HG Jr. Clifton, NJ, Oxford Health Care, 1988, pp 25–42

Mendez MF, Doss RC, Taylor JL, et al: Depression in epilepsy: relationship to seizures and anticonvulsant therapy. J Nerv Ment Dis 181:444–447, 1993

Metrakos K, Metrakos JD: Genetics of convulsive disorders, II: genetics and encephalographic studies in centrencephalic epilepsy. Neurology 11:454–483, 1961

Neppe VM, Kaplan C: Short-term treatment of atypical spells with carbamazepine. Clin Neuropharmacol 11:287–289, 1988

Neppe VM, Tucker GJ: Modern perspectives on epilepsy in relation to psychiatry: behavioral disturbances of epilepsy. Hosp Community Psychiatry 39:389–396, 1988

Neppe VM, Tucker GJ, Wilensky AJ: Fundamentals of carbamazepine use in neuropsychiatry. J Clin Psychiatry 49 (suppl 4):4–6, 1988

Neppe VM, Bowman B, Sawchuk KSLJ: Carbamazepine for atypical psychosis with episodic hostility: a preliminary study. J Nerv Ment Dis 179:339–340, 1991

Nilsson L, Ahlbom A, Farahmand BY, et al: Risk factors for suicide in epilepsy: a case control study. Epilepsia 43:644–651, 2002

Novak J, Corke P, Fairley N: "Petit mal status" in adults. Dis Nerv Syst 32:245–248, 1971

Perucca E, Manzo L, Crema A: Pharmacokinetic interactions between antiepileptic and psychotropic drugs, in The Psychopharmacology of Epilepsy. Edited by Trimble MR. Chichester, UK, Wiley, 1985, pp 95–105

Pincus JH, Tucker GJ: Behavioral Neurology, 3rd Edition. New York, Oxford University Press, 1985

Popkin M, Tucker GJ: Mental disorders due to a general medical condition and substance-induced disorders: mood, anxiety, psychotic, catatonic, and personality disorders, in DSM-IV Source Book. Edited by Widiger T, Frances J, Pincus HA, et al. Washington, DC, American Psychiatric Press, 1994, pp 243–276

Popli A, Kando J, Pillay S, et al: Occurrence of seizures related to psychotropic medication among psychiatric inpatients. Psychiatr Serv 46:486–488, 1995

Post RM, Uhde TW, Joffe RT, et al: Anticonvulsant drugs in psychiatric illness: new treatment alternatives and theoretical implications, in The Psychopharmacology of Epilepsy. Edited by Trimble MR. Chichester, UK, Wiley, 1985, pp 141–171

Preskorn SH, Fast GA: Tricyclic antidepressant–induced seizures and plasma drug concentration. J Clin Psychiatry 53:160–162, 1992

Prueter C, Norra C: Mood disorders and their treatment in patients with epilepsy. J Neuropsychiatry Clin Neurosci 17:20–28, 2005

Pulliainen V, Jokelainen M: Effects of phenytoin and carbamazepine on cognitive functions in newly diagnosed epileptic patients. Acta Neurol Scand 89:81–86, 1994

Regan KJ, Banks GK, Beran RG: Therapeutic recreation programmes for children with epilepsy. Seizure 2:195–200, 1993

Rodin EA: Psychomotor epilepsy and aggressive behavior. Arch Gen Psychiatry 28:210–213, 1973

Rosenstein DL, Nelson JC, Jacobs SC, et al: Seizures associated with antidepressants: a review. J Clin Psychiatry 54:289–299, 1993

Roth M, Harper M: Temporal lobe epilepsy and the phobic anxiety–depersonalization syndrome, II: practical and theoretical considerations. Compr Psychiatry 3:215–226, 1962

Ryback R, Gardner E: Limbic system dysrhythmia: a diagnostic EEG procedure utilizing procaine activation. J Neuropsychiatry Clin Neurosci 3:321–329, 1991

Sackeim HA: The anticonvulsant hypothesis of the mechanisms of action of ECT: current status. J ECT 15:5–26, 1999

Sadler M, Goodwin J: The sensitivity of various electrodes in the detection of epileptiform potentials (EPs) in patients with partial complex (PC) seizures (letter). Epilepsia 27:627, 1986

Schiffer R: Epilepsy, psychosis, and forced normalization (editorial). Arch Neurol 44:253, 1987

Schoenenberger R, Tonasijevic M, Jha A, et al: Appropriateness of antiepileptic drug level monitoring. JAMA 274:1622–1626, 1995

Shukla G, Bhatia M, Vivekanandhan S: Serum prolactin levels for differentiation of nonepileptic versus true seizures: limited utility. Epilepsy Behav 5:517–521, 2004

Silver JM, Hales RE, Yudofsky SC: Psychopharmacology of depression in neurologic disorders. J Clin Psychiatry 51:33–39, 1990

Slater E, Beard AW, Glithero E: The schizophrenialike psychoses of epilepsy. Br J Psychiatry 109:95–150, 1963

Thomas M, Jankovic J: Psychogenic movement disorders: diagnosis and management. CNS Drugs 18:437–452, 2004

Thomas P, Zifkin B, Migneco O, et al: Nonconvulsive status epilepticus of frontal origin. Neurology 52:1174–1183, 1999

Tojek TM, Lumley M, Barkley G, et al: Stress and other psychosocial characteristics of patients with psychogenic nonepileptic seizures. Psychosomatics 41:221–226, 2000

Toone BK, Garralda ME, Ron MA: The psychoses of epilepsy and the functional psychoses: a clinical and phenomenological comparison. Br J Psychiatry 141:256–261, 1982

Trimble MR: The relationship between epilepsy and schizophrenia: a biochemical hypothesis. Biol Psychiatry 12:299–304, 1977

Trimble MR: The effects of anticonvulsant drugs on cognitive abilities. Pharmacol Ther 4:677–685, 1979

Trimble MR: Cognitive hazards of seizure disorders. Epilepsia 29 (suppl 1):S19–S24, 1988

Trimble MR, Thompson PJ: Anticonvulsant drugs, cognitive impairment, and behavior. Epilepsia 24(suppl):S55–S63, 1983

Tucker GJ: Current diagnostic issues in neuropsychiatry, in Neuropsychiatry. Edited by Fogel BS, Schiffer RB. Baltimore, MD, Williams & Wilkins, 1996, pp 1009–1014

Von Meduna L: Die Konvulsionstherapie der Schizophrenia. Halle, Germany, Marhold, 1937

Vukmir RB: Does serum prolactin indicate the presence of seizure in the emergency department patient? J Neurol 251:736–739, 2004

Willert C, Spitzer C, Kusserow S, et al: Serum neuron-specific enolase, prolactin, and creatine kinase after epileptic and psychogenic non-epileptic seizures. Acta Neurol Scand 109:318–323, 2004

Zwil AS, Pelchat RJ: ECT in the treatment of patients with neurological and somatic disease. Int J Psychiatry Med 24:1–29, 1994

6

Cerebrovascular Disorders

Robert G. Robinson, M.D.

Sergio E. Starkstein, M.D., Ph.D.

Stroke is the most common serious neurological disorder in the world and is the leading cause of long-term disability. Stroke accounts for half of all the acute hospitalizations for neurological disease, and according to the American Heart Association, 795,000 new strokes occur annually and 6.5 million survivors of stroke live in the United States, with 10% of individuals older than 75 years being stroke survivors (Lloyd-Jones et al. 2010). The neuropsychiatric complications of cerebrovascular disease include a wide range of emotional and cognitive disturbances. In this chapter, we discuss emotional disorders associated with stroke.

Poststroke Depression

Diagnosis

To diagnose poststroke depression (PSD), researchers in most studies have used structured interviews and diagnostic criteria defined by DSM-IV-TR (American Psychiatric Association 2000) or Research Diagnostic Criteria (Aben et al. 2002; Cassidy et al. 2004; Morris et al. 1990). Poststroke major depression is categorized in DSM-IV-TR as "mood disorder due to stroke with major depressive-like episode" (American Psychiatric Association 2000, pp. 404–405). For patients with less severe forms of depression, there are "research criteria" in DSM-IV-TR for minor depression (i.e., subsyndromal major depression; the diagnosis requires depression or anhedonia with at least one but fewer than four additional symptoms of major depression) or, alternatively, a diagnosis of mood disorder due to stroke with depressive features (i.e., depressed mood but criteria for major depression not met).

Phenomenology

Lipsey et al. (1986) examined the frequency of depressive symptoms in a group of 43 patients with major PSD compared with that in a group of 43 age-matched patients with "functional" depression (i.e., depression with no known brain pathology). The main finding was that both groups showed almost identical profiles of symptoms, including those that were not part of the diagnostic criteria. More than 50% of the patients who met the diagnostic criteria for major PSD reported sadness, anxiety, tension, loss of interest and concentration, sleep disturbances with early morning awakening, loss of appetite with weight loss, difficulty concentrating and thinking, and thoughts of death.

Prevalence

In recent years, a large number of studies around the world have examined the prevalence of PSD. In general, these studies have found similar rates of major and minor depression among patients hospitalized for acute stroke, patients in rehabilitation hospitals, and patients in outpatient clinics. Based on 2,769 patients, the mean frequency of major depression among patients in acute and rehabilitation hospitals was 21.6% for major depression and 20% for minor depression (Robinson 2006). Among 2,108 patients studied in community settings, however, the mean prevalence rates were 14% for major depression and 9.1% for minor depression (Robinson 2006).

Duration

A series of 142 acute stroke patients were prospectively studied in a 2-year longitudinal study of PSD (Robinson 2006). At the time of the initial in-hospital evaluation, 19% of the patients had the DSM-IV-TR diagnosis of major depression, whereas 25% had minor depression. Of those with major depression, 47% still had major depression at the 6-month follow-up evaluation, whereas only 11% of the original group still had major depression at 1-year follow-up, and none were still depressed at 2 years. In contrast, however, patients with minor depression had a less favorable prognosis; more than 50% of the patients with in-hospital minor depression continued to have major or minor depression throughout the 2-year follow-up. In addition, about 30% of patients who were not depressed in the hospital became depressed after discharge. Thus, the natural course of major depression appeared to be between 6 months and 1 year, whereas the duration of minor depression was more variable, and in many cases the patients appeared to be chronically depressed.

Morris et al. (1990) found that among a group of 99 patients in a stroke rehabilitation hospital in Australia, those with major depression had a mean duration of major depression of 40 weeks, whereas those with adjustment disorders (minor depression) had a mean duration of depression of only 12 weeks. These findings confirm that poststroke major depression has a duration of approximately 9–12 months but suggest that the course is more variable among patients with minor depression.

Relationship to Lesion Variables

The relationship between depressive disorder and lesion location has been perhaps the most controversial area of research in the field of poststroke mood disorder. Although establishing an association between specific clinical symptoms and lesion location is one of the fundamental goals of clinical practice in neurology, this has rarely been done in the context of psychiatric disorders.

The first study to report a significant correlation of clinical to pathological variables in PSD was an investigation by Robinson and Szetela (1981) of 29 patients with left hemisphere brain injury secondary to stroke ($n=18$) or to traumatic brain injury ($n=11$). Lesions were localized by computed tomography (CT), and a significant inverse correlation was found between the severity of depression and the distance of the anterior border of the lesion from the frontal pole ($r=0.76$). This surprising finding led to a number of subsequent examinations of this phenomenon in other populations. A meta-analysis by Narushima et al. (2003) found eight independent studies of severity of depression and proximity of the stroke lesion to the right or left frontal pole done within the first 6 months following stroke. In total, 163 patients had an overall correlation coefficient of −0.53 using fixed and −0.59 using random model assumptions ($P<0.001$). In the right hemisphere, however, a total of 106 patients had nonsignificant correlations between severity of depression and distance of the lesions from the right frontal pole ($r=−0.20$, fixed model; $r=−0.23$, random model) (Narushima et al. 2003).

On the basis of the finding that PSD and lesion location are dependent on time since stroke, Robinson (2003) conducted a meta-analysis of studies conducted within 2 months following stroke, comparing the frequency of major depression among patients with left anterior versus left posterior lesions and left anterior versus right anterior lesions. There were 128 patients in the left anterior versus left posterior comparison, with a fixed model odds ratio (OR) of 2.29 (95% confidence interval [CI] = 1.6–3.4, $P<0.001$) and random model OR of 2.29 (95% CI = 1.5–3.4, $P<0.001$). Similarly, the comparison of left and right anterior lesions had ORs of 2.18 (fixed model: 95% CI = 1.4–3.3, $P<0.001$) and 2.16 (random model: 95% CI = 1.3–3.6, $P<0.004$).

The results of Robinson's (2003) study suggest that the failure of other investigators to replicate the association of left anterior lesion location with increased frequency of depression may in most cases be related to time since stroke. The lateralized effect of left anterior lesions on both major and minor depression is a phenomenon of the acute poststroke period, when the patients are less than 2 months poststroke. In a review, Bhogal et al. (2004) concluded that the association between left hemisphere lesion location and PSD was dependent on whether the patients were inpatients versus community patients (OR = 1.36, 95% CI = 1.05–1.76, $P<0.05$) or acute patients versus chronic patients (OR acute = 2.14, 95% CI = 1.5–3.04, $P<0.05$).

Premorbid Risk Factors

The studies reviewed in the previous subsection, "Relationship to Lesion Variables," indicate that although significant proportions of patients with left anterior or right posterior lesions develop PSD, not every patient with a lesion in these locations develops a depressive mood. This observation raises the question of why clinical variability occurs and why some but not all patients with lesions in these locations develop depression.

Starkstein et al. (1988b) examined these questions by comparing 13 patients with major PSD with 13 stroke patients without depression, all of whom had lesions of the same size and location. Eleven pairs of patients had left hemisphere lesions; two pairs had right hemisphere lesions. Patients with major PSD, however, had significantly more subcortical atrophy ($P < 0.05$), as measured both by the ratio of third ventricle to brain (i.e., the area of the third ventricle divided by the area of the brain at the same level) and by the ratio of lateral ventricle to brain (i.e., the area of the body of the lateral ventricle contralateral to the brain lesion divided by the brain area at the same level). It is likely that the subcortical atrophy preceded the stroke. Thus, a mild degree of subcortical atrophy may be one of the premorbid risk factors that increases the risk of developing major depression following a stroke.

Relationship to Physical Impairment

Numerous investigators have reported a significant association between depression and functional physical impairment (i.e., activities of daily living [ADL]). Of 18 studies involving 3,281 patients, 15 (83%) found a statistically significant relationship between PSD and severity of impairment in ADL (Robinson 2006). This association, however, might be construed as the severe functional impairment producing depression or, alternatively, the severity of depression influencing the severity of functional impairment. Studies, in fact, support both interpretations.

In addition to depression influencing physical recovery from stroke, the timing of treatment of depression affects physical recovery. Narushima and Robinson (2003) compared 34 patients who received antidepressant treatment with either nortriptyline (100 mg/day) or fluoxetine (40 mg/day) for 12 weeks beginning 19–25 days after stroke with 28 patients who received the same antidepressant treatment but began 140 (± 28 SD) days poststroke. During the period from 6 to 24 months following stroke, with the two groups matched for time since stroke, there was a significant group×time interaction. The early-treatment group continued to show gradual recovery in ADL over 2 years, whereas the late-treatment group showed gradual deterioration between the 12- and 24-month follow-ups (Narushima and Robinson 2003).

Finally, in a recent study, Mikami et al. (in press) found that compared with patients given placebo, patients who took fluoxetine or nortriptyline for

3 months following stroke experienced significantly better physical recovery from stroke, as measured by the Rankin Scale. This effect of fluoxetine and nortriptyline was independent of depression, age, rehabilitation therapy, and stroke severity. Thus, antidepressants may augment physical recovery even in the absence of depression.

Relationship to Cognitive Impairment

Although numerous investigators have reported that elderly patients with functional major depression have intellectual deficits that improve with treatment of depression, this issue was first examined in patients with PSD by Robinson et al. (1986). Patients with major depression after a left hemisphere infarct were found to have significantly lower (more impaired) scores on the Mini-Mental State Examination (MMSE; Folstein et al. 1975) than did a comparable group of nondepressed patients. Both the size of patients' lesions and their depression scores correlated independently with severity of cognitive impairment. MMSE findings in stroke patients with or without major depression, grouped by infarct location, from three separate studies are shown in Figure 6–1.

In a study by Starkstein et al. (1988b), stroke patients with and without major depression were matched for lesion location and volume. Of 13 patients with major PSD, 10 had an MMSE score lower than that of their matched control subjects, 2 had the same score, and only 1 had a higher score ($P<0.001$). Thus, even when patients were matched for lesion size and location, depressed patients were more cognitively impaired.

Jorge et al. (2010) examined cognitive recovery in patients within 3 months of stroke, but without PSD, who were given escitalopram ($n=43$) or placebo ($n=45$) using double-blind methods or nonblinded Problem Solving Therapy (PST) ($n=41$). After 1 year of treatment, patients given escitalopram had a significantly greater recovery in total score on the Repeatable Battery for the Assessment of Neuropsychological Studies, as well as improvements in delayed memory and immediate memory. These findings indicate that escitalopram may augment cognitive (particularly memory) recovery from stroke, independent of depression.

Mechanism of Poststroke Depression

Although the cause of PSD remains unknown, one of the mechanisms that has been hypothesized to play an etiological role is dysfunction of the biogenic

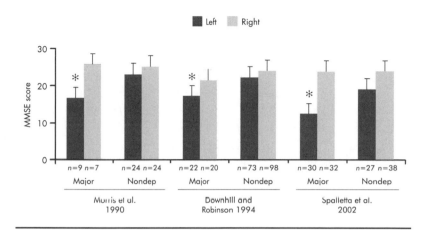

Figure 6–1.   Mini-Mental State Examination (MMSE) scores following acute stroke in three studies among patients with major or no mood disturbance grouped according to the hemisphere of ischemia.

In all three studies, there was a significant difference between patients with major depression (Major) after left hemisphere stroke and nondepressed (Nondep) patients with similar lesions. Major depression after right hemisphere lesions did not lead to the same phenomenon. Error bars represent the standard deviation divided by the square root of N.
$*P=0.001$.
Source.   Reprinted from Robinson RG: *The Clinical Neuropsychiatry of Stroke,* 2nd Edition. Cambridge, UK, Cambridge University Press, 2006. Used with permission.

amine system. The noradrenergic and serotonergic cell bodies are located in the brain stem and send ascending projections through the medial forebrain bundle to the frontal cortex. The ascending axons then arc posteriorly and run longitudinally through the deep layers of the cortex, arborizing and sending terminal projections into the superficial cortical layers (Morrison et al. 1979). Lesions that disrupt these pathways in the frontal cortex or the basal ganglia may affect many downstream fibers. On the basis of these neuroanatomical facts and the clinical finding that severity of depression correlates with proximity of the lesion to the frontal pole, Robinson et al. (1984) suggested that PSD may be the consequence of depletions of norepinephrine and/or serotonin produced by lesions in the frontal lobe or basal ganglia.

Spalletta et al. (2006) hypothesized that proinflammatory cytokines resulting from ischemic brain damage may explain why ischemic lesions lead to depletions of biogenic amines. Stroke is known to produce release of cytokines such as intracellular anthocyanin 1 (AN1) or interleukin-1β (IL-1β), both of which have been found to be elevated in deceased individuals over age 60 years who had a history of major depression compared with control subjects. Cytokines have been shown to activate the enzyme indole 2,3-dioxygenase (IDO), which catabolizes tryptophan, leading to decreased levels of serotonin (Capuron and Dantzer 2003). Thus, depletion of serotonin induced by cytokines may trigger depressions following stroke.

Treatment of Poststroke Depression

At the time of this writing, eight placebo-controlled randomized double-blind treatment studies had been published on the efficacy of single-antidepressant treatment of PSD (Table 6–1). In the first study, Lipsey et al. (1984) examined 14 patients treated with nortriptyline and 20 patients given placebo. The 11 patients treated with nortriptyline who completed the 6-week study showed significantly greater improvement in their Hamilton Rating Scale for Depression (Ham-D) scores than did 15 placebo-treated patients ($P<0.01$). In another double-blind controlled trial, in which the selective serotonin reuptake inhibitor (SSRI) citalopram was used, improvement in Ham-D scores was significantly greater over 6 weeks in patients receiving active treatment ($n=27$ completers) than in the placebo group ($n=32$ completers) (Andersen et al. 1994a). At both 3 and 6 weeks, the group receiving active treatment had significantly lower Ham-D scores than did the group receiving placebo. This study established for the first time the efficacy of an SSRI in the treatment of PSD.

Electroconvulsive therapy has also been reported to be effective for treating PSD (Murray et al. 1986). It causes few side effects and no neurological deterioration. Psychostimulants have also been reported in open-label trials to be effective for the treatment of PSD. Additionally, psychological treatment using cognitive-behavioral therapy (CBT) in 123 stroke patients was found by Lincoln and Flannaghan (2003) to be no more effective than an attention (i.e., placebo) treatment ($n=39$ CBT completers; $n=43$ placebo completers).

In a double-blind study by Robinson et al. (2008), 176 nondepressed patients began treatment within 3 months following stroke. After 1 year of treatment with escitalopram (10 mg for patients age 65 or younger; 5 mg for patients over age 65), PST, or placebo, patients given placebo were 4.5 times more likely to develop first-episode depression than were patients given escitalopram (i.e., 22.4% placebo, 8.5% escitalopram; $P=0.001$) and 2.2 times more likely than patients given PST (22.4% placebo, 11.9% PST; $P=0.001$), even after controlling for age, sex, treatment site, and severity of impairment. This study demonstrates that PSD can be prevented in most patients.

Psychosocial Adjustment

Thompson et al. (1989) examined 40 stroke patients and their caregivers an average of 9 months after the occurrence of stroke. They found that a lack of meaningfulness in life and overprotection by the caregiver were independent predictors of depression. Kotila et al. (1998) examined depression after stroke as part of the FINNSTROKE Study. This study examined the effect of active rehabilitation programs after discharge, together with support and social activities, on the frequency of depression among patients and caregivers 3 months and 1 year after stroke. At both 3 months and 1 year, the frequency of depression was significantly lower among patients receiving active outpatient treatment than among patients without active rehabilitation programs (at 3 months, 41% and 54%, respectively; at 1 year, 42% and 55%, respectively). The rate of depression among caregivers was significantly greater at 1 year in districts without active rehabilitation programs than in districts with them ($P=0.036$). Greater severity of impairment as measured by the Rankin Scale (Rankin 1957) was also associated with increased depression among caregivers 3 months after stroke.

Poststroke Mania

Among 366 patients with bipolar disorder, Cassidy and Carroll (2002) found that late-onset mania (i.e., after age 47) was significantly associated with risk factors for vascular disease.

Phenomenology of Secondary Mania

Starkstein et al. (1988a) examined a series of 12 consecutive patients who met DSM-III (American Psychiatric Association 1980) criteria for an organic affective syndrome, manic type. These patients, who developed mania after a stroke, traumatic brain injury, or tumors, were compared with patients with functional mania (i.e., those with no known neuropathology) (Starkstein et al. 1987).

Table 6–1.   Double-blind placebo-controlled studies of poststroke depression

Study	N	Medication (n) (maximum dose)	Duration	Evaluation method	Results	Response rate	Completion rate
Lipsey et al. 1984	34	Nortriptyline (14) (100 mg), placebo (20)	6 weeks	Ham-D, ZDS	Nortriptyline> placebo, intention to treat and efficacy	100% nortriptyline, 33% placebo	11 of 14 nortriptyline, 15 of 20 placebo
Reding et al. 1986	27	Trazodone (7) (200 mg), placebo (9)	32±6 days	ZDS	Trazodone>placebo on Barthel ADL scores for patients with abnormal DST	NR	NR
Andersen et al. 1994b	66	Citalopram (33) (20 mg, 10 mg> 65 years), placebo (33)	6 weeks	Ham-D, MES	Intention-to-treat response rates: citalopram> placebo	61% citalopram, 29% placebo	26 of 33 citalopram, 31 of 33 placebo
Grade et al. 1998	21	Methylphenidate (10) (30 mg), placebo (11)	3 weeks	Ham-D	Intention-to-treat response rates: methylphenidate> placebo	NR	9 of 10 methyl- phenidate, 10 of 11 placebo
Wiart et al. 2000	31	Fluoxetine (16) (20 mg), placebo (15)	6 weeks	MADRS	Intention-to-treat response rates: fluoxetine> placebo	62% fluoxetine, 33% placebo	14 of 16 fluoxetine, 15 of 15 placebo

Table 6–1. Double-blind placebo-controlled studies of poststroke depression *(continued)*

Study	N	Medication (n) (maximum dose)	Duration	Evaluation method	Results	Response rate	Completion rate
Robinson et al. 2000	56	Fluoxetine (23) (40 mg), nortriptyline (16) (100 mg), placebo (17)	12 weeks	Ham-D	Intention-to-treat response rates: nortriptyline> placebo= fluoxetine= placebo	14% fluoxetine, 77% nortriptyline, 31% placebo	14 of 23 fluoxetine, 13 of 16 nortriptyline, 13 of 17 placebo
Fruehwald et al. 2003	54	Fluoxetine (28) (20 mg), placebo (26)	12 weeks	BDI, Ham-D	Ham-D>15 fluoxetine=placebo Ham-D scores	69% fluoxetine Ham-D<13, 75% placebo	26 of 28 fluoxetine, 24 of 26 placebo
Rampello et al. 2005	31	Reboxetine (16) (4 mg), placebo (15)	16 weeks	BDI, Ham-D	Reboxetine>placebo for PSD patients with retardation	NR	NR

Note. ADL=activities of daily living; BDI=Beck Depression Inventory; DST=dexamethasone suppression test; Ham-D=Hamilton Rating Scale for Depression; MADRS=Montgomery-Åsberg Depression Rating Scale; MES=Melancholia Scale; NR=not reported; PSD=poststroke depression; ZDS=Zung Self-Rating Depression Scale.
Source. Adapted from Robinson RG, Starkstein SE: "Neuropsychiatric Aspects of Cerebrovascular Disorders, in *Essentials of Neuropsychiatry and Behavioral Neurosciences*, 2nd Edition. Edited by Yudofsky SC, Hales RE. Washington, DC, American Psychiatric Publishing, 2010, pp. 299–322. Used with permission. Copyright © 2010 American Psychiatric Association.

The two groups of patients showed similar frequencies of elation, pressured speech, flight of ideas, grandiose thoughts, insomnia, hallucinations, and paranoid delusions. Thus, the symptoms of mania that occurred after brain damage (secondary mania) appeared to be the same as those found in patients with mania without brain damage (primary mania).

Lesion Location

Robinson et al. (1988) reported on 17 patients with secondary mania. Most had right hemisphere lesions involving either cortical limbic areas, such as the orbitofrontal cortex and the basotemporal cortex, or subcortical nuclei, such as the head of the caudate or the thalamus. The frequency of right hemisphere lesions was significantly greater in patients with secondary mania than in patients with major depression, who tended to have left frontal or basal ganglia lesions.

Risk Factors

Not every patient with a lesion in limbic areas of the right hemisphere will develop secondary mania. Therefore, there must be risk factors for this disorder. Studies thus far have identified two such factors. One is a family genetic vulnerability for mood disorder (Robinson et al. 1988), and the other is a mild degree of subcortical atrophy as determined by increased ventricle-to-brain ratios. The subcortical atrophy probably preceded the stroke, but its cause remains unknown (Starkstein et al. 1987).

Although the mechanism of secondary mania remains unknown, both lesion studies and metabolic studies suggest that the right basotemporal cortex may play an important role. A combination of biogenic amine system dysfunction and release of tonic inhibitory input into the basotemporal cortex and lateral limbic system may lead to the production of mania.

Treatment of Secondary Mania

Although no systematic treatment studies of secondary mania have been conducted, reports have suggested several potentially useful treatment modalities. Bakchine et al. (1989) carried out a double-blind placebo-controlled treatment study in a single patient with secondary mania. Clonidine (0.6 mg/day) rapidly reversed the manic symptoms, whereas carbamazepine (1,200 mg/day) was associated with no mood changes and levodopa (375 mg/day) was associated with an increase in manic symptoms. In other treatment studies, however, the anticonvulsants valproic acid and carbamazepine as well as neuroleptics and lithium therapy have been reported to be useful in treating secondary mania (Starkstein et al. 1991). None of these treatments, however, have been evaluated in double-blind placebo-controlled studies.

Poststroke Bipolar Disorder

Although some patients have one or more manic episodes after brain injury, other manic patients also have depression after brain injury. In an effort to examine the crucial factors in determining which patients have bipolar as opposed to unipolar disorder, Starkstein et al. (1991) examined 19 patients with the diagnosis of secondary mania. The bipolar (manic-depressive) group consisted of patients who, after the occurrence of the brain lesion, met DSM-III-R (American Psychiatric Association 1987) criteria for organic mood syndrome, mania, followed or preceded by organic mood syndrome, depressed. The unipolar mania group consisted of patients who met the criteria for mania described previously (i.e., DSM-III-R organic mood syndrome, mania), not followed or preceded by depression. All patients had CT scan evidence of vascular, neoplastic, or traumatic brain lesion and no history of other neurological, toxic, or metabolic conditions.

Patients in the bipolar group were found to have significantly greater intellectual impairment as measured by MMSE scores ($P<0.05$). Almost half of the patients in the bipolar group had recurrent episodes of depression, whereas approximately one-fourth of patients in both the unipolar and bipolar groups had recurrent episodes of mania.

Of the 7 patients with bipolar disorder, 6 had lesions restricted to the right hemisphere, which involved the head of the caudate nucleus (2 patients); the thalamus (3 patients); and the head of the caudate nucleus, the dorsolateral frontal cortex, and the basotemporal cortex (1 patient). The remaining patient developed bipolar illness after surgical removal of a pituitary adenoma. In contrast to the primarily subcortical lesions in the bipolar group, 8 of 12 patients in the unipolar mania group had lesions restricted to the right hemisphere, which involved the basotemporal cortex (6 patients), orbitofrontal cortex (1 patient), and head of the caudate nucleus (1 patient). The remaining 4 patients had bilateral lesions involving the orbitofrontal cortex (3 patients) and the orbitofrontal white matter (1 patient) (Starkstein et al. 1991).

This study suggests that patients with bipolar disorder tend to have sub-cortical lesions (mainly involving the right head of the caudate or the right thalamus), whereas patients with pure mania tend to show a higher frequency of cortical lesions (particularly in the right orbitofrontal and right basotemporal cortices).

Poststroke Anxiety Disorder

Castillo et al. (1993) found that 78 patients (27%) of a group of 288 patients hospitalized with an acute stroke met DSM-III-R criteria for generalized anxiety disorder (GAD), excluding the 6-month duration criteria. Most patients with GAD also had major or minor depression (i.e., 58 of 78 patients with GAD also had depression). Depression plus anxiety was associated with left cortical lesions, whereas anxiety alone was associated with right hemisphere lesions. In a 2-year follow-up in a subgroup of 142 of these 288 patients, Castillo et al. (1995) found that 32 (23%) developed GAD after the initial in-hospital evaluation (i.e., between 3 and 24 months after stroke). Early-onset but not late-onset GAD was associated with a history of psychiatric disorder, including alcohol abuse, and early-onset anxiety had a mean duration of 1.5 months, whereas delayed-onset GAD had a mean duration of 3 months.

Aström (1996) examined 71 acute stroke patients for anxiety disorder and followed these patients over 3 years. The strongest correlates of GAD were the absence of social contacts outside the family and dependence of patients on others to perform their primary ADL. These factors were significantly more common in the GAD than in the non-GAD population 3 months, 1 year, 2 years, and 3 years after stroke.

Shimoda and Robinson (1998) examined the effect of GAD on outcome in patients with stroke. A group of 142 patients examined during hospitalization for acute stroke and followed for 2 years were diagnosed with GAD ($n=9$), major depressive disorder alone ($n=10$), both GAD and major depression ($n=10$), or neither GAD nor depression ($n=36$). An examination of the effect of GAD and major depression at the time of the initial hospital evaluation on recovery in ADL at short-term follow-up (3–6 months) demonstrated a significant effect of major depression but no significant effect of GAD and no interaction. At long-term follow-up (1–2 years), however, there was a significant interaction between major depression and GAD to inhibit recovery in ADL.

In a treatment study, Kimura and Robinson (2003) examined the effect of nortriptyline on GAD comorbid with PSD. The study included 29 patients who met criteria for GAD (17 with comorbid major depression, 10 with minor depression, and 2 with no depression). A repeated-measures analysis of variance of Hamilton Anxiety Scale (Ham-A; Hamilton 1959) scores using an intention-to-treat analysis demonstrated a significant group×time interaction ($P=0.002$) (i.e., the nortriptyline group improved more quickly than the placebo group). Planned comparisons revealed that the nortriptyline group was significantly more improved than the placebo group at nortriptyline dosages of 50 mg, 75 mg, and 100 mg. Nine of 13 (69%) in the nortriptyline-treated group had a greater than 50% reduction in Ham-A scores, whereas only 3 of 14 placebo-treated patients (21%) had a similar reduction ($P=0.017$). After patients received 50 mg of nortriptyline for 2–3 weeks, their scores improved 39% on the Ham-A but only 14% on the Ham-D ($P=0.03$). This finding suggests that anxiety symptoms were responding more rapidly than depressive symptoms.

Poststroke Psychosis

The phenomenon of hallucinations and delusions in patients who have experienced stroke has been called *agitated delirium, acute atypical psychosis, peduncular hallucinosis, release hallucinations,* and *acute organic psychosis.* In a study of acute organic psychosis occurring after stroke lesions, Rabins et al. (1991) found a very low prevalence of psychosis among stroke patients (only 5 in more than 300 consecutive admissions). All 5 of these patients, however, had right hemisphere lesions, primarily involving frontoparietal regions. When compared with 5 age-matched patients with cerebrovascular lesions in similar locations but no psychosis, patients with secondary psychosis had significantly greater subcortical atrophy, as manifested by significantly larger areas of both the frontal horn of the lateral ventricle and the body of the lateral ventricle (measured on the side contralateral to the brain lesion) (Rabins et al. 1991). Several investigators have also reported a high frequency of seizures among patients with secondary psychosis (Levine and Finklestein 1982). These seizures usually started after the occurrence of the brain lesion but before the onset of psychosis. The study by Rabins et al. (1991) found seizures in 3 of 5 patients with poststroke psychosis, compared with 0 of 5 poststroke, nonpsychiatric control subjects.

Rabins et al. (1991) hypothesized that three factors may be important in the mechanism of organic hallucinations: 1) a right hemisphere lesion involving the temporoparietal cortex, 2) seizures, and/or 3) subcortical brain atrophy.

Poststroke Apathy

Apathy is the absence or lack of motivation as manifested by decreased motor function, cognitive function, emotional feeling, and interest. It has been reported frequently among patients with brain injury. Using the Apathy Scale, Starkstein et al. (1993a) examined a consecutive series of 80 patients with single-stroke lesions and no significant impairment in comprehension. Of the 80 patients, 9 (11%) showed apathy as their only psychiatric disorder, whereas another 11% had both apathy and depression. The only demographic correlate of apathy was age, because apathetic patients (with or without depression) were significantly older than nonapathetic patients. In addition, apathetic patients showed significantly more severe deficits in ADL, and a significant interaction was noted between depression and apathy on ADL scores, with the greatest impairment found in patients who were both apathetic and depressed.

Poststroke Catastrophic Reaction

Catastrophic reaction is a term coined by Goldstein (1939) to describe the "inability of the organism to cope when faced with physical or cognitive deficits" and is expressed by anxiety, tears, aggressive behavior, swearing, displacement, refusal, renouncement, and sometimes compensatory boasting. Starkstein et al. (1993b) assessed a consecutive series of 62 patients using the Catastrophic Reaction Scale, which was developed to assess the existence and severity of catastrophic reactions. This scale has been demonstrated to be a reliable instrument in the measurement of symptoms of catastrophic reaction.

Catastrophic reactions occurred in 12 of 62 (19%) consecutive patients with acute stroke lesions. Three major findings emerged from this study. First, patients with catastrophic reactions were found to have a significantly higher frequency of familial and personal history of psychiatric disorders (mostly depression) than were patients without catastrophic reactions. Second, catastrophic reaction was not significantly more frequent among patients with aphasia (33%) than among those without (66%). This finding does not support the contention that catastrophic reactions are an understandable psychological response of "frustrated" aphasic patients (Gainotti 1972). Third, 9 of the 12 patients with catastrophic reaction also had major depression, 2 had minor depression, and only 1 was not depressed. On the other hand, among the 50 patients without catastrophic reactions, 7 had major depression, 6 had minor depression, and 37 were not depressed. Thus, catastrophic reaction is a comorbid condition that occurs in some but not all patients with PSD or that may characterize a subgroup of PSD patients.

Poststroke Pathological Emotions (Pseudobulbar Affect)

Pathological emotion is a common complication of stroke lesions. It is characterized by sudden, easily provoked episodes of crying that, although frequent, generally occur in appropriate situations and are accompanied by a congruent mood change. Pathological laughing and crying is a more severe form of emotional lability and is characterized by episodes of laughing and/or crying that are not appropriate to the context. They may appear spontaneously or may be elicited by nonemotional events, and they do not correspond to underlying emotional feelings. These disorders have also been termed *emotional incontinence* and *pseudobulbar affect*.

Robinson et al. (1993) examined the clinical correlates and treatment of emotional lability (including pathological laughter and crying) in patients with either acute or chronic stroke. They developed a Pathological Laughter and Crying Scale (PLACS) to assess the existence and severity of emotional lability. The total daily doses of nortriptyline were 25 mg for 1 week, 50 mg for 2 weeks, 70 mg for 1 week, and 100 mg for the last 2 weeks of the study. A total of 28 patients completed the 6-week protocol. Patients receiving nortriptyline showed significant improvements in PLACS scores compared with the patients receiving placebo. These differences were statistically significant both at 4 and at 6 weeks. Although a significant improvement in depression scores was also observed, improvements in PLACS scores were significant for both depressed and nondepressed patients with pathological laughing and crying, indicating that treatment response was not simply related to an improvement in depression.

In double-blind treatment studies of pathological emotion, both fluoxetine (Brown et al. 1998) and sertraline (Burns et al. 1999) have been shown to significantly reduce the frequency of crying episodes.

Conclusion

Numerous emotional and behavioral disorders can occur after cerebrovascular lesions. Major depression occurs in 21.6% of patients hospitalized for stroke, and minor depression occurs in another 20% (Robinson 2006). Major depression is significantly associated with left frontal and left basal ganglia lesions during the acute stroke period and may be successfully treated with nortriptyline or citalopram. Effective treatment of depression has been shown with nortriptyline, fluoxetine, or citalopram. Antidepressant treatment of nondepressed patients has been shown to prevent depression and augment physical and cognitive recovery.

Mania is a rare complication of stroke and is strongly associated with right hemisphere damage involving the orbitofrontal cortex, basotemporal cortex, thalamus, or basal ganglia. Risk factors for mania include a family history of psychiatric disorders and subcortical atrophy. Bipolar disorders are associated with subcortical lesions of the right hemisphere, whereas mania without depression results from right cortical lesions.

GAD, which is present in about 27% of stroke patients (Castillo et al. 1993, 1995), is associated with depression in the majority of cases. The few patients who have poststroke anxiety and no depression have a high frequency of alcoholism and lesions of the right hemisphere. Apathy is present in about 20% of stroke patients. It is associated with older age, more severe deficits in ADL, and a significantly higher frequency of lesions involving the posterior limb of the internal capsule. A controlled treatment study demonstrated that poststroke GAD can be treated effectively with nortriptyline (Lipsey et al. 1984).

Psychotic disorders are rare complications of stroke lesions. Poststroke hallucinations are associated with right hemisphere temporoparietal lesions, subcortical brain atrophy, and seizures.

Catastrophic reactions occur in about 20% of stroke patients (Starkstein et al. 1993b). These reactions are not related to the severity of impairments or the presence of aphasia but may represent a symptom for one clinical type of poststroke major depression. Pathological laughing and crying is another common complication of stroke lesions that may sometimes coexist with depression and may be successfully treated with nortriptyline, citalopram, fluoxetine, or sertraline.

Recommended Readings

Robinson RG: The Clinical Neuropsychiatry of Stroke, 2nd Edition. Cambridge, UK, Cambridge University Press, 2006

Whyte EM, Mulsant BH: Poststroke depression: epidemiology, pathophysiology and biological treatment. Biol Psychiatry 52:253–264, 2002

References

Aben I, Verhey F, Lousberg R, et al: Validity of the Beck Depression Inventory, Hospital Anxiety and Depression Scale, SCL-90, and Hamilton Depression Rating Scale as screening instruments for depression in stroke patients. Psychosomatics 43:386–393, 2002

American Psychiatric Association: Diagnostic and Statistical Manual of Mental Disorders, 3rd Edition. Washington, DC, American Psychiatric Association, 1980

American Psychiatric Association: Diagnostic and Statistical Manual of Mental Disorders, 3rd Edition, Revised. Washington, DC, American Psychiatric Association, 1987

American Psychiatric Association: Diagnostic and Statistical Manual of Mental Disorders, 4th Edition, Text Revision. Washington, DC, American Psychiatric Association, 2000

Andersen G, Vestergaard K, Riis J: Citalopram for post-stroke pathological crying. Lancet 3422:837–839, 1993

Andersen G, Vestergaard K, Lauritzen L: Effective treatment of poststroke depression with the selective serotonin reuptake inhibitor citalopram. Stroke 25:1099–1104, 1994a

Andersen G, Vestergaard K, Riis JO, et al: Incidence of post-stroke depression during the first year in a large unselected stroke population determined using a valid standardized rating scale. Acta Psychiatr Scand 90:190–195, 1994b

Aström M: Generalized anxiety disorder in stroke patients: a 3-year longitudinal study. Stroke 27:270–275, 1996

Bakchine S, Lacomblez L, Benoit N, et al: Manic-like state after bilateral orbitofrontal and right temporoparietal injury: efficacy of clonidine. Neurology 39:777–781, 1989

Bhogal SK, Teasell R, Foley N, et al: Lesion location and poststroke depression: systematic review of the methodological limitations in the literature. Stroke 35:794–802, 2004

Brown KW, Sloan RL, Pentland B: Fluoxetine as a treatment for post-stroke emotionalism. Acta Psychiatr Scand 98:455–458, 1998

Burns A, Russell E, Stratton-Powell H, et al: Sertraline in stroke-associated lability of mood. Int J Geriatr Psychiatry 14:681–685, 1999

Capuron L, Dantzer R: Cytokines and depression: the need for a new paradigm. Brain Behav Immun 17 (suppl 1):S119–S124, 2003

Cassidy E, O'Connor R, O'Keane V: Prevalence of post-stroke depression in an Irish sample and its relationship with disability and outcome following inpatient rehabilitation. Disabil Rehabil 26:71–77, 2004

Cassidy F, Carroll BJ: Vascular risk factors in late onset mania. Psychol Med 32:359–362, 2002

Castillo CS, Starkstein SE, Fedoroff JP, et al: Generalized anxiety disorder after stroke. J Nerv Ment Dis 181:100–106, 1993

Castillo CS, Schultz SK, Robinson RG: Clinical correlates of early onset and late-onset poststroke generalized anxiety. Am J Psychiatry 152:1174–1179, 1995

Downhill JE Jr, Robinson RG: Longitudinal assessment of depression and cognitive impairment following stroke. J Nerv Ment Dis 182:425–431, 1994

Folstein MF, Folstein SE, McHugh PR: "Mini-mental state": a practical method for grading the cognitive state of patients for the clinician. J Psychiatr Res 12:189–198, 1975

Fruehwald S, Gatterbauer E, Rehak P, et al: Early fluoxetine treatment of post-stroke depression: a three-month double-blind placebo-controlled study with an open-label long-term follow up. J Neurol 250:347–351, 2003

Gainotti G: Emotional behavior and hemispheric side of the brain. Cortex 8:41–55, 1972

Goldstein K: The Organism: A Holistic Approach to Biology Derived From Pathological Data in Man. New York, American Books, 1939

Grade C, Redford B, Chrostowski J, et al: Methylphenidate in early poststroke recovery: a double-blind, placebo-controlled study. Arch Phys Med Rehabil 79:1047–1050, 1998

Hamilton M: The assessment of anxiety states by rating. Br J Med Psychol 32:50–55, 1959

Jorge RE, Acion L, Moser D, et al: Escitalopram enhancement of cognitive recovery following stroke. Arch Gen Psychiatry 67:187–196, 2010

Kimura M, Robinson RG: Treatment of poststroke generalized anxiety disorder comorbid with poststroke depression: merged analysis of nortriptyline trials. Am J Geriatr Psychiatry 11:320–327, 2003

Kotila M, Numminen H, Waltimo O, et al: Depression after stroke: results of the FINNSTROKE Study. Stroke 29:368–372, 1998

Levine DN, Finklestein S: Delayed psychosis after right temporoparietal stroke or trauma: relation to epilepsy. Neurology 32:267–273, 1982

Lincoln NB, Flannaghan T: Cognitive behavioral psychotherapy for depression following stroke: a randomized controlled trial. Stroke 34:111–115, 2003

Lipsey JR, Robinson RG, Pearlson GD, et al: Nortriptyline treatment of post-stroke depression: a double-blind study. Lancet 1:297–300, 1984

Lipsey JR, Spencer WC, Rabins PV, et al: Phenomenological comparison of poststroke depression and functional depression. Am J Psychiatry 143:527–529, 1986

Lloyd-Jones D, Adams RJ, Brown TM, et al: Heart disease and stroke statistics—2010 update: a report from the American Heart Association. Circulation 121:e46–e215

Mikami K, Jorge RE, Adams HP Jr, et al: Effect of antidepressants on the course of disability following stroke. Am J Geriatr Psychiatry (in press)

Morris PLP, Robinson RG, Raphael B: Prevalence and course of depressive disorders in hospitalized stroke patients. Int J Psychiatry Med 20:349–364, 1990

Morrison JH, Molliver ME, Grzanna R: Noradrenergic innervation of cerebral cortex: widespread effects of local cortical lesions. Science 205:313–316, 1979

Murray GB, Shea V, Conn DK: Electroconvulsive therapy for poststroke depression. J Clin Psychiatry 47:258–260, 1986

Narushima K, Robinson RG: The effect of early versus late antidepressant treatment on physical impairment associated with poststroke depression: is there a time-related therapeutic window? J Nerv Ment Dis 191:645–652, 2003

Narushima K, Kosier JT, Robinson RG: A reappraisal of post-stroke depression, intra- and inter-hemispheric lesion location using meta-analysis. J Neuropsychiatry Clin Neurosci 15:422–430, 2003

Rabins PV, Starkstein SE, Robinson RG: Risk factors for developing atypical (schizophreniform) psychosis following stroke. J Neuropsychiatry Clin Neurosci 3:6–9, 1991

Rampello L, Alvano A, Chiechio S, et al: An evaluation of efficacy and safety of reboxetine in elderly patients affected by "retarded" post-stroke depression: a random, placebo-controlled study. Arch Gerontol Geriatr 40:275–285, 2005

Rankin J: Cerebral vascular accidents in patients over the age of 60, III: diagnosis and treatment. Scott Med J 2:254–268, 1957

Reding MJ, Orto LA, Winter SW, et al: Antidepressant therapy after stroke: a double-blind trial. Arch Neurol 43:763–765, 1986

Robinson RG: The controversy over post-stroke depression and lesion location. Psychiatr Times 20:39–40, 2003

Robinson RG: The Clinical Neuropsychiatry of Stroke, 2nd Edition. Cambridge, UK, Cambridge University Press, 2006

Robinson RG, Szetela B: Mood change following left hemispheric brain injury. Ann Neurol 9:447–453, 1981

Robinson RG, Kubos KL, Starr LB, et al: Mood disorders in stroke patients: importance of location of lesion. Brain 107:81–93, 1984

Robinson RG, Bolla-Wilson K, Kaplan E, et al: Depression influences intellectual impairment in stroke patients. Br J Psychiatry 148:541–547, 1986

Robinson RG, Boston JD, Starkstein SE, et al: Comparison of mania with depression following brain injury: causal factors. Am J Psychiatry 145:172–178, 1988

Robinson RG, Parikh RM, Lipsey JR, et al: Pathological laughing and crying following stroke: validation of a measurement scale and a double-blind treatment study. Am J Psychiatry 150:286–293, 1993

Robinson RG, Schultz SK, Castillo C, et al: Nortriptyline versus fluoxetine in the treatment of depression and in short term recovery after stroke: a placebo controlled, double-blind study. Am J Psychiatry 157:351–359, 2000

Robinson RG, Jorge RE, Moser DJ, et al: Escitalopram and problem-solving therapy for prevention of poststroke depression: a randomized controlled trial. JAMA 299:2391–2400, 2008

Shimoda K, Robinson RG: Effects of anxiety disorder on impairment and recovery from stroke. J Neuropsychiatry Clin Neurosci 10:34–40, 1998

Spalletta G, Guida G, De Angelis D, et al: Predictors of cognitive level and depression severity are different in patients with left and right hemispheric stroke within the first year of illness. J Neurol 249:1541–1551, 2002

Spalletta G, Bossù P, Ciaramella A, et al: The etiology of post-stroke depression: a review of the literature and a new hypothesis involving inflammatory cytokines. Mol Psychiatry 11:984–991, 2006

Starkstein SE, Pearlson GD, Boston J, et al: Mania after brain injury: a controlled study of causative factors. Arch Neurol 44:1069–1073, 1987

Starkstein SE, Boston JD, Robinson RG: Mechanisms of mania after brain injury: 12 case reports and review of the literature. J Nerv Ment Dis 176:87–100, 1988a

Starkstein SE, Robinson RG, Price TR: Comparison of patients with and without poststroke major depression matched for size and location of lesion. Arch Gen Psychiatry 45:247–252, 1988b

Starkstein SE, Fedoroff JP, Berthier MD, et al: Manic depressive and pure manic states after brain lesions. Biol Psychiatry 29:149–158, 1991

Starkstein SE, Fedoroff JP, Price TR, et al: Apathy following cerebrovascular lesions. Stroke 24:1625–1630, 1993a

Starkstein SE, Fedoroff JP, Price TR, et al: Catastrophic reaction after cerebrovascular lesions: frequency, correlates, and validation of a scale. J Neurol Neurosurg Psychiatry 5:189–194, 1993b

Thompson SC, Sobolew-Shobin A, Graham MA, et al: Psychosocial adjustment following stroke. Soc Sci Med 28:239–247, 1989

Wiart L, Petit H, Joseph PA, et al: Fluoxetine in early poststroke depression: a double-blind placebo-controlled study. Stroke 31:1829–1832, 2000

7

Brain Tumors

Trevor R. P. Price, M.D.

Kenneth L. Goetz, M.D.

Mark R. Lovell, Ph.D.

The annual incidence of primary brain tumors is 9.0 per 100,000, and that of metastatic brain tumors is 8.3 per 100,000. Evidence suggests that the overall incidence of brain tumors and the proportion of brain tumors that are malignant have been increasing since 1990 in industrialized countries (Jukich et al. 2001; Olney et al. 1996).

Brain tumors are typically classified according to whether they are primary or metastatic, as well as by location and histological cell type. Most primary tumors are either meningiomas or, more frequently, gliomas. The most common metastatic lesions are from lung and breast malignancies. Seventy percent of all tumors are supratentorial, with occurrence by lobe (Figure 7–1). This distribution is influenced to some degree by tumor histology (Table 7–1).

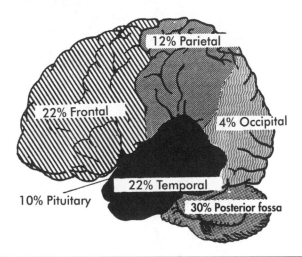

Figure 7–1.   Relative frequency of intracranial brain tumors according to location in the adult.

Source.   Reprinted from Lohr JB, Cadet JL: "Neuropsychiatric Aspects of Brain Tumors," in *The American Psychiatric Press Textbook of Neuropsychiatry.* Edited by Talbott JA, Hales RE, Yudofsky SC. Washington, DC, American Psychiatric Press, 1987, p. 355. Used with permission. Copyright © 1987 by American Psychiatric Press.

Age is also a determining factor for the frequency of various tumor types. In children, astrocytomas are most common, followed by medulloblastomas (Radhakrishnan et al. 1994). Gliomas are more often seen in the middle-aged population, and meningiomas increase in incidence among elderly people (Radhakrishnan et al. 1994). Metastatic tumors are more frequent in the elderly population and occur with greater frequency than primary brain tumors.

According to Kocher et al. (1984), primary brain tumors are up to 10 times more common among psychiatric patients than among psychiatrically healthy control subjects. Also, mental changes and behavioral symptoms, including confusion and various other neuropsychiatric symptoms, are more frequent early indicators of primary brain tumors than are classic physical manifestations such as headaches, seizures, and focal neurological signs.

Although the various tumor classifications may eventually turn out to be important in understanding the occurrence of neuropsychiatric symptoms associated with brain tumors, no large-scale, detailed studies have yet carefully examined correlations between such symptoms and various tumor characteristics. Knowledge of the neuropsychiatric and neuropsychological concomitants of brain tumors is based on a relatively small number of clinical case reports and uncontrolled case series from the older neurological and neurosurgical literature. Much of the discussion that follows draws on these sources.

General Neuropsychiatric and Neuropsychological Considerations

Patients with central nervous system (CNS) tumors can present with mental symptoms that are virtually indistinguishable from those of patients with primary psychiatric disorders (Jarquin-Valdivia 2004; Madhusoodanan et al. 2004). These symptoms run the gamut from those of major depression and schizophrenia to those of personality disorders and conversion syndromes. Over the years, many clinicians and researchers have hypothesized the existence of a predictable relationship between tumor location and neuropsychiatric phenomenology. Some studies have supported the generally held belief that depression is more common in patients with frontal lobe tumors but psychosis is more common in patients with temporal lobe neoplasms (Filley and Kleinschmidt-DeMasters 1995; Wellisch et al. 2002). Most of the older, autopsy-related studies did not strongly support this hypothesis and often concluded that the observed behavior changes were of no localizing value (Keschner et al. 1938; Selecki 1965). The nature and severity of psychiatric dysfunction accompanying tumors are probably determined by other factors that are as important as or even more important than anatomical location, because neuroanatomical substrates of particular behaviors tend not to be localized to single lobes or specific anatomical locations.

The best examples of these nonlocalized substrates are behaviors mediated by tumors involving the limbic system, which includes the temporal lobes and portions of the frontal lobes; the hypothalamus; and the midbrain. Tumors affecting any of these structures may produce similar psychopathology. Furthermore, even lesions outside the limbic system may produce similar behavior changes, attributable to limbic release or disinhibition, through diaschisis or disconnection syndromes. Limbic tumors often have been associated with depression, affective flattening, apathy, agitation, assaultive behavior, and even a

Table 7–1.   Distribution of intracranial tumors, by brain area, in the adult

Brain area	Tumor type
Brain stem	Astrocytoma, anaplastic astrocytoma, glioblastoma multiforme
Cerebellopontine angle	Acoustic schwannoma
	Meningioma
	Epidermoid cyst
	Choroid plexus papilloma
	Glomus juglare tumor
Cerebellum	Hemangioblastoma
	Metastatic carcinoma
	Astrocytoma
	Medulloblastoma
Cerebral hemisphere	Astrocytoma, anaplastic astrocytoma, glioblastoma multiforme
	Meningioma
	Metingioma
	Metastatic carcinoma
	Vascular malformation
	Oligodendroglioma
	Ependymoma
	Sarcoma
Corpus callosum	Astrocytoma, anaplastic astrocytoma, glioblastoma multiforme
	Oligodendroglioma
	Lipoma
Fourth ventricle	Ependymoma
	Choroid plexus papilloma
	Meningioma
Lateral ventricle	Ependymoma
	Meningioma
	Subependymoma
	Choroid plexus papilloma

Table 7–1. Distribution of intracranial tumors, by brain area, in the adult *(continued)*

Brain area	Tumor type
Optic chiasm and nerve	Meningioma
	Astrocytoma
Pineal region	Germ cell neoplasm
Pituitary region	Pituitary adenoma
	Craniopharyngioma
	Meningioma
	Germ cell neoplasm
Region of the foramen magnum	Meningioma
	Schwannoma
	Neurofibroma
Region about the third ventricle	Astrocytoma, anaplastic astrocytoma, glioblastoma multiforme
	Oligodendroglioma
	Ependymoma
	Pilocytic astrocytoma
Third ventricle	Colloid cyst
	Ependymoma

Source. Burger et al. 1991.

variety of psychotic symptoms. In one study of patients with tumors in or near limbic system structures who had initially been admitted to psychiatric hospitals (Malamud 1967), the patients were found to share similar psychopathology regardless of the actual structures involved.

A study by Starkstein et al. (1988) of patients who developed mania after a variety of brain lesions, including tumors, also illustrates the difficulty of trying to associate specific kinds of psychiatric symptoms with the anatomical location of tumors. Although there was an overall predominance of right-sided involvement, lesions occurred in the frontal, temporoparietal, and temporooccipital lobes, as well as in the cerebellum, thalamus, and pituitary. The authors concluded that the unifying aspect in all of these lesions was not their anatomical location but rather the interconnection of the involved structures with the orbitofrontal cortex. This finding underscores the need for formulating more sophisticated localization models in which both neuroanatomical location and connectivity are considered as they relate to focal brain lesions.

Other factors also may influence presenting symptoms and thereby diminish the localizing value of a particular behavior change. Increased intracranial pressure is a nonspecific consequence of CNS tumors in general and has been implicated in behavior changes such as apathy, depression, irritability, and agitation, as well as changes in consciousness. In a study of lesions involving the occipital lobes, Allen (1930) concluded that most observed mental changes were due to increases in intracranial pressure rather than effects of the tumors themselves.

Another factor is the patient's premorbid level of functioning, which often has a significant effect on the nature of the clinical presentation. Tumors often cause an exaggeration of the individual's previous predominant character traits and coping styles. The behavior changes associated with a brain tumor usually represent a complex combination of the patient's premorbid psychiatric status, tumor-associated mental symptoms, and adaptive or maladaptive responses to the psychological stress of having been diagnosed with a brain tumor.

According to Lishman (1987), rapidly growing tumors are more commonly associated with severe, acute psychiatric symptoms, such as agitation or psychosis, as well as with more obvious cognitive dysfunctions. Patients with slow-growing tumors are more likely to present with vague personality changes, apathy, or depression, often without associated cognitive changes. Multiple tumor foci also tend to produce behavioral symptoms with greater frequency than do single lesions.

In general, the factors that most significantly influence symptom formation appear to be the extent of tumor involvement, the rapidity of the tumor's growth, and the tumor's propensity to cause increased intracranial pressure. In addition, the patient's premorbid psychiatric history, level of functioning, and characteristic psychological coping mechanisms may play a significant contributing role in determining the nature of the patient's particular symptoms. In fact, lesion location may often play a relatively minor role.

Although lesion location is probably not the most important factor in determining the occurrence of specific types of neuropsychiatric symptoms, some reports suggest that brain lesions in certain locations may be associated with increased frequency of psychiatric symptoms. For example, although Keschner et al. (1936) found no overall difference in the types of behavioral symptoms associated with tumors of the frontal and temporal lobes, they did find that to a small degree, complex visual and auditory hallucinations were more common among patients with tumors of the temporal lobe and that "facetiousness" was more frequently found among those with tumors of the frontal lobe. Behavior changes are twice as likely to occur among patients with supratentorial tumors as among those with infratentorial tumors (Keschner et al. 1938). Likewise, mental changes tend to be early symptoms in 18% of patients with supratentorial tumors but in only 5% of those with infratentorial tumors. Psychiatric disturbances also were found to be more common among patients with tumors of the frontal and temporal lobes than in those with tumors of the parietal or occipital lobes.

Psychotic symptoms tend to be particularly frequent among patients with tumors of the temporal lobes and pituitary gland and much less common among those with occipital and cerebellar tumors, although this finding seems to depend on the particular study being reviewed (Davison and Bagley 1969).

Despite limitations, the literature taken as a whole seems to support a higher frequency of behavior changes among patients with lesions of the frontal and temporal lobes, as well as those with lesions involving deep midline structures. Similarly, bilateral tumors and those with multifocal involvement appear to be more frequently associated with neuropsychiatric symptoms.

Neuropsychiatric and Neuropsychological Symptoms and Brain Tumor Location

In the discussion that follows, we review the range of neuropsychiatric and neuropsychological signs and symptoms that have been reported to co-occur preferentially with brain tumors involving various anatomical structures, including the frontal, temporal, parietal, and occipital lobes; the diencephalon; the corpus callosum; the pituitary; and the posterior fossa.

Tumors of the Frontal Lobe

Neuropsychiatric and Behavioral Manifestations

Tumors of the frontal lobes are frequently associated with behavioral symptoms. One study reported mental changes in as many as 90% of cases (Strauss and Keschner 1935). Of these patients, 43% manifested such changes early in the course of their illness.

Injuries to the frontal lobes have been associated with three kinds of clinical syndromes (Cummings 1993). Orbitofrontal syndrome is characterized by changes in personality. These patients typically present with irritability and lability. Cognitively, patients with this syndrome often have poor judgment and a lack of insight into their behavior. Conversely, patients with injury to the frontal convexities, the so-called dorsolateral prefrontal syndrome, often present with apathy, indifference, and psychomotor retardation. Such patients have difficulty initiating or persisting in behavioral activities, have problems with sustained attention and/or sequencing, and may show perseverative behavior (Goldberg 1986). These deficits may not be apparent on standard intellectual or neuropsychological assessments but usually become apparent with more specific tests of executive functioning, such as the Wisconsin Card Sorting Test (Goldberg 1986; Heaton 1985). Finally, an anterior cingulate syndrome has been described. Patients with this syndrome may be akinetic, with mutism and an inability to respond to commands.

Most patients with tumors of the frontal lobe present with combinations of symptoms, probably due in part to the fact that tumors of the frontal lobe are rarely confined to a single subregion and may cause effects on other areas, both directly and indirectly via pressure effects and edema, as well as by diaschisis and disconnection. It is therefore difficult to find descriptions of these three syndromes in pure form when reviewing the literature on frontal lobe neoplasms. Psychiatric symptoms also appear to be more common in patients with lesions of the anterior frontal lobe than in those with lesions of the posterior frontal lobe, suggesting that tumor location on the anteroposterior gradient within the frontal lobe may play a role in determining clinical presentation (Gautier-Smith 1970).

Anxiety has been noted to increase with frontal tumor progression (Kaplan and Miner 1997). Affective symptoms are common and can include depression, irritability, apathy, and euphoria. Often, psychomotor retardation with aspontaneity, hypokinesia, or akinesia is present. In one study of 25 patients with frontal lobe tumors (Direkze et al. 1971), 20% had initially presented to psychiatric units with what appeared to be mood disturbances. In their study of 85 patients, Strauss and Keschner (1935) reported affective symptoms in 63%, of whom 30% presented with euphoria and 4% presented with hypomania. Although these authors found no correlation between clinical presentations and laterality of lesions, Belyi (1987) noted that patients with right frontal lesions tended to present with euphoria, whereas those with left frontal lesions tended to present with akinesia, abulia, and depressed affect. Lampl et al. (1995) reported psychiatric symptoms only in patients with right frontal as opposed to left frontal meningiomas. Burns and Swerdlow (2003) reported pedophilia and constructional apraxia signs and symptoms occurring in association with a right orbitofrontal tumor.

Changes in personality have been found in up to 70% of patients with frontal lobe tumors (Strauss and Keschner 1935). Personality changes, which have been described as "characteristic" of frontal lobe disease (Pincus and Tucker 1978), include irresponsibility, childishness, facetiousness, disinhibition, and indifference toward others, as well as inappropriate sexual behavior. Although these behaviors are consistent with descriptions of the characteristic features of orbitofrontal syndrome, similar "frontal lobe" personality changes have been described in patients with temporal lobe and diencephalic lesions, probably as a result of the rich, reciprocal interconnections that link the temporal, limbic, and frontal regions.

Psychotic symptoms occur with some regularity in patients with frontal lobe tumors. Strauss and Keschner (1935) reported a 10% incidence of both delusions and hallucinations in their series. Other psychotic symptoms reported in patients with frontal lobe tumors have included paranoid ideation and ideas of reference. Typically, delusions secondary to intracranial tumors are less complex than those that occur as part of the delusional systems of patients with schizophrenia. Likewise, simple rather than complex hallucinations and visual rather than auditory hallucinations tend to occur in patients with brain tumors.

Neuropsychological Manifestations

Cognitively, patients with tumors of the frontal region of the brain, and of the prefrontal area in particular, often present with significant behavior changes in the absence of obvious intellectual decline or focal neurological dysfunction. In such patients, previously acquired cognitive skills are often preserved, and performance on formal intelligence testing may be quite adequate. More sophisticated neuropsychological assessment of executive functioning, however, often detects profound deficits in the individual's ability to organize, initiate, and direct personal behavior (Lezak 1995; Teuber 1972).

Tumors of the frontal lobes also can result in significant deficits in attentional processes. In addition, tumors of the posterior frontal lobe can lead to expressive (Broca's) aphasia when the lesion is localized to the dominant hemisphere (Benson 1979) or to aprosody when the lesion is localized to the anterior nondominant hemisphere (Ross 1988).

Tumors of the Temporal Lobe

Neuropsychiatric and Behavioral Manifestations

In any discussion of the psychiatric and behavioral symptoms associated with tumors of the temporal lobe, it is important to distinguish between seizure-associated and non-seizure-associated symptoms and, within the former category, ictal and interictal phenomena. Ictal phenomena are discussed in Chapter 5, "Seizure Disorders." In this section, we confine our discussion to non-seizure-associated and interictal symptoms due to temporal lobe tumors.

Patients with temporal lobe tumors have been noted to have a high frequency of schizophrenia-like illnesses. Malamud (1967) reported that 6 (55%) of 11 patients with temporal lobe tumors initially presented with a diagnosis of schizophrenia. Selecki (1965) reported that an initial diagnosis of schizophrenia had been made in 2 of his 9 patients with temporal lobe tumors, and he reported auditory hallucinations in 5. More recently, Roberts et al. (1990) reported that gangliogliomas, neoplastic hamartomatous lesions that preferentially involve the left medial temporal lobes, are frequently found in patients with delayed-onset, schizophrenia-like psychoses associated with chronic temporal lobe epilepsy.

Patients with temporal lobe dysfunction due to tumors or other causes often present with psychotic symptoms that are somewhat atypical for classic schizophrenia. Supporting the association between psychotic symptomatology and temporal lobe tumors is the work of Davison and Bagley (1969), who reviewed the cases of 77 psychotic patients with known brain neoplasms and found that tumors of the temporal lobes were most frequent.

Other studies, however, have not confirmed the apparent high frequency of psychotic syndromes in patients with temporal lobe tumors. Keschner et al. (1936) studied 110 such patients and found that only 2 had complex hallucinations. In another study (Mulder and Daly 1952), only 4 (4%) of 100 patients with temporal lobe tumors had psychotic symptoms. Strobos (1953) noted complex auditory hallucinations in only 1 (1.6%) of his 62 patients with temporal lobe tumors. He found complex visual hallucinations in 5 (8%) and simple olfactory or gustatory hallucinations in 19 (31%), although these hallucinations almost invariably immediately preceded the onset of seizures.

Neuropsychiatric symptoms associated with temporal lobe tumors tend to be similar to those seen in patients with frontal lobe tumors and may include depressed mood with apathy and irritability and euphoric, expansive mood with hypomania or mania.

Personality change has been described in more than 50% of patients with temporal lobe tumors and may be an early symptom thereof (Keschner et al. 1936). Other personality changes commonly caused by brain tumors include affective lability, episodic behavioral dyscontrol, intermittent anger, irritability, euphoria, and facetiousness (Lishman 1987).

Anxiety symptoms appear to be commonly associated with temporal lobe tumors. Mulder and Daly (1952) noted anxiety in 36 (36%) of their 100 patients. Two cases of panic attacks in patients with right temporal lobe tumors have been reported (Drubach and Kelly 1989; Ghadirian et al. 1986).

Neuropsychological Manifestations

Tumors of the temporal lobes can also result in neuropsychological and cognitive deficits. Verbal or nonverbal memory functioning may be affected, depending on the cerebral hemisphere involved. Dysfunction of the dominant temporal lobe is often associated with deficits in the ability to learn and remember verbal information, whereas nondominant temporal lobe dysfunction is often associated with deficits in acquiring and retaining nonverbal (i.e., visuospatial) information (Bauer et al. 1993; Butters and Milotis 1979). Tumors of the dominant temporal lobe also may result in receptive (Wernicke's) aphasia, whereas tumors of the nondominant lobe may lead to disruption of the discrimination of nonspeech sounds (Spreen et al. 1965).

Tumors of the Parietal Lobe

Neuropsychiatric and Behavioral Manifestations

In general, tumors of the parietal lobe are relatively "silent" with respect to psychiatric symptoms (Critchley 1964). Schlesinger (1950) found affective symptoms in only 5 (16%) of 31 patients with parietal lobe tumors. The affective symptoms in these patients were predominantly depression and apathy, rather than euphoria or mania. In case reports, authors have reported on depression in a woman with a left parietal lesion (Madhusoodanan et al. 2004) and mania in patients with right parietal tumors (Khouzam et al. 1994; Salazar-Calderon Perriggo et al. 1993).

Psychotic symptoms also appear to be less common in patients with parietal lobe tumors. Selecki (1965), however, reported episodes of "paranoid psychosis" in 2 of the 7 patients with parietal lobe tumors in his series. Cotard's syndrome, involving the denial of one's own existence, has been reported in a patient with a left parietal astrocytoma (Bhatia 1993).

Neuropsychological Manifestations

In general, parietal lobe tumors are more likely to lead to cognitive than to psychiatric symptoms. Tumors of the anterior parietal lobes may result in abnormalities of sensory perception in the contralateral hand. Inability of the individual to perceive objects placed in the hand (astereognosis) is common and may have localizing value with regard to the contralateral parietal cortex. Difficulty in recognizing shapes, letters, and numbers drawn on the hand (agraphesthesia) is common and may aid in localizing neoplasms to the parietal lobes. Apraxias also may be present. Parietal lobe tumors, particularly when localized to the nondominant hemisphere, may interfere with the ability to decipher visuospatial information (Warrington and Rabin 1970).

Tumors of the dominant parietal lobe may lead to dysgraphia, acalculia, finger agnosia, and right-left confusion (Gerstmann's syndrome) and often affect reading and spelling. Individuals with parietal lobe tumors often present with a marked lack of awareness or even frank denial of their neurological and neuropsychiatric difficulties. Such phenomena are referred to as *anosognosia* or *neglect syndrome*. Because of the often bizarre neurological complaints and atypical symptoms that may accompany parietal lobe tumors, patients with these lesions are often thought to have psychiatric problems and often initially receive misdiagnoses of either a conversion disorder or some other type of somatization disorder (Jones and Barklage 1990).

Tumors of the Occipital Lobe

Neuropsychiatric and Behavioral Manifestations

Patients with tumors of the occipital lobe also may present with psychiatric symptoms, although they are less likely to do so than are patients with tumors of the frontal or temporal lobes (Keschner et al. 1938). In 1930, Allen found psychiatric symptoms in 55% of a large series (*N*=40) of patients with occipital lobe tumors. In 17% of these patients, behavioral symptoms had been the presenting complaint. The most characteristic finding was visual hallucinations, which were present in 25%. These hallucinations tended to be simple and unformed and were frequently merely flashes of light. Only 2 patients had complex visual hallucinations.

Other symptoms that have been observed in patients with occipital lobe tumors include agitation, irritability, suspiciousness, and fatigue. Keschner et al. (1938) observed affective symptoms in 5 (45%) of 11 patients with occipital lobe tumors. Three (27%) of these patients were dysphoric, and 2 (18%) presented with euphoria or facetiousness.

Neuropsychological Manifestations

Tumors of the occipital lobes may cause significant and characteristic difficulties in cognitive and perceptual functions. A typical finding in patients with occipital lobe neoplasms is homonymous hemianopsia. Inability to recognize items visually (visual agnosia) also may be seen (Lezak 1995). Inability to recognize familiar faces (prosopagnosia) also may accompany neoplastic lesions in the occipital lobes, particularly when the lesions are bilateral (Meadows 1974).

Diencephalic Tumors

Neuropsychiatric and Behavioral Manifestations

Tumors of the diencephalon typically involve regions that are part of or closely contiguous to the limbic system. These lesions also interrupt the various cortical-striatal-pallidal-thalamic-cortical loops, which affect many frontal lobe functions (Alexander and Crutcher 1990). It is therefore not surprising that these lesions are often associated with psychiatric and behavioral disturbances. For example, Malamud (1967) reported diagnoses of schizophrenia in 4 of 7 patients with tumors involving structures near the third ventricle. Cairns and Mosberg (1951) reported "emotional instability" and psychosis in patients with colloid cysts of the third ventricle. Burkle and Lipowski (1978) also reported depression, affective flattening, and withdrawal in a patient with a colloid cyst of the third ventricle. Personality changes similar to those seen in patients with frontal lobe disease (Gutmann et al. 1990), akinetic mutism (Cairns et al. 1941), catatonia (Neuman et al. 1996), or obsessive-compulsive disorder (Gamazo-

Garrán et al. 2002) have all been reported in patients with diencephalic or deep midline tumors.

Hypothalamic tumors have been associated with disorders of eating behavior, including hyperphagia (Coffey 1989), and with symptoms that are indistinguishable from those of anorexia nervosa (Lin et al. 2003). Chipkevitch (1994) reported on 21 cases in the literature in which patients with brain lesions presented with symptoms consistent with a diagnosis of anorexia nervosa. Eleven (52%) of these patients had tumors of the hypothalamus. In 8 of these patients, surgical resection or radiation treatment led to improvement in the symptoms of anorexia. Patients with lesions of the hypothalamus also can present with hypersomnia and daytime somnolence.

Neuropsychological Manifestations

Neoplasms originating in subcortical brain regions often have their most significant effects on memory. These lesions often result in significant impairment in the retrieval of learned material. Detailed neuropsychological evaluations of patients with subcortical tumors may identify a pattern of "subcortical dementia" characterized by a general slowing of thought processes, forgetfulness, apathy, abulia, and depression and an impaired ability to manipulate acquired knowledge (Cummings 1990). Tumors in this area also may lead indirectly to more diffuse, generalized cognitive dysfunction by interfering with the normal circulation of cerebrospinal fluid, causing hydrocephalus.

Tumors of the Corpus Callosum

Tumors of the corpus callosum, especially involving the genu and splenium (Schlesinger 1950), have been associated with behavioral symptoms in up to 90% of patients (Selecki 1964). Although a broad array of behavior changes, including psychosis and personality changes, have been reported, affective symptoms appear to be particularly common with tumors involving this area. In one study, patients with corpus callosum tumors were compared with patients with other types of tumors; significantly more depression was found in the group with tumors of the corpus callosum (Nasrallah and McChesney 1981). Tanaghow et al. (1989) described a patient with a corpus callosum tumor without focal neurological findings who had initially presented with atypical features of depression and prominent cognitive deficits.

Pituitary Tumors

Patients with pituitary tumors often present with behavior changes resulting from upward extension of the tumor to other structures, particularly those in the diencephalon. This is a common occurrence in patients with craniopharyngiomas, who sometimes present with disorders of sleep or temperature regulation, clinical phenomena that are ordinarily more common with tumors of the hypothalamus. Anorexia nervosa syndromes also have been reported in patients with craniopharyngiomas (Chipkevitch 1994).

Tumors of the pituitary also can result in endocrine disturbances, which can cause neuropsychiatric symptoms. Basophilic adenomas are commonly associated with Cushing's syndrome, which is likewise often associated with affective lability, depression, or psychotic symptoms. Patients with acidophilic adenomas often present with acromegaly, which has been associated, although infrequently, with both anxiety and depression (Avery 1973).

Like patients with brain tumors involving other anatomical locations, patients with pituitary tumors have been reported to experience the entire spectrum of psychiatric symptoms, from depression and apathy (Weitzner et al. 2005) to paranoia. White and Cobb (1955), in a review of 5 patients with pituitary lesions, reported delusions and hallucinations in 3 patients (60%). In a study by Russell and Pennybacker (1961), 8 (33%) of 24 patients had severe mental disturbances that dominated their clinical picture, and 3 (13%) had initially presented to psychiatric hospitals for diagnosis and treatment.

Tumors of the Posterior Fossa

Although infratentorial and posterior fossa lesions are less common overall, patients with these lesions have been reported to have all of the psychiatric and behavioral disturbances that have been described in patients with supratentorial tumors. In one series, psychiatric and behavioral symptoms were found in 76% of patients with lesions of the posterior fossa and included paranoid delusions and affective disorders (Wilson and Rupp 1946). Pollack et al. (1996) also reported affective disorders, psychosis, personality change, and somatization in their small series. Cases of mania also have been noted (e.g., Greenberg and Brown 1985). Tumors of the posterior fossa have been reported to be associated with irritability, apathy, hypersomnolence, and auditory hallucinations (Cairns 1950). Visual hallucinations have been reported in conjunction with tumors compressing the midbrain (Dunn and Weisberg 1983; Nadvi and van Dellen 1994), and manic or mixed states have been described in 3 adults with acoustic neuroma (Kalayam et al. 1994). Overanxious disorder with school phobia was reported in a 12-year-old boy with a fourth-ventricle tumor (Blackman and Wheler 1987). The anxiety symptoms were alleviated by surgical removal of the tumor.

Clinical Diagnosis

General Clinical Characteristics of Patients With Brain Tumors

The most characteristic clinical feature of CNS tumors is the progressive appearance of focal neurological signs and symptoms in addition to neuropsychiatric symptoms. The latter are actually more frequent than the neurological signs and symptoms in early brain tumors and may include changes in personality and affect, altered sensorium, and cognitive and memory dysfunction. The specific constellation of clinical phenomena encountered and the rapidity with which they progress depend on the tumor's type, size, location, and rate of growth; whether it is benign or malignant; and, if the latter, how aggressive it is and whether there is associated cerebral edema, increased intracranial pressure, and hydrocephalus.

Typical neurological signs and symptoms associated with brain tumors include headaches (25%–35%), nausea and vomiting (33%), seizures (20%–50%), papilledema, and visual changes, including field cuts and diplopia. Focal motor and sensory changes are of considerable value in localizing the tumor.

Suspecting a Brain Tumor in a Psychiatric Patient

Although recognition of brain tumors in patients presenting with characteristic focal neurological signs and symptoms should not ordinarily be problematic, diagnosing a brain tumor promptly and accurately may be quite difficult in a patient presenting with predominantly psychiatric and behavioral symptoms. However, the occurrence of one or more of the following five signs and symptoms in a known psychiatric patient or in a patient presenting for the first time with psychiatric symptoms should heighten the clinician's index of suspicion regarding the possibility of a brain tumor:

1. Seizures, especially if of new onset in an adult and if focal or partial, with or without secondary generalization. Seizures may be the initial neurological manifestation of a tumor in up to 50% of cases.
2. Headaches, especially those that are of new onset; that are generalized and dull (i.e., nonspecific); that are of increasing severity and/or frequency; or that are positional, nocturnal, or present immediately on awakening.
3. Nausea and vomiting, especially in conjunction with headaches.
4. Sensory changes: visual changes such as loss or diminution of vision, visual field defects, or diplopia; auditory changes such as tinnitus or hearing loss, especially when unilateral; and vertigo.
5. Other focal neurological signs and symptoms, such as localized weakness, localized sensory loss, paresthesias or dysesthesias, ataxia, and incoordination.

The clinician should bear in mind that nausea and vomiting, visual field defects, papilledema, and other focal neurological signs and symptoms may not be seen until very late, especially with "silent" tumors, such as meningiomas or slow-growing astrocytomas, and other kinds of tumors occurring in relatively "silent" locations (see next subsection).

Diagnostic Evaluation

A comprehensive, careful, and detailed history of the nature and time course of both psychiatric and neurological signs and symptoms is the cornerstone of diagnosis. This should be supplemented by careful physical and neurological examinations, appropriate brain imaging and electrodiagnostic studies, and bedside neurocognitive assessment, including the Mini-Mental State Examination (MMSE), as well as formal neuropsychological testing.

All psychiatric patients, and particularly those in whom the psychiatrist is considering a brain tumor in the differential diagnosis, should have full and careful physical, neurological, and mental status examinations. It is important to be aware that despite repeated careful clinical examinations, some brain tumors may not become clinically apparent until relatively late in their course. Such tumors often involve the anterior frontal lobes, corpus callosum, nondominant parietal and temporal lobes, and posterior fossa, the so-called silent regions.

Treatment of Psychiatric and Behavioral Symptoms Due to Brain Tumors

Pharmacological Management

Primary Psychiatric Disorders

The psychopharmacological management of brain tumor patients with preexisting primary psychiatric illnesses should follow the same general therapeutic principles that apply to tumor-free patients with similar disorders. However, the psychiatrist needs to be cognizant of the potential need to make downward adjustments in medication dosage and to use drugs that are less likely to cause delirium in patients with brain tumors, given these patients' increased susceptibility to many of the side effects of psychotropic medications. This vigilance is especially important for patients who are in the immediate postoperative period or are receiving chemotherapy or radiation therapy. Lithium, low-potency antipsychotic drugs, tertiary amine tricyclic antidepressants (TCAs), and antiparkinsonian agents all have significant dose-related deliriogenic potential when given individually, and especially when they are given in combination or with other potentially deliriogenic agents. The psychiatrist may need to substitute an atypical antipsychotic, carbamazepine, valproic acid, lamotrigine, oxcarbazepine, gabapentin, or a benzodiazepine, such as lorazepam or clonazepam, for lithium in patients with mania; a newer-generation heterocyclic or secondary amine TCA, a selective serotonin reuptake inhibitor (SSRI), or one of the newer, novel-structured antidepressants for tertiary amine TCAs in patients with depression; or one of the atypical antipsychotics for standard neuroleptics in patients with schizophrenia.

Another significant concern is the potential for some drugs to precipitate seizures, especially in patients with brain tumors. Neuroleptics, antidepressants, and lithium all can lower seizure threshold to varying degrees. Although the available data are inconclusive, standard neuroleptics such as molindone and fluphenazine, and possibly haloperidol (Mendez et al. 1984), are among the older antipsychotic drugs that are believed to carry the smallest risk for seizures, whereas low-potency agents such as chlorpromazine and clozapine are associated with an increased frequency of seizures (Stoudemire et al. 1993). In general, the atypical antipsychotics are believed to have a lower likelihood of precipitating seizures and thus offer an important therapeutic advantage over the old-line antipsychotics. Among the antidepressants, maprotiline and bupropion appear to have the greatest seizure-inducing potential (Dubovsky 1992). It is not clear which antidepressants carry the smallest overall risk, but the SSRIs have been reported to have a low likelihood of precipitating seizures. In acutely manic patients with brain tumors, for whom lithium might otherwise be the drug of choice, carbamazepine, valproic acid, oxcarbazepine, lorazepam, clonazepam, and gabapentin—all of which have anticonvulsant properties—may be preferable alternatives.

The psychiatrist should also bear in mind that patients with brain tumors who have psychiatric disorders and are also taking anticonvulsants for a known seizure diathesis should be monitored carefully for the adequacy of anticonvulsant blood levels and should have their anticonvulsant dosage increased or decreased as appropriate when psychotropic agents are given. Certain of these medications have epileptogenic effects, as well as the potential for decreasing or increasing anticonvulsant blood levels.

Mental Symptoms and Disorders

The psychopharmacological treatment of organic mental symptoms and syndromes caused by cerebral tumors follows the same general principles as the drug treatment of phenomenologically similar symptoms due to primary psychiatric illnesses. In treating secondary psychiatric symptoms pharmacologically in patients with brain tumors, some important caveats must be borne in mind. Patients with psychiatric symptoms that are a direct consequence of a brain tumor frequently respond favorably to medications but will frequently tolerate them only in significantly lower dosages. Thus, side-effect profiles of psychotropic drugs being considered for the treatment of patients with brain tumors must be very carefully considered, especially with regard to sedative, extrapyramidal, deliriogenic, and epileptogenic effects and potential drug interactions.

Psychotic Disorders

First-generation antipsychotic medications may be beneficial in treating the hallucinations, delusions, and thought content and process disturbances that may accompany tumor-associated psychotic syndromes. High-potency antipsychotics, which have fewer nonneurological side effects than do the low-potency antipsychotics, are generally preferable if one of the standard neuroleptics is to be used; however, the former more often cause extrapyramidal symptoms, which may be more severe and persistent in patients with brain tumors. In patients with "organic" psychotic disorders, the therapeutically effective antipsychotic dosage is often lower than that required for the treatment of primary "functional" psychoses. Thus, as little as 1–5 mg, rather than 10–20 mg, of haloperidol per day (or equivalent dosages of other antipsychotics) may be effective. The atypical antipsychotics have been reported to be effective in patients with other psychotic syndromes associated with neurological disorders and have, as a result of their low side-effect profile, generally been well tolerated. Thus, the atypical antipsychotics may well turn out to be the treatment of choice in brain tumor patients with psychotic symptoms. When initiating treatment with antipsychotics, the psychiatrist should "start low and go slow." This precept is especially true for elderly patients, in whom effective antipsychotic dosages may be lower than in younger patients.

Antiparkinsonian agents, such as benztropine, trihexyphenidyl, and orphenadrine, are effective in the treatment of extrapyramidal side effects resulting from the use of neuroleptics in patients with brain tumors. However, in such patients, these agents have a greater likelihood of causing or contributing to the occurrence of anticholinergic delirium when they are used in conjunction with low-potency neuroleptics and/or tertiary amine TCAs. Thus, their use generally should be avoided unless a clear-cut clinical indication exists, and the dosage of antiparkinsonian agents should be minimized when these other drugs are used. Diphenhydramine or amantadine for dystonic and parkinsonian symptoms and benzodiazepines or β-blockers for akathisia can be effective alternatives and have less potential for causing delirium.

Mood Disorders

Antidepressant medications are often effective in the treatment of depressive mood disorders in patients with brain tumors. Standard TCAs are useful, but currently the SSRIs, newer-generation heterocyclic antidepressants, and secondary amine TCAs are often used preferentially. The SSRIs are relatively expensive, but they are therapeutically effective and do not cause delirium, do have a favorable side-effect profile, and often may be effective in such patients. Methylphenidate has been shown to be effective (Masand et al. 1991) and to have a rapid onset of action (Woods et al. 1986) in patients with brain tumors. Because methylphenidate is generally well tolerated and does not lower the seizure threshold, its use as an antidepressant in patients with brain tumors is increasing.

Monoamine oxidase inhibitors may be effective when other antidepressants are not. They do not ordinarily pose an undue risk in patients with brain tumors, but the clinician must bear in mind that the cognitive impairment that often occurs in such patients may interfere with their ability to maintain a tyramine-free diet.

If single-antidepressant regimens are ineffective, various combinations may work. When pharmacological treatments have failed, electroconvulsive therapy (ECT) or repetitive transcranial magnetic stimulation with appropriate precautions should be given serious consideration.

Mood disorders with manic features due to brain tumors, although relatively rare, generally respond to lithium in the usual therapeutic range of 0.8–1.2 mEq/L. For patients in whom seizures have been a part of the clinical picture, however, carbamazepine, valproate, oxcarbazepine, lorazepam, clonazepam, gabapentin, and—in cases in which drug therapy has been ineffective—ECT may be preferable alternatives.

Newer treatment approaches, including vagus nerve stimulation and transcranial magnetic stimulation, have shown promise in early clinical trials with a variety of mood disorders, including depression, mania (Berman et al. 2000; Grisaru et al. 1998; Rush et al. 2000), and psychotic symptoms (Hoffman et al. 1999). Clarification of their future role in the treatment of brain tumor patients with depression and other neuropsychiatric syndromes awaits further research.

Anxiety Disorders

Anxiety symptoms caused either directly or indirectly by brain tumors should not be treated with neuroleptics unless psychotic features are present. The benzodiazepines are often effective and have the added benefit of possessing anticonvulsant properties. However, benzodiazepines may induce delirium in patients with organic brain disease, including brain tumors. This argues for the preferential use of short-acting agents in lower dosages, especially in older patients. Other disadvantages of benzodiazepines include their abuse potential and their occasional propensity (especially with the varieties that have long half-lives) to cause seemingly paradoxical reactions, characterized by increased arousal and agitation. Buspirone, which is free of these potentially negative effects, should be considered as an alternative to the benzodiazepines.

Its main drawbacks are its delayed onset and an only modest degree of anxiolytic action. Hydroxyzine, SSRIs, or low dosages of tertiary amine TCAs, such as doxepin or amitriptyline, also may have beneficial anxiolytic effects in some patients. Finally, panic attacks associated with temporal lobe tumors may respond to carbamazepine, valproate, or primidone, as well as to the usual antidepressant and antianxiety drugs.

Delirium

Delirium in patients with brain tumors may be associated with a wide variety of psychiatric and behavioral symptoms. Hallucinations (especially visual) and delusions are common in patients with delirium and often respond to symptomatic treatment with low dosages of haloperidol, other high-potency neuroleptics, or one of the atypical antipsychotics, while the underlying causes of the delirium are being sought and treated.

Personality Changes

Mood lability may be associated with personality changes due to a brain tumor and may respond to lithium, carbamazepine, or other mood stabilizers. Some patients with frontal lobe syndromes associated with tumors respond to carbamazepine, as do some patients with temporal lobe tumors who present with associated interictal aggression and violent behavior. Patients with brain tumors who have impulse dyscontrol and rageful, explosive episodes, like patients with intermittent explosive disorders due to other medical and neurological conditions, may respond to empirical therapeutic trials of anticonvulsants, such as carbamazepine, valproic acid, or phenytoin; psychotropics, including lithium; high-potency neuroleptics; or stimulants or β-blockers.

Psychotherapeutic Management

Supportive psychotherapy geared to the patient's current overall functional status, psychosocial situation, interpersonal and family relationships, cognitive capacities, and emotional needs is a very important element in the treatment of any brain tumor patient. The often devastating psychological stress of initially receiving a brain tumor diagnosis and then having to undergo various invasive, painful, and potentially debilitating diagnostic studies and subsequent treatments for it can trigger in the patient both the recurrence of preexisting primary psychiatric disorders and the de novo appearance of reactive psychiatric symptoms. Likewise, the diagnosis and treatment of a brain tumor in a loved one is enormously stressful for families. Under any clinical scenario, supportive psychotherapy for patients and supportive psychoeducation and therapeutic interventions for their families are likely to be well received and very helpful for both and should play a major role in overall clinical management.

Ideally, supportive psychotherapy for both the patient and the family or significant others should focus primarily on concrete, reality-based cognitive and psychoeducational issues relating to diagnosis, treatment, and prognosis of the patient's brain tumor. Psychotherapeutic interactions with the patient should be geared to the patient's cognitive capacities. Over time, the focus of psychotherapy often shifts to the effect of the illness on the patient's emotional and functional status, its effect on the family, the real and imagined challenges of coping with actual or anticipated functional disabilities, and the difficult processes of dealing with anticipatory grief related to potential losses and eventual death. Patients vary widely in their capacity to adjust to and cope with the potentially devastating consequences of brain tumors, and the success of their adjustment and adaptation greatly depends on the flexibility of their premorbid coping abilities. Some patients may appear to be little affected, whereas others may experience severe and even overwhelming symptoms of anxiety and depression. These latter patients may experience greater difficulty continuing to function optimally in their usual work and family roles and may need more aggressive psychotherapeutic and psychopharmacological interventions.

Cognitive Rehabilitation

In addition to psychopharmacological and psychotherapeutic treatments, cognitive, occupational, and vocational rehabilitative interventions can be very helpful for patients whose tumors, or the treatments they have received for them, have produced behavioral, cognitive, or functional sequelae. Such sequelae can be identified and quantified by comparing preoperative with postoperative results on the Halstead-Reitan Neuropsychological Test Battery (Reitan and Wolfson 1993) or other comprehensive neuropsychological test batteries and various functional assessment tools. Serial testing at intervals during the patient's postoperative rehabilitation allows for objective documentation of neuropsychological and functional deficits and allows for objective monitoring of improvement or deterioration over time. Thus, in general, neuropsychological and functional assessments should be a standard part of the pretreatment evaluation and posttreatment follow-up of patients receiving treatment for brain tumors.

Cognitive, occupational, and vocational rehabilitative strategies can be developed that will seek to address deficits in intellectual, language, visuospatial, memory, and neurocognitive functioning, as well as vocational functioning and ability to carry out activities of daily living, resulting from a brain tumor. In addition, behavioral techniques have been successfully applied to problematic behaviors resulting from insults to the brain. Such interventions may be used alone or in conjunction with other therapies. For a more detailed discussion of these various approaches, see Chapter 12, "Cognitive Rehabilitation and Behavior Therapy for Patients With Neuropsychiatric Disorders."

Conclusion

Brain tumors often are associated with a broad range of psychiatric, behavioral, and neurocognitive symptoms. The differential diagnosis of any patient who has acute or progressive changes in behavior, personality, or cognitive function should include a brain tumor, especially if any focal neurological signs and symptoms are present. In addition to assessment of psychiatric and behavioral symptoms, a full neuropsychiatric evaluation should include physical, neurological, and mental status examinations (e.g., MMSE); appropriate brain imaging and other neurodiagnostic studies; and formal neuropsychological testing, particularly when there is any question of neurocognitive dysfunction on bedside testing with the MMSE.

The nature, frequency, and severity of psychiatric symptoms observed in patients with brain tumors depend on the combined effects of several clinical factors, including the type, location, size, rate of growth, and malignancy of the tumor, as well as the connectivity of affected neurons. In general, behavioral symptoms associated with smaller, slower-growing, less aggressive tumors are most likely to be misdiagnosed as psychiatric in origin, particularly when they occur in "silent" regions of the brain, which do not give rise to focal neurological signs or symptoms.

Although tumors of the frontal lobe, temporal lobe, and diencephalon appear to be most commonly associated with psychiatric and behavioral symptoms, the variation in symptoms that may occur with each of these types of tumors is exceedingly broad. In general, the relationship between particular neuropsychiatric symptoms and specific anatomical locations of the brain tumors that are causing them is not very consistent.

Optimal treatment of tumor-associated psychiatric, neuropsychiatric, and neuropsychological dysfunctions is multifaceted and dependent on the coordinated interventions of a multidisciplinary treatment team. The psychopharmacological treatment of psychiatric and behavioral syndromes should follow the same general principles as those for treatment of corresponding primary psychiatric disorders. However, the choice of drugs and the dosages may require modification because many of the psychotropic agents can induce seizures or delirium, and patients with brain tumors are more vulnerable to these and other side effects of psychotropic medications.

Adjunctive supportive psychotherapy for both the patient and the family is very important, as are psychosocial and psychoeducational interventions tailored to their specific needs. Such psychotherapeutic and psychosocial interventions must be carefully integrated with psychopharmacological, rehabilitative (neurocognitive, physical, occupational, vocational), and behavioral treatment approaches as clinically indicated. In turn, all of these must be coordinated with the neurosurgeon's ongoing treatment interventions to optimize the patient's overall medical and surgical management. With well-planned integration and coordination of these multiple complementary therapeutic approaches, both the quantity and the quality of the patient's life may be substantially enhanced.

Recommended Readings

Cummings J: Clinical Neuropsychiatry. Orlando, FL, Grune & Stratton, 1985

Feinberg T, Frank M (eds): Behavioral Neurology and Neuropsychology. New York, McGraw-Hill, 1997

Jobe TH, Gaviria M: Clinical Neuropsychiatry. Oxford, UK, Blackwell Science, 1997

Kandel E, Schwartz J, Jessel T: Principles of Neural Science, 4th Edition. New York, McGraw-Hill, 2000

Lishman A, Malden MA: Organic Psychiatry: The Psychological Consequences of Cerebral Disorders, 3rd Edition. Oxford, UK, Blackwell Science, 1998

Mesulam M: Principles of Behavioral Neurology. Philadelphia, PA, FA Davis, 1986

Strub R, Black FW: Neurobehavioral Disorders: A Clinical Approach. Philadelphia, PA, FA Davis, 1988

References

Alexander GE, Crutcher MD: Functional architecture of basal ganglia circuits: neural substrates of parallel processing. Trends Neurosci 13:266–271, 1990

Allen IM: A clinical study of tumours involving the occipital lobe. Brain 53:194–243, 1930

Avery TL: A case of acromegaly and gigantism with depression. Br J Psychiatry 122:599–600, 1973

Bauer RM, Tobias B, Valenstein E: Amnesic disorders, in Clinical Neuropsychology, 3rd Edition. Edited by Heilman KM, Valenstein E. New York, Oxford University Press, 1993, pp 523–578

Belyi BI: Mental impairment in unilateral frontal tumors: role of the laterality of the lesion. Int J Neurosci 32:799–810, 1987

Benson DF: Aphasia, Alexia, and Agraphia. New York, Churchill Livingstone, 1979

Berman RM, Narasimhan M, Sanacora G, et al: A randomized clinical trial of repetitive transcranial magnetic stimulation in the treatment of major depression. Biol Psychiatry 47:332–337, 2000

Bhatia MS: Cotard's syndrome in parietal lobe tumor. Indian Pediatr 30:1019–1021, 1993

Blackman M, Wheler GH: A case of mistaken identity: a fourth ventricular tumor presenting as school phobia in a 12 year old boy. Can J Psychiatry 32:584–587, 1987

Burkle FM, Lipowski ZJ: Colloid cyst of the third ventricle presenting as psychiatric disorder. Am J Psychiatry 135:373–374, 1978

Burger PC, Scheithauer BW, Vogel FS: Surgical Pathology of the Nervous System and Its Coverings, 3rd Edition. New York, Churchill Livingstone, 1991

Burns JM, Swerdlow RH: Right orbitofrontal tumor with pedophilia symptom and constructional apraxia sign. Arch Neurol 60:437–440, 2003

Butters N, Milotis P: Amnestic disorders, in Clinical Neuropsychology. Edited by Heilman KM, Valenstein E. New York, Oxford University Press, 1979, pp 403–439

Cairns H: Mental disorders with tumours of the pons. Folia Psychiatr Neurol Neurochir Neerl 53:193–203, 1950

Cairns H, Mosberg WH: Colloid cysts of the third ventricle. Surg Gynecol Obstet 92:545–570, 1951

Cairns H, Oldfield RC, Pennybacker JB, et al: Akinetic mutism with an epidermoid cyst of the 3rd ventricle. Brain 64:273–290, 1941

Chipkevitch E: Brain tumors and anorexia nervosa syndrome. Brain Dev 16:175–179, 1994

Coffey RJ: Hypothalamic and basal forebrain germinoma presenting with amnesia and hyperphagia. Surg Neurol 31:228–233, 1989

Critchley M: Psychiatric symptoms and parietal disease: differential diagnosis. Proc R Soc Med 57:422–428, 1964

Cummings JL: Subcortical Dementia. New York, Oxford University Press, 1990

Cummings JL: Frontal-subcortical circuits and human behavior. Arch Neurol 50:873–880, 1993

Davison K, Bagley CR: Schizophrenia-like psychoses associated with organic disorders of the central nervous system: a review of the literature, in Current Problems in Neuropsychiatry: Schizophrenia, Epilepsy, the Temporal Lobe (Br J Psychiatry Spec Publ No 4). Edited by Harrington RN. London, Headley Brothers, 1969, pp 126–130

Direkze M, Bayliss SG, Cutting JC: Primary tumours of the frontal lobe. Br J Clin Pract 25:207–213, 1971

Drubach DA, Kelly MP: Panic disorder associated with a right paralimbic lesion. Neuropsychiatry Neuropsychol Behav Neurol 2:282–289, 1989

Dubovsky SL: Psychopharmacological treatment in neuropsychiatry, in The American Psychiatric Press Textbook of Neuropsychiatry. Edited by Yudofsky SC, Hales RE. Washington, DC, American Psychiatric Press, 1992, pp 663–701

Dunn DW, Weisberg LA: Peduncular hallucinations caused by brainstem compression. Neurology 33:1360–1361, 1983

Filley CM, Kleinschmidt-DeMasters BK: Neurobehavioral presentations of brain neoplasms. West J Med 163:19–25, 1995

Gamazo-Garrán P, Soutullo CA, Ortuño F: Obsessive-compulsive disorder secondary to brain dysgerminoma in an adolescent boy: a positron emission tomography case report. J Child Adolesc Psychopharmacol 12:259–263, 2002

Gautier-Smith P: Parasagittal and Falx Meningiomas. London, Butterworths, 1970

Ghadirian AM, Gauthier S, Bertrand S: Anxiety attacks in a patient with a right temporal lobe meningioma. J Clin Psychiatry 47:270–271, 1986

Goldberg E: Varieties of perseverations: comparison of two taxonomies. J Clin Exp Neuropsychol 6:710–726, 1986

Greenberg DB, Brown GL: Mania resulting from brain stem tumor: single case study. J Nerv Ment Dis 173:434–436, 1985

Grisaru N, Chudakov B, Yaroslavsky Y, et al: Transcranial magnetic stimulation in mania: a controlled study. Am J Psychiatry 155:1608–1610, 1998

Gutmann DH, Grossman RI, Mollman JE: Personality changes associated with thalamic infiltration. J Neurooncol 8:263–267, 1990

Heaton RK: Wisconsin Card Sorting Test. Odessa, FL, Psychological Assessment Resources, 1985

Hoffman RE, Boutros NN, Berman RM, et al: Transcranial magnetic stimulation of left temporoparietal cortex in three patients reporting hallucinated "voices." Biol Psychiatry 46:130–132, 1999

Jarquin-Valdivia AA: Psychiatric symptoms and brain tumors: a brief historical overview. Arch Neurol 61:1800–1804, 2004

Jones JB, Barklage NE: Conversion disorder: camouflage for brain lesions in two cases. Arch Intern Med 150:1343–1345, 1990

Jukich PJ, McCarthy BJ, Surawicz TS, et al: Trends in incidence of primary brain tumors in the United States, 1985–1994. Neuro Oncol 3:141–151, 2001

Kalayam B, Young RC, Tsuboyama GK: Mood disorders associated with acoustic neuromas. Int J Psychiatry Med 24:31–43, 1994

Kaplan CP, Miner ME: Anxiety and depression in elderly patients receiving treatment for cerebral tumours. Brain Inj 11:129–135, 1997

Keschner M, Bender MB, Strauss I: Mental symptoms in cases of tumor of the temporal lobe. Arch Neurol Psychiatry 35:572–596, 1936

Keschner M, Bender MB, Strauss I: Mental symptoms associated with brain tumor: a study of 530 verified cases. J Am Med Assoc 110:714–718, 1938

Khouzam HR, Emery PE, Reaves B: Secondary mania in late life. J Am Geriatr Soc 42:85–87, 1994

Kocher R, Linder M, Stula D: [Primary brain tumors in psychiatry] (in German). Schweiz Arch Neurol Neurochir Psychiatr 135:217–227, 1984

Lampl Y, Barak Y, Achiron A, et al: Intracranial meningiomas: correlation of peritumoral edema and psychiatric disturbances. Psychiatry Res 58:177–180, 1995

Lezak MD: Neuropsychological Assessment, 3rd Edition. New York, Oxford University Press, 1995

Lin L, Lioa SC, Lee YJ, et al: Brain tumor presenting as anorexia nervosa in a 19-year-old man. J Formos Med Assoc 102:737–740, 2003

Lishman WA: Organic Psychiatry: The Psychological Consequences of Cerebral Disorder. New York, Oxford University Press, 1987

Madhusoodanan S, Danan D, Brenner R, et al: Brain tumor and psychiatric manifestations: a case report and brief review. Ann Clin Psychiatry 16:111–113, 2004

Malamud N: Psychiatric disorder with intracranial tumors of limbic system. Arch Neurol 17:113–123, 1967

Masand P, Murray GB, Pickett P: Psychostimulants in post-stroke depression. J Neuropsychiatry Clin Neurosci 3:23–27, 1991

Meadows JC: The anatomical basis of prosopagnosia. J Neurol Neurosurg Psychiatry 37:489–501, 1974

Mendez MF, Cummings JL, Benson DF: Epilepsy: psychiatric aspects and use of psychotropics. Psychosomatics 25:883–894, 1984

Mulder DW, Daly D: Psychiatric symptoms associated with lesions of temporal lobe. J Am Med Assoc 150:173–176, 1952

Nadvi SS, van Dellen JR: Transient peduncular hallucinations secondary to brain stem compression by a medulloblastoma. Surg Neurol 41:250–252, 1994

Nasrallah HA, McChesney CM: Psychopathology of corpus callosum tumors. Biol Psychiatry 16:663–669, 1981

Neuman E, Rancurel G, Lecrubier Y, et al: Schizophreniform catatonia in 6 cases secondary to hydrocephalus with subthalamic mesencephalic tumor associated with hypodopaminergia. Neuropsychobiology 34:76–81, 1996

Olney JW, Farber NB, Spitznagel E, et al: Increasing brain tumor rates: is there a link to aspartame? J Neuropathol Exp Neurol 55:1115–1123, 1996

Pincus JH, Tucker GJ: Behavioral Neurology, 2nd Edition. New York, Oxford University Press, 1978

Pollack L, Klein C, Rabey JM, et al: Posterior fossa lesions associated with neuropsychiatric symptomatology. Int J Neurosci 87:119–126, 1996

Radhakrishnan K, Bohnen NI, Kurland LT: Epidemiology of brain tumors, in Brain Tumors: A Comprehensive Text. Edited by Morantz RA, Walsh JW. New York, Marcel Dekker, 1994, pp 1–18

Reitan RM, Wolfson D: The Halstead-Reitan Neuropsychological Test Battery: Theory and Clinical Interpretation. Tucson, AZ, Neuropsychology Press, 1993

Roberts GW, Done DJ, Bruton C, et al: A "mock up" of schizophrenia: temporal lobe epilepsy and schizophrenia-like psychosis. Biol Psychiatry 28:127–143, 1990

Ross E: Prosody and brain lateralization: fact vs. fancy or is it all just semantics? Arch Neurol 45:338–339, 1988

Rush AJ, George MS, Sackheim HA, et al: Vagus nerve stimulation (VNS) for refractory depressions: a multicenter study. Biol Psychiatry 47:276–286, 2000

Russell RW, Pennybacker JB: Craniopharyngioma in the elderly. J Neurol Neurosurg Psychiatry 24:1–13, 1961

Salazar-Calderon Perriggo VH, Oommen KJ, Sobonya RE: Silent solitary right parietal chondroma resulting in secondary mania. Clin Neuropathol 12:325–329, 1993

Schlesinger B: Mental changes in intracranial tumors and related problems. Confin Neurol 10:225–263, 1950

Selecki BR: Cerebral mid-line tumours involving the corpus callosum among mental hospital patients. Med J Aust 2:954–960, 1964

Selecki BR: Intracranial space-occupying lesions among patients admitted to mental hospitals. Med J Aust 1:383–390, 1965

Spreen O, Benton A, Fincham R: Auditory agnosia without aphasia. Arch Neurol 13:84–92, 1965

Starkstein SE, Boston JD, Robinson RG: Mechanisms of mania after brain injury: 12 case reports and review of the literature. J Nerv Ment Dis 176:87–100, 1988

Stoudemire A, Fogel BS, Gulley LR, et al: Psychopharmacology in the medical patient, in Psychiatric Care of the Medical Patient. Edited by Stoudemire A, Fogel BS. New York, Oxford University Press, 1993, pp 155–206

Strauss I, Keschner M: Mental symptoms in cases of tumor of the frontal lobe. Arch Neurol Psychiatry 33:986–1005, 1935

Strobos RRJ: Tumors of the temporal lobe. Neurology 3:752–760, 1953

Tanaghow A, Lewis J, Jones GH: Anterior tumour of the corpus callosum with atypical depression. Br J Psychiatry 155:854–856, 1989

Teuber HL: Unity and diversity of frontal lobe functions. Acta Neurobiol Exp (Wars) 32:615–656, 1972

Warrington EK, Rabin P: Perceptual matching in patients with cerebral lesions. Neuropsychologia 8:475–487, 1970

Weitzner MA, Kanfer S, Booth-Jones M: Apathy and pituitary disease: it has nothing to do with depression. J Neuropsychiatry Clin Neurosci 17:159–166, 2005

Wellisch DK, Kaleita TA, Freeman D, et al: Predicting major depression in brain tumor patients. Psychooncology 11:230–238, 2002

White J, Cobb S: Psychological changes associated with giant pituitary neoplasms. Arch Neurol Psychiatry 74:383–396, 1955

Wilson G, Rupp C: Mental symptoms associated with extramedullary posterior fossa tumors. Trans Am Neurol Assoc 71:104–107, 1946

Woods SW, Tesar GE, Murray GB, et al: Psychostimulant treatment of depressive disorders secondary to medical illness. J Clin Psychiatry 47:12–15, 1986

8

HIV-1 Infection of the Central Nervous System

Brian Giunta, M.D., Ph.D.

Jun Tan, M.D., Ph.D.

Francisco Fernandez, M.D.

HIV infection is a major health and social issue. In this chapter, we outline neuropathological and neurobehavioral aspects of HIV infection of the central nervous system (CNS), as well as clinical management of patients with this infection.

CNS Pathology Resulting Directly From HIV

Brain infection by HIV can result in HIV-associated neurocognitive disorders (HAND) that range from asymptomatic neurocognitive impairment to HIV-1-associated dementia (HAD) (Antinori et al. 2007). Gross brain examination reveals that the white matter, subcortical structures (basal ganglia, thalamus, temporolimbic structures), cortex (Wiley et al. 1991), and spinal cord are commonly involved in HAD, as demonstrated by vacuolar myelopathy, atrophy, and multinucleated giant cells (McArthur et al. 2005). Although neurons are not productively infected by HIV (Weis et al. 1993), they sustain neurotoxic effects. The HIV epidemic is extending into older age brackets and is commonly characterized by pathology resembling that of Alzheimer's disease, including increased brain amyloid-β deposition (Achim et al. 2004; Green et al. 2005) and decreased cerebrospinal fluid (CSF) β-amyloid levels (Brew et al. 2005).

Once HIV enters the CNS, a complex cascade of events can occur to cause neural injury, which is thought to result in the various neurobehavioral syndromes (Gartner 2000). Lipton and Gendleman (1995) described these events. First, in the process of binding to a CD4$^+$ receptor–containing cell, HIV glycoprotein gp120 irreversibly binds to a calcium channel and increases intracellular free calcium (Stefano et al. 1993). HIV gp120 also induces the cell to increase neurotoxin production and may alter brain glucose metabolism, which could lead to brain dysfunction (Lipton and Gendleman 1995). Second, after the virus enters the cell and incorporates its genome into the host's genome, it can induce the infected macrophage to release more injurious compounds in the presence of other stimulators, such as other CNS infectious by-products and cytokines produced in response to infections by other immunologically active cells. Lipton and Gendleman (1995) described these compounds as including glutamate-like substances such as quinolinic acid; free radicals such as superoxide anions; other cytokines such as tumor necrosis factor (TNF)–α, interleukin-1–β, and interferon-γ; and eicosanoids such as arachidonic acid. Additionally, gp120 and certain fragment peptides are powerful activators of N-methyl-D-aspartate (NMDA) receptors of the CNS, the mechanism associated with neuroexcitotoxicity (Gemignani et al. 2000). In sum, these molecular mechanisms, although not the sole cause of neural demise and brain dysfunction in HIV infection, all contribute to neurocellular injury by several mechanisms, including increased intracellular calcium and increased concentrations of the toxic inorganic compound nitric oxide.

Importantly, other HIV proteins can cause neural dysfunction and death through other pathways, which may act in concert or separately from the above-mentioned gp120-mediated process. Indeed, in addition to gp120, several

HIV-related provirus products can trigger apoptosis (Maccarrone et al. 2000; Shiramizu et al. 2005). TNF-α can be produced by gp120 binding to macrophages, which may lead to this process (Sekigawa et al. 1995). Apoptosis is also induced in neurons by the HIV transactivator (Tat) protein (Li et al. 1995). Inhibition of these processes can be applied to HAND treatment.

CNS Neuropathology Due to Opportunistic Infections and Neoplasia

When severe neurological disease, opportunistic infections, or malignancies arise, the patient's condition meets criteria for AIDS. Immunocompromise is reflected by clinical and laboratory markers—namely, fewer than 200 CD4+ cells/mm^3. Additionally, syphilis and tuberculosis are increasingly found as coinfections in patients with AIDS. These disorders must be considered in the differential diagnosis of CNS infection (Brew et al. 1988; Neuenburg et al. 2002). Proper diagnosis and aggressive treatment of the cause of the neurological problem are important to postpone mortality and restore CNS function. CNS involvement can result from opportunistic viruses such as those listed in Table 8–1 (Bredesen et al. 1988).

Direct Assessment of CNS Injury in HIV Disease

Neuroimaging Findings

Computed tomography (CT) and magnetic resonance imaging (MRI) may be the most common neurodiagnostic imaging tests used (Bakshi 2004). Both show atrophy and can help to define pathological entities such as ring-enhancing lesions and white matter involvement. MRI is superior to CT in showing areas of focal high-signal intensities in subcortical white and gray matter by the T2-weighted signal. T1 relaxation times have not indicated structural differences between older HIV-infected patients and control subjects (Freund-Levi et al. 1989). MRI also has not proven useful in depicting structural correlates of neurologically asymptomatic HIV infection (Post et al. 1991). MRI, however, has disclosed neurostructural changes in medically symptomatic but neurologically asymptomatic HIV-positive patients.

Table 8–1.   Central nervous system conditions associated with HIV infection and AIDS

HIV-associated disorders

HIV-1-associated cognitive/motor complex

   HIV-1-associated dementia

   HIV-1-associated minor cognitive/motor disorder

   HIV-1-associated myelopathy

Opportunistic viral infections

Cytomegalovirus

Herpes simplex virus, types 1 and 2

Herpes zoster virus

Papovavirus (progressive multifocal leukoencephalopathy)

Adenovirus type 2

Other opportunistic infections of the CNS

Toxoplasma gondii

Cryptococcus neoformans

Candida albicans

Aspergillus fumigatus

Coccidioides immitis

Mucormycosis

Rhizopus species

Acremonium alabamensis

Histoplasma capsulatum

Mycobacterium tuberculosis

Mycobacterium avium-intracellulare

Listeria monocytogenes

Nocardia asteroides

Table 8–1. Central nervous system conditions associated with HIV infection and AIDS *(continued)*

Neoplasms

Primary CNS lymphoma

Metastatic lymphoma

Metastatic Kaposi's sarcoma

Cerebrovascular pathology

Infarction

Hemorrhage

Vasculitis

Adverse effects of treatments for HIV and
  AIDS-related disorders

Source.   Adapted from Bredesen et al. 1988.

Imaging reflecting CNS function, such as positron emission tomography (PET) (Pomara et al. 2001), single-photon emission computed tomography (SPECT) (Sacktor et al. 1995), magnetic resonance spectroscopy (MRS) (Tucker et al. 2004), functional MRI (Navia and Gonzalez 1997), and regional cerebral blood flow (rCBF), has shown regional functional abnormalities in HIV infection (Tucker et al. 2004). These imaging modalities have established themselves as sensitive to different aspects of functioning: PET reflects metabolism; SPECT, functional MRI, and rCBF reflect brain perfusion; and MRS reflects biochemical function and dysfunction.

Cerebrospinal Fluid Findings

The CSF of HIV-infected patients having fever with or without altered mental status or with complaints about mental functioning should be evaluated quickly for signs of opportunistic infection (Buffet et al. 1991) (see Table 8–1). Specific CSF findings indicating HIV infection include virions and HIV-specific antibody; however, neither correlates with the severity of HAND (Reboul et al. 1989). CSF β_2-microglobulin has shown some specificity in differentiating HAD from multiple sclerosis and other CNS disorders (Carrieri et al. 1992). The level of quinolinic acid, an excitotoxin and NMDA receptor agonist, is related to severity of dementia and clinical status (Heyes et al. 1991). CSF quinolinic acid levels were found to correlate with regional brain atrophy as quantified by MRI, whereas CSF β_2-microglobulin levels were not (Heyes et al. 2001).

Neurobehavioral Assessment of HIV Infection of the CNS

The current criteria for HAND delineate three neurocognitive disorders: asymptomatic neurocognitive impairment (ANI), minor neurocognitive disorder (MND), and HAD (Antinori et al. 2007). ANI is a subclinical condition (*not* a formal disorder) marked by cognitive decline in two or more domains of neuropsychological testing but without significant decline in functional status. For MND, the following must be present: ANI deficits plus, at most, a minor functional impairment in activities of daily living and no other known etiology for the symptoms. For HAD, MND criteria must be met plus at least a moderate level of functional status impairment, a lack of clouding of consciousness (i.e., delirium), and no support for another etiology accounting for these symptoms.

The earliest level of cognitive impairment is subclinical; impairment at this level ranges from a decrement in previous level of functioning in attention, speed of information processing, memory, abstraction, and fine motor skills to formal test-defined deficits in some of these domains. These deficits may impart no observable effects on activities of daily living or on functional performance and are thus termed *asymptomatic neurocognitive impairment* and account for more than 20% of asymptomatic HIV-1–infected individuals (Wilkie et al. 1990). ANI, as measured by formal cognitive testing, doubles with advanced disease (Heaton et al. 1995, 2009). Another estimated 20%–30% of asymptomatic HIV-1–infected individuals may meet these criteria (Goodkin et al. 2001).

Indications of MND may be mild and are frequently attributed to the systemic illness or a psychosocial reaction to HIV infection. Many patients will be cognizant of their own mental and physical sluggishness and personality changes, and affective symptoms may occur concomitantly. Dysphoria due to the seriousness of the illness or induced by medications or affective disturbances could theoretically cause cognitive difficulties—for example, pseudodementia of depression—but Heaton et al. (2009) reported that the level of cognitive dysfunction is not correlated with mood disorder, and the level of cognitive impairment surpasses that expected from distraction due to affective causes.

Dementia's persistent cognitive impairment differentiates it from delirium, and HAND are characterized by both cortical and subcortical signs and symptoms that may progress from ANI to HAD. Fully developed HAD is commonly marked by severe dementia (multiple cognitive areas, aphasia and/ or mutism, severe frontal lobe symptoms, and psychomotor slowing), intense distractibility, and disorientation. Affective and behavioral symptoms include severe behavioral disinhibition, mania, psychosis, and severe depression. Motor abnormalities, such as ataxia, spasticity, hyperreflexia, and incontinence of bladder and bowel, can also occur.

Van Gorp et al. (1989) reported that psychomotor tasks, such as the Digit Symbol and Block Design subtests of the Wechsler Adult Intelligence Scale and the Trail Making Test Part B from the Halstead-Reitan Neuropsychological Test Battery, and memory tasks, such as the delayed Visual Reproduction subtest from the Wechsler Memory Scale and delayed recall in the Rey-Osterrieth Complex Figure Test, were most affected in the early stages of HIV-associated cognitive impairment. We and others have found that tasks detecting psychomotor and neuromotor disturbances in HIV-related neural dysfunction, such as visuomotor reaction time (Dunlop et al. 1992) and fine motor dexterity, are also sensitive measures for the early detection of impairment. Such tasks may be more vulnerable to the effects of HIV than is central processing speed. Other areas of cognitive function that are assessed by neuropsychological batteries include aphasia, apraxia, and other complex language-associated functioning; verbal abstract reasoning and problem solving; and perceptual functioning of the different sensory modalities. If the patient's lack of stamina or another situation precludes an extensive battery, the following comprehensive but briefer battery is recommended (Selnes et al. 1991):

- *Attention and memory*—Digit Span subtest from Wechsler Adult Intelligence Scale—Revised, and Rey Auditory-Verbal Learning Test
- *Language*—Controlled Oral Word Association Test from Benton Multilingual Aphasia Examination
- *Executive/psychomotor function*—Symbol Digit Modalities Test, Trail Making Test Parts A and B, and Grooved Pegboard test

The HIV Dementia Scale (HDS; Power et al. 1995) has been proposed to discriminate patients with HIV infection and dementia from patients with HIV infection but not dementia. Nonneurologically trained examiners may omit the saccadic eye movement examination portion, and the HDS retains the ability to discriminate grossly among mild-moderate and moderate-severe dementia (Skolasky et al. 1998). Importantly, neuropsychological impairment is related to functional deficits that may lead to medication noncompliance, further emphasizing the importance of objective cognitive assessment in addition to measures of cognitive complaints and other self-report measures (Heaton et al. 2004).

Treatment of HIV Infection of the CNS

Primary Therapy: Antivirals

For a detailed review of the primary and secondary salvage therapeutic strategies for the treatment of HIV/AIDS, the reader is referred to guidelines published by the U.S. Department of Health and Human Services (DHHS) for the use of antiretroviral therapies in adults and children (DHHS Panel on Antiretroviral Guidelines for Adults and Adolescents 2009). No specific guidelines exist for treating cognitive impairment and HAD. However, available studies suggest that the main thrust of treatment should be to produce virological suppression of both plasma and CNS compartments.

Zidovudine is a potent reverse transcriptase inhibitor in vitro and reduces morbidity by decreasing the number of serious complications in patients with AIDS as well as in asymptomatic patients (Fischl et al. 1987). It also attenuates the symptomatic course of HAND (Yarchoan et al. 1987) and penetrates the brain at a level at which one-half can be recovered from CSF (Wong et al. 1992). Dosages may need to be high (up to 2,000 mg/day) to maintain therapeutic CNS levels, because zidovudine is cleared from the brain via active transport (Wang and Sawchuk 1995; Wong et al. 1993). Clinicians should keep this finding in mind when calculating the maintenance dosage of zidovudine in the patient with subjective complaints consistent with HIV-1-associated minor cognitive/motor disorder or HAD.

In addition to zidovudine, other antivirals such as nevirapine, indinavir, lopinavir, amprenavir, abacavir, stavudine, emtricitabine, darunavir, and raltegravir penetrate the blood-brain barrier and reach sufficient CSF levels to inhibit HIV replication in the brain (Brew 2010). Several studies have demonstrated that higher CSF levels of these agents are associated with greater improvements in global neuropsychological test results (Cysique et al. 2009; Letendre et al. 2010). Zidovudine, nevirapine, and indinavir remain the agents with the best blood-brain barrier penetration and potential for CNS prophylaxis (Letendre et al. 2010).

Adjunctive Therapy: Additional Biological and Pharmacological Interventions

Neuroinflammation from excitotoxicity and chemokine/cytokine overexpression is the common final pathway in HAD. Certain calcium channel blockers (e.g., flunarizine) were protective against gp120 toxicity in vitro. For example, nimodipine (30–60 mg orally 4–6 times per day) is used to regulate neuron-injuring intracellular calcium increments (Dreyer et al. 1990). Other calcium channel blockers had no or minimal effect (Harbison et al. 1991).

Galantamine is a potent allosteric potentiating ligand of nicotinic acetylcholine receptors (Samochocki et al. 2003; Santos et al. 2002) and cholinesterase inhibitors (Shytle et al. 2004). Giunta et al. (2004) showed that nicotine in the presence of galantamine synergistically attenuates HIV-1 gp120/interferon-γ–induced microglial activation, as evidenced by decreased TNF-α and nitric oxide releases. This finding suggests a novel therapeutic combination to treat or prevent the onset of HAD through this modulation of the microglia inflammation mechanism.

Epigallocatechin gallate (EGCG), the major component of green tea, has been reported to have neuroprotective properties (Mandel et al. 2004). Most important, Kawai et al. (2003) reported that EGCG directly binds to the CD4 receptor and interferes with HIV-1 gp120 binding at the target cell surface. Giunta et al. (2006) found that EGCG treatment of primary neurons from normal mice reduced HAD-like neuronal injury mediated by interferon-γ and/or HIV-1 viral proteins gp120 and Tat, as evidenced by decreased lactate dehydrogenase release and increased ratio of Bcl-xL to Bax protein. In addition, primary neurons derived from Stat1-deficient mice were largely resistant to HAD-like neuronal damage. In accord with these findings, EGCG also attenuated Alzheimer's disease–like neuropathology damage in vitro and in vivo (Giunta et al. 2008;

Rrapo et al. 2009). Taken together, these data suggest that green tea–derived EGCG possibly represents a novel therapeutic approach for the prevention and treatment of HAD and its Alzheimer's disease–like pathology.

Adjuvant Therapy: Psychopharmacological Enhancement of Function

Adjuvant therapy in the form of psychostimulant treatment can help improve functioning in cognitive domains (also see "Depression" subsection in next section of chapter). Early data indicated that methylphenidate significantly improved verbal rote memory, rate of cognitive tracking, and rate of mental set shifting (Fernandez et al. 1988a, 1988b), as demonstrated by improvement of scores on neuropsychological instruments into the normal range. Subsequent investigations (Angrist et al. 1991) confirmed this effect. Possible support for the efficacy of psychostimulants may come from their enhancement of dopaminergic functioning in neural populations that subtend attention or concentration, memory retrieval, and speed of cognitive processing (Fernandez and Levy 1990).

Manifestations and Treatment of Specific HIV-Related Neuropsychiatric Disorders

The range of HIV-related neuropsychiatric disorders includes most of the major mental disorders listed in DSM-IV-TR (American Psychiatric Association 2000). The most common psychiatric effects are those "due to general medical conditions," such as delirium and psychosis; dementia; mood disorder, including depression and mania; and stress syndromes such as anxiety disorders (Fernandez 1989; Fernandez et al. 1989b, 1995; Goodkin 2009).

Delirium and Psychosis

Delirium is the most prevalent and frequently undiagnosed neuropsychiatric disorder; up to 30% of hospitalized medical-surgical patients have undetected delirium. In the post-HAART (highly active antiretroviral therapy) era, delirium is reported in 20% of patients (O'Dowd and McKegney 1990). Timely pharmacological intervention may help to suppress the delirium symptoms; however, in a study by Fernandez et al. (1989b), complete reversal of delirium occurred in only 37% of the patients with AIDS.

In the only double-blind placebo-controlled study comparing haloperidol, chlorpromazine, and lorazepam treatment of delirium, Breitbart et al. (1996) found that lorazepam worsened the delirious process; in terms of antipsychotic treatments, haloperidol and chlorpromazine were roughly equally effective. The atypical antipsychotics risperidone (Singh et al. 1997) and olanzapine have been used with success at various dosages to target psychotic symptoms. Olanzapine's affinity for the cytochrome P450 (CYP) 3A4 isoenzyme system may be problematic for patients taking specific protease inhibitors (Sockalingam et al. 2005). A trial of other atypical antipsychotics may be warranted, but there is little experience to date with these agents (Stolar et al. 2005).

Fernandez et al. (1989a) reported on the safety and efficacy of intravenous haloperidol treatment for delirium; haloperidol was either administered alone or combined with lorazepam with or without hydromorphone for agitated patients with delirium. Neuroleptic malignant syndrome is the most ominous potential adverse effect (Breitbart et al. 1988); however, in our experience, this syndrome is rare in this population.

Psychosis associated with HIV infection has been less frequently studied. The differential diagnosis of psychotic symptoms in an HIV-seropositive patient includes delirium, HAD, mania (which may be due to HIV infection), recurrence of premorbid psychotic illnesses, psychoactive substance intoxication, HAART medication toxicities (particularly with efavirenz; Lowenhaupt et al. 2007), and general medical conditions manifesting with psychotic symptoms. The same atypical antipsychotic medications are effective in treating psychotic symptoms no matter what the etiology.

Depression

Disorders with depressed mood are highly prevalent in patients with HIV (Goodkin 2009). Marzuk et al. (1988) reported that the relative risk of suicide in men with AIDS was 36.3 times that for men without an AIDS diagnosis and 66.2 times that of the general population. Although pharmacotherapy is the most rapid intervention for remission of depression, specific guidelines for drug selection are conspicuously absent.

The low-anticholinergic tricyclic antidepressants (TCAs) may be useful for treating depression in HIV-infected patients because these drugs have less risk than the highly anticholinergic TCAs for exacerbating cognitive deficits. The choice of a particular TCA should be guided by its specific action and side effects (Richelson 1988) in relation to the patient's depressive symptoms and medical condition (Fernandez and Levy 1991). The therapeutic dosage of a TCA may be lower (e.g., 10–75 mg) for an HIV-infected patient with neuropsychiatric impairment than for a noninfected person.

In general, all non-TCA agents are effective and lack significant anticholinergic, histaminergic, adrenergic, and cardiac side effects. However, most do inhibit the biochemical activity of drugs that metabolize the isoenzyme CYP 2D6 or 3A4. Citalopram (Currier et al. 2004), escitalopram, venlafaxine, and mirtazapine are the weakest 2D6 and 3A isoenzyme inhibitors (Greenblatt et al. 1998). Clinicians may use these agents with low affinity for the 2D6 and 3A isoenzyme system in HIV-related depression while carefully monitoring the co-administration of prescribed and over-the-counter medications.

Bupropion has both noradrenergic and dopaminergic effects and has been used effectively in HIV/AIDS patients with depression (Maldonado et al. 2000). It has been associated with seizures and should be used cautiously in patients with neurological disease or avoided altogether (Maldonado et al. 2000).

Nefazodone is a serotonin receptor antagonist and serotonin reuptake inhibitor that works at the serotonin type 2 receptor site. It also is a minor noradrenergic reuptake inhibitor. Because of its affinity for CYP and its propensity for hepatotoxicity, nefazodone should be avoided in the treatment of depression in patients with HIV/AIDS (Stolar et al. 2005).

Methylphenidate (Fernandez and Levy 1991; Fernandez et al. 1988a, 1988b; Holmes et al. 1989) and dextroamphetamine (Wagner and Rabkin 2000) are especially effective in treating depression or subclinical depression symptoms in patients with HIV/AIDS (Breitbart et al. 2001). In HIV-infected patients without cognitive impairment, methylphenidate treatment yielded a remission of depression symptoms that was statistically indistinguishable from that achieved with the TCA desipramine (Fernandez et al. 1995). The usual methylphenidate dosage is 5–20 mg taken in the morning, at midmorning, and in early afternoon to avoid disturbing nighttime sleep (Fernandez et al. 1989a).

Hypogonadism in the context of HIV can present as depression. Hormone replacement therapy with testosterone was reported effective in men (Rabkin et al. 2004) and in women (Miller et al. 1998). Because hormone replacement therapy in patients with neurobehavioral impairments may cause irritability, rage, and violent behavior, it should be used with caution.

Depressed HIV-infected patients with psychotic symptoms or an organic mood disturbance, or for whom pharmacological treatment has failed or is not possible (due to other concomitant medications), may benefit from electroconvulsive therapy (ECT) (Weiner 1983). However, ECT may increase confusion in some encephalopathic HIV-infected patients (Schaerf et al. 1989).

Mania

Acute mania with HIV disease may be the result of premorbid bipolar disorder; brain lesions from HIV, opportunistic infections, or AIDS-related neoplasms; or medications (McGowan et al. 1991; O'Dowd and McKegney 1988; Wright et al. 1989).

Treatment of mania in HIV-infected patients is similar to that in non-HIV-infected patients. Lithium has been found useful in the treatment of secondary mania due to zidovudine (O'Dowd and McKegney 1988). Close monitoring of levels and blood chemistry is essential for avoidance of toxicity in debilitated patients or those with the wasting syndrome. Monitoring is especially critical when infectious complications occur, such as with cryptosporidium infection or other causes of severe diarrhea, or with other severe fluid losses. Even when dosages are used to maintain therapeutic serum concentrations of 0.5–1.0 mEq/L, patients with advanced disease cannot tolerate treatment with lithium.

Valproate also has been approved as a treatment for mania (McElroy et al. 1992). It may be tried cautiously in patients whose renal or electrolyte status makes lithium use problematic. There is a single report of valproic acid decreasing intracellular glutathione concentration and stimulating HIV (Melton et al. 1997). We have retrospectively evaluated our valproate-treated patients' medical records and have not found any increases in viral load to suggest that this is a clinically relevant concern.

No clinical reports are yet available on the efficacy of newer antiepileptic agents such as gabapentin, lamotrigine, and topiramate in treating HIV-related mania. Of these, lamotrigine is the only U.S. Food and Drug Administration–approved medication for maintenance therapy in bipolar affective disorder and therefore may be equally effective in HIV-related mania. It is safe to use in the context of HIV.

Although atypical antipsychotics may be used in patients with HIV, concerns regarding extrapyramidal side effects, especially in patients with CNS involvement, may deter the use of these medications (Goodkin 2009).

Anxiety and Insomnia

The stresses associated with treatment of HIV elicit anxiety (Fernandez 1989; Perry et al. 1992), especially for patients predisposed to anxiety disorders. Anxiety disorders of any type often respond to supportive therapy, cognitive-behavioral therapy, progressive muscular relaxation training, self-hypnosis, cognitive imagery, and biofeedback without anxiolytic pharmacotherapy. Anxiolytic agents may help the patient to function better in all aspects of daily living. However, the automatic use of benzodiazepines as anxiolytics is risky in cases of severe anxiety or restlessness, because these compounds may further compromise the patient's coping capacity and may be disinhibiting.

Anxiety and insomnia may result from treatment with zidovudine, efavirenz, or steroids, or be secondary to the effects of HIV on the CNS. In patients with these conditions, brief pharmacotherapy with short- to intermediate-acting benzodiazepines is warranted (Fernandez 1988). Alprazolam for anxiety and triazolam and estazolam for insomnia should be avoided in patients receiving HAART because of the drugs' affinity for CYP 3A4. Chronic use of benzodiazepines may be appropriate in some patients. If so, we advocate use of clonazepam tablets or wafers. If tolerance develops in these patients, 50–200 mg of trazodone at bedtime may be combined with or substituted for the benzodiazepine. Although the β-blocker propranolol is often useful for healthy individuals who are anxious or phobic, it has a propensity to result in hypotensive episodes, particularly in patients who may have undiagnosed HIV-related dysautonomia (Lin-Greenberger and Taneja-Uppal 1987). Antihistamines, such as hydroxyzine, have low efficacy for anxiolysis unless the anxiety is accompanied by specific respiratory problems.

Studies of the effectiveness of the nonbenzodiazepine anxiolytic buspirone (Kastenholz and Crismon 1984) in HIV-infected patients indicate its value when immediate anxiolysis is not essential. Buspirone's anxiolytic effects lack excessive sedation or potential for dependence. It should be prescribed with caution for HIV-infected patients with CNS impairment, and its use should be monitored closely because buspirone-related dyskinesias (Strauss 1988) may be more easily elicited in HIV-infected patients than in noninfected patients with anxiety. Cases of possible buspirone-related mania have been reported (McDaniel et al. 1990; Price and Bielefeld 1989).

Nonbenzodiazepines in use for insomnia include zolpidem, zaleplon, and eszopiclone (Sharma et al. 2005). Zolpidem is a nonbenzodiazepine sedative-hypnotic, and it is the most prescribed agent in HIV-related insomnia. Zolpidem is primarily a substrate of CYP 3A4. Clinically significant interactions may occur with concurrent use of CYP 3A4 inhibitors and inducers such as ritonavir, delavirdine, and nevirapine. Zaleplon is a short-acting nonbenzodiazepine sedative-hypnotic. Zaleplon is primarily metabolized by aldehyde oxidase to form 5-oxo-zaleplon. To a lesser extent, zaleplon is metabolized by the hepatic isoenzyme CYP 3A4, and all its metabolites are inactive. However, antiretroviral protease inhibitors may increase the levels of zaleplon. Although clinical data do not exist, and this interaction is not expected to require routine zaleplon dosage adjustment, the clinician should remain vigilant for possible problems. Eszopiclone is a nonbenzodiazepine hypnotic agent that is a pyrrolopyrazine derivative of the cyclopyrrolone class. Eszopiclone is metabolized by CYP 3A4 and 2E1 via demethylation and oxidation. Inhibitors of CYP 3A4, such as the protease inhibitors, will result in an increase in the levels of eszopiclone. Clinical experience with eszopiclone in patients with HIV-related insomnia is limited.

Conclusion

The neuropsychiatric complications of HIV infection are a perplexing assortment of neurological, neurocognitive, and affective/behavioral effects. Thus, health care providers should maintain a high index of suspicion of even the most subtle of behavioral symptoms in previously asymptomatic persons, because several means of investigation (e.g., electrophysiological, neuropsychological) have disclosed that neurological involvement may occur early in the course of the disease. As the AIDS epidemic continues, these symptoms may arise in individuals other than those in the initial high-risk categories, and a careful history of possible exposure must be included in any workup of unusual cognitive, neurological, or neuropsychiatric symptoms fitting the pattern described in this chapter. If the etiology is found to be HIV related, then prompt aggressive treatment of the conditions, perhaps with innovative measures, is warranted, to maintain as optimal a quality of life as can be promoted, for as long as possible.

Recommended Readings

American Psychiatric Association: Practice Guideline for the Treatment of Patients With HIV/AIDS. November 2000. Available at: http://www.psychiatryonline. com/pracGuide/pracGuideChapToc_4.aspx. Accessed April 11, 2011.

Fernandez F, Ruiz P (eds): Psychiatric Aspects of HIV/AIDS. Philadelphia, PA, Lippincott Williams & Wilkins, 2006

Goodkin K (ed): The Spectrum of Neuro-AIDS Disorders. Washington, DC, ASM Press, 2008

References

Achim CL, Masliah E, Schindelar J, et al: Immunophilin expression in the HIV-infected brain. J Neuroimmunol 157:126–132, 2004

American Psychiatric Association: Diagnostic and Statistical Manual of Mental Disorders, 4th Edition, Text Revision. Washington, DC, American Psychiatric Association, 2000

Angrist B, D'Hollosy M, Sanfilipo M, et al: Central nervous system stimulants as symptomatic treatments for AIDS-related neuropsychiatric impairment. J Clin Psychopharmacol 12:268–272, 1991

Antinori A, Arendt G, Becker JT, et al: Updated research nosology for HIV-associated neurocognitive disorders. Neurology 69:1789–1799, 2007

Bakshi R: Neuroimaging of HIV and AIDS related illnesses: a review. Front Biosci 9:632–646, 2004

Bredesen DE, Levy RM, Rosenblum ML: The neurology of human immunodeficiency virus infection. Q J Med 68:665–677, 1988

Breitbart W, Marotta RF, Call P: AIDS and neuroleptic malignant syndrome. Lancet 2:1488–1489, 1988

Breitbart W, Marotta RF, Platt MM, et al: A double-blind trial of haloperidol, chlorpromazine, and lorazepam in the treatment of delirium in hospitalized patients. Am J Psychiatry 153:231–237, 1996

Breitbart W, Rosenfeld B, Kaim M, et al: A randomized, double-blind, placebo-controlled trial of psychostimulants for the treatment of fatigue in ambulatory patients with human immunodeficiency virus disease. Arch Intern Med 161:411–420, 2001

Brew BJ: Benefit or toxicity from neurologically targeted antiretroviral therapy? Clin Infect Dis 50:930–932, 2010

Brew BJ, Sidtis JJ, Petito CK, et al: The neurologic complications of AIDS and human immunodeficiency virus infection, in Advances in Contemporary Neurology. Edited by Plum F. Philadelphia, PA, FA Davis, 1988, pp 1–49

Brew BJ, Pemberton L, Blennow K, et al: CSF amyloid beta42 and tau levels correlate with AIDS dementia complex. Neurology 65:1490–1492, 2005

Buffet R, Agut H, Chieze F, et al: Virological markers in the cerebrospinal fluid from HIV-1-infected individuals. AIDS 5:1419–1424, 1991

Carrieri PB, Indaco A, Maiorino A, et al: Cerebrospinal fluid beta-2-microglobulin in multiple sclerosis and AIDS dementia complex. Neurol Res 14:282–283, 1992

Currier MB, Molina G, Kato M: Citalopram treatment of major depressive disorder in Hispanic HIV and AIDS patients: a prospective study. Psychosomatics 45:210–216, 2004

Cysique L, Vaida F, Letendre S, et al: Dynamics of cognitive change in impaired HIV-positive patients initiating antiretroviral therapy. Neurology 73:342–348, 2009

DHHS Panel on Antiretroviral Guidelines for Adults and Adolescents: Guidelines for the use of antiretroviral agents in HIV-1–infected adults and adolescents. Washington, DC, U.S. Department of Health and Human Services. December 1, 2009. Available at: http://www.aidsinfo.nih.gov/ContentFiles/AdultandAdolescentGL.pdf. Accessed February 24, 2010.

Dreyer EB, Kaiser PK, Offermann JT, et al: HIV-1 coat protein neurotoxicity prevented by calcium channel antagonists. Science 248:364–367, 1990

Dunlop O, Bjørklund RA, Abedelnoor M, et al: Five different tests of reaction time evaluated in HIV seropositive men. Acta Neurol Scand 8:260–266, 1992

Fernandez F: Psychiatric complications in HIV-related illnesses, in American Psychiatric Association AIDS Primer. Washington, DC, American Psychiatric Press, 1988

Fernandez F: Anxiety and the neuropsychiatry of AIDS. J Clin Psychiatry 50(suppl):9–14, 1989

Fernandez F, Levy JK: Adjuvant treatment of HIV dementia with psychostimulants, in Behavioral Aspects of AIDS and Other Sexually Transmitted Diseases. Edited by Ostrow D. New York, Plenum, 1990, pp 279–286

Fernandez F, Levy JK: Psychopharmacotherapy of psychiatric syndromes in asymptomatic and symptomatic HIV infection. Psychiatr Med 9:377–393, 1991

Fernandez F, Adams F, Levy JK, et al: Cognitive impairment due to AIDS-related complex and its response to psychostimulants. Psychosomatics 29:38–46, 1988a

Fernandez F, Levy JK, Galizzi H: Response of HIV-related depression to psychostimulants: case reports. Hosp Community Psychiatry 39:628–631, 1988b

Fernandez F, Holmes VF, Levy JK, et al: Consultation-liaison psychiatry and HIV-related disorders. Hosp Community Psychiatry 40:146–153, 1989a

Fernandez F, Levy JK, Mansell PWA: Management of delirium in terminally ill AIDS patients. Int J Psychiatry Med 19:165–172, 1989b

Fernandez F, Levy JK, Sampley HR, et al: Effects of methylphenidate in HIV-related depression: a comparative trial with desipramine. Int J Psychiatry Med 25:53–67, 1995

Fischl MA, Richman DD, Grieco MH, et al: The efficacy of azidothymidine (AZT) in the treatment of patients with AIDS and AIDS-related complex: a double-blind, placebo-controlled study. N Engl J Med 317:185–191, 1987

Freund-Levi Y, Saaf J, Wahlund L-O, et al: Ultra low field brain MRI in HIV transfusion infected patients. Magn Reson Imaging 7:225–230, 1989

Gartner S: HIV infection and dementia. Science 287:602–604, 2000

Gemignani A, Paudice P, Pittaluga A, et al: The HIV-1 coat protein gp120 and some of its fragments potently activate native cerebral NMDA receptors mediating neuropeptide release. Eur J Neurosci 12:2839–2846, 2000

Giunta B, Ehrhart J, Townsend K, et al: Galantamine and nicotine have a synergistic effect on inhibition of microglial activation induced by HIV-1 gp120. Brain Res Bull 64:165–170, 2004

Giunta B, Obregon D, Hou H, et al: EGCG mitigates neurotoxicity mediated by HIV-1 proteins gp120 and Tat in the presence of IFN-gamma: role of JAK/STAT1 signaling and implications for HIV-associated dementia. Brain Res 1123:216–225, 2006

Giunta B, Zhou Y, Hou H, et al: HIV-1 TAT inhibits microglial phagocytes of Aβ peptide. Int J Clin Exp Pathol 1(3):260–275, 2008

Goodkin K: Psychiatric aspects of HIV spectrum disease. Focus 7:303–310, 2009

Goodkin K, Baldewicz TT, Wilkie FL, et al: Cognitive-motor impairment and disorder in HIV-1 infection. Psychiatr Ann 31:37–44, 2001

Green DA, Masliah E, Vinters HV, et al: Brain deposition of beta-amyloid is a common pathologic feature in HIV positive patients. AIDS 19:407–411, 2005

Greenblatt DJ, von Moltke LL, Harmatz JS, et al: Drug interactions with newer antidepressants: role of human cytochromes P450. J Clin Psychiatry 59 (suppl 15):19–27, 1998

Harbison MA, Kim S, Gillis JM, et al: Effect of the calcium channel blocker verapamil on human immunodeficiency virus type 1 replication in lymphoid cells. J Infect Dis 164:43–60, 1991

Heaton RK, Grant I, Butters N, et al: The HNRC 500: neuropsychology of HIV infection at different disease stages. J Int Neuropsychol Soc 1:231–251, 1995

Heaton RK, Marcotte TD, Rivera Mindt M, et al: The impact of HIV-associated neuropsychological impairment on everyday functioning. J Int Neuropsychol Soc 10:317–331, 2004

Heaton RK, Grant I, Butters N, et al: The HNRC 500–neuropsychology of HIV infection at different disease stages. J Int Neuropsychol Soc 1:231–251, 2009

Heyes MP, Brew BJ, Martin A, et al: Quinolinic acid in cerebrospinal fluid and serum in HIV-1 infection: relationship to clinical neurological status. Ann Neurol 29:202–209, 1991

Heyes MP, Ellis RJ, Ryan L, et al: Elevated cerebrospinal fluid quinolinic acid levels are associated with region-specific cerebral volume loss in HIV infection. Brain 124 (pt 5):1033–1042, 2001

Holmes VF, Fernandez F, Levy JK: Psychostimulant response in AIDS-related complex patients. J Clin Psychiatry 50:5–8, 1989

Kastenholz KV, Crismon ML: Buspirone, a novel nonbenzodiazepine anxiolytic. Clin Pharmacol Ther 3:600–607, 1984

Kawai K, Tsuno NH, Kitayama J, et al: Epigallocatechin gallate, the main component of tea polyphenol, binds to CD4 and interferes with gp120 binding. J Allergy Clin Immunol 112:951–957, 2003

Letendre S, FitzSimons C, Ellis R, et al: Correlates of CSF viral loads in 1,221 volunteers in the CHARTER Cohort. Paper presented at the 17th Conference on Retroviruses and Opportunistic Infections, San Francisco, CA, February 2010

Li CJ, Friedman DJ, Wang C, et al: Induction of apoptosis in uninfected lymphocytes by HIV-1 Tat protein. Science 268:429–431, 1995

Lin-Greenberger A, Taneja-Uppal N: Dysautonomia and infection with the human immunodeficiency virus (letter). Ann Intern Med 106:167, 1987

Lipton SA, Gendleman HE: Dementia associated with the acquired immunodeficiency syndrome. N Engl J Med 332:934–940, 1995

Lowenhaupt EA, Matson K, Qureishi B, et al: Psychosis in a 12-year-old HIV-positive girl with an increased serum concentration of efavirenz. Clin Infect Dis 45:e128–e130, 2007

Maccarrone M, Bari M, Corasaniti MT, et al: HIV-1 coat glycoprotein gp120 induces apoptosis in rat brain neocortex by deranging the arachidonate cascade in favor of prostanoids. J Neurochem 75:196–203, 2000

Maldonado JL, Fernandez F, Levy JK: Acquired immunodeficiency syndrome, in Psychiatric Management of Neurological Disease. Edited by Lauterbach EC. Washington, DC, American Psychiatric Press, 2000, pp 271–295

Mandel S, Weinreb O, Amit T, et al: Cell signaling pathways in the neuroprotective actions of the green tea polyphenol (–)-epigallocatechin-3-gallate: implications for neurodegenerative diseases. J Neurochem 88:1555–1569, 2004 [erratum in J Neurochem 89:527, 2004]

Marzuk PM, Tierney H, Tardiff K, et al: Increased risk of suicide in persons with AIDS. JAMA 259:1333–1337, 1988

McArthur JC, Brew B, Nath A: Neurological complications of HIV infection. Lancet Neurol 4:543–555, 2005

McDaniel SJ, Ninan PT, Magnuson JV: Possible induction of mania by buspirone. Am J Psychiatry 147:125–126, 1990

McElroy SL, Keck PE JR, Pope HG Jr, et al: Valproate in the treatment of bipolar disorder: literature review and clinical guidelines. J Clin Psychopharmacol 12::42S–52S, 1992

McGowan I, Potter M, George RJD, et al: HIV encephalopathy presenting as hypomania. Genitourin Med 67:420–424, 1991

Melton ST, Kirkwood CK, Ghaemi SN: Pharmacotherapy of HIV dementia. Ann Pharmacother 31:457–473, 1997

Miller K, Corcoran C, Armstrong C, et al: Transdermal testosterone administration in women with acquired immunodeficiency syndrome wasting: a pilot study. J Clin Endocrinol Metab 83:2717–2725, 1998

Navia BA, Gonzalez RG: Functional imaging of the AIDS dementia complex and the metabolic pathology of the HIV-1-infected brain. Neuroimaging Clin N Am 7:431–445, 1997

Neuenburg JK, Brodt HR, Herndier GB, et al: HIV-related neuropathology, 1985–1999: rising prevalence of HIV encephalopathy in the era of highly active antiretroviral therapy. J Acquir Immune Defic Syndr 31:171–177, 2002

O'Dowd MA, McKegney FP: Manic syndrome associated with zidovudine. JAMA 260:3587–3588, 1988

O'Dowd MA, McKegney FP: AIDS patients compared to others seen in psychiatric consultation. Gen Hosp Psychiatry 12:50–55, 1990

Perry S, Fishman B, Jacobsberg L, et al: Relationships over 1 year between lymphocyte subsets and psychosocial variables among adults with infection by human immunodeficiency virus. Arch Gen Psychiatry 49:396–401, 1992

Pomara N, Crandall DT, Chois SJ, et al: White matter abnormalities in HIV-1 infection: a diffusion tensor imaging study. Psychiatry Res 106:15–24, 2001

Post MJD, Berger JR, Quencer RM: Asymptomatic and neurologically symptomatic HIV-seropositive individuals: prospective evaluation with cranial MR imaging. Radiology 178:131–139, 1991

Power C, Selnes OA, Grim JA, et al: HIV Dementia Scale: a rapid screening test. J Acquir Immune Defic Syndr Hum Retrovirol 8:273–278, 1995

Price WA, Bielefeld M: Buspirone induced mania. J Clin Psychopharmacol 9:150–151, 1989

Rabkin JG, Wagner JG, McElhiney MC, et al: Testosterone versus fluoxetine for depression and fatigue in HIV/AIDS patients: a placebo controlled trial. J Clin Psychopharmacol 24:379–385, 2004

Reboul J, Schuller E, Pialoux G, et al: Immunoglobulins and complement components in 37 patients infected by HIV-1 virus: comparison of general (systemic) and intrathecal immunity. J Neurol Sci 89:243–252, 1989

Richelson E: Synaptic pharmacology of antidepressants: an update. McLean Hospital Journal 13:67–88, 1988

Rrapo E, Zhu Y, Tian J, et al: Green-tea EGCG reduces GFAP associated neuronal loss in HIV-1 Tat transgenic mice. Am J Transl Res 1(1):72–79, 2009

Sacktor N, Prohovnik I, Van Heertum RL, et al: Cerebral single-photon emission computed tomography abnormalities in human immunodeficiency virus type 1–infected gay men without cognitive impairment. Arch Neurol 52:607–611, 1995

Samochocki M, Hoffle A, Fehrenbacher A, et al: Galantamine is an allosterically potentiating ligand of neuronal nicotinic but not of muscarinic acetylcholine receptors. J Pharmacol Exp Ther 305:1024–1036, 2003

Santos MD, Alkondon M, Pereira EF, et al: The nicotinic allosteric potentiating ligand galantamine facilitates synaptic transmission in the mammalian central nervous system. Mol Pharmacol 61:1222–1234, 2002

Schaerf FW, Miller RS, Lipsey JR, et al: ECT for major depression in four patients infected with human immunodeficiency virus. Am J Psychiatry 146:782–784, 1989

Sekigawa I, Koshino K, Hishikawa T, et al: Inhibitory effect of the immunosuppressant FK506 on apoptotic cell death induced by HIV-1 gp120. J Clin Immunol 15:312–317, 1995

Selnes OA, Jacobson L, Machado AM, et al: Normative data for a brief neuropsychological screening battery. Percept Mot Skills 73:539–550, 1991

Sharma SM, McDaniel JS, Sheehan NL: General principles of pharmacotherapy for the patient with HIV infection, in HIV and Psychiatry: Training and Resource Manual. Edited by Citron K, Brouillette M-J, Beckett A. Cambridge, UK, Cambridge University Press, 2005, pp 56–87

Shiramizu B, Gartner S, Williams A, et al: Circulating proviral HIV DNA and HIV-associated dementia. AIDS 19:45–52, 2005

Shytle RD, Mori T, Townsend K, et al: Cholinergic modulation of microglial activation by alpha 7 nicotinic receptors. J Neurochem 89:337–343, 2004

Singh AN, Golledge H, Catalan J: Treatment of HIV-related psychotic disorders with risperidone: a series of 21 cases. J Psychosom Res 42:489–493, 1997

Skolasky RL, Esposito DR, Selnes OA, et al: Modified HIV Dementia Scale: accurate staging of HIV-associated dementia: neuroscience of HIV infection (abstract). J Neurovirol 4(suppl):366, 1998

Sockalingam S, Parekh N, Bogoch II, et al: Delirium in the postoperative cardiac patient: a review. J Card Surg 20:560–567, 2005

Stefano GB, Smith EM, Cadet P, et al: HIV gp120 alteration of DAMA and IL-1 alpha induced chemotaxic responses in human and invertebrate immunocytes. J Neuroimmunol 43:177–184, 1993

Stolar A, Catalano G, Hakala SM, et al: Mood disorders and psychosis in HIV, in HIV and Psychiatry: Training and Resource Manual. Edited by Citron K, Brouillette M-J, Beckett A. Cambridge, UK, Cambridge University Press, 2005, pp 88–109

Strauss A: Oral dyskinesia associated with buspirone use in an elderly woman. J Clin Psychiatry 49:322–323, 1988

Tucker K, Robertson KR, Lin W, et al: Neuroimaging in human immunodeficiency virus infection. J Neuroimmunol 157:153–162, 2004

Van Gorp WG, Miller E, Satz P, et al: Neuropsychological performance in HIV-1 immunocompromised patients (abstract). J Clin Exp Neuropsychol 11:35, 1989

Wagner GJ, Rabkin J: Effects of dextroamphetamine on depression and fatigue in men with HIV: a double-blind, placebo-controlled trial. J Clin Psychiatry 61:436–440, 2000

Wang Y, Sawchuk RJ: Zidovudine transport in the rabbit brain during intravenous and intracerebroventricular infusion. J Pharm Sci 84:871–876, 1995

Weiner RD: ECT in the physically ill. J Psychiatr Treat Eval 5:457–462, 1983

Weis S, Haug H, Budka H: Neuronal damage in the cerebral cortex of AIDS brains: a morphometric study. Acta Neuropathol 85:185–189, 1993

Wiley CA, Masliah E, Morey M, et al: Neocortical damage during HIV infection. Ann Neurol 29:651–657, 1991

Wilkie FL, Eisdorfer C, Morgan R, et al: Cognition in early human immunodeficiency virus infection. Arch Neurol 47:433–440, 1990

Wong SL, Wang Y, Sawchuk RJ: Analysis of zidovudine distribution to specific regions in rabbit brain using microdialysis. Pharm Res 9:332–338, 1992

Wong SL, Van Bell K, Sawchuk RJ: Distributional transport kinetics of zidovudine between plasma and brain extracellular fluid/cerebrospinal fluid in the rabbit: investigation of the inhibitory effect of probenecid utilizing microdialysis. J Pharmacol Exp Ther 264:899–909, 1993

Wright JM, Sachdev PS, Perkins RJ, et al: Zidovudine-related mania. Med J Aust 150:339–341, 1989

Yarchoan R, Berg G, Brouwers P, et al: Response of human-immunodeficiency-virus-associated neurological disease to 3′-azido-3′-deoxythymidine. Lancet 1:132–135, 1987

9

Dementias Associated With Motor Dysfunction

Alan J. Lerner, M.D.
David Riley, M.D.

The dementias associated with motor system dysfunction are diverse disorders. Depending on where the primary pathology occurs in the motor system (basal ganglia, cerebellum, or motor neuron), symptoms can include abnormal movements, incoordination, or weakness, in addition to the neuropsychiatric features. In contrast, in primary degenerative dementias such as Alzheimer's disease (AD) and variably in frontotemporal dementia (FTD), motor signs are relatively incidental and usually become prominent only in later stages of the disease (see Chapter 10, "Alzheimer's Disease and Other Dementing Illnesses").

In this chapter, we review Huntington's disease (HD), Parkinson's disease (PD), progressive supranuclear palsy (PSP), and other conditions in which movement or motor disorders are cardinal clinical features. The specific etiologies of

287

these diseases are often unknown, the understanding of genetic and molecular pathogenesis is incomplete, and clinical features frequently overlap among different conditions, making a clear nosology difficult.

The combination of motor, cognitive, and behavioral abnormalities is particularly stressful for patients, family members, and professional caregivers because of the multifaceted impairment in quality of life. Medications available to treat the motor symptoms may aggravate cognitive and behavioral dysfunction. Motor impairments themselves can create special difficulties in neuropsychiatric and neuropsychological testing.

Dementia classification depends on proper understanding of essential clinical and biological features. One early approach was the distinction between cortical and subcortical dementias (Albert et al. 1974). AD and behavioral variant FTD (formerly called Pick's disease) were considered prototypical cortical dementias, with predominantly neocortical pathology and clinical symptoms such as aphasia, apraxia, and agnosia. In contrast, patients with subcortical dementias (e.g., HD, PD, PSP) were said to show prominent deficits in processing speed, memory dysfunction, and affective changes. However, dementias cannot be easily classified into these two large categories because of overlap in site of pathology and symptomatology (Apaydin et al. 2002; Mayeux et al. 1983; Whitehouse 1986).

Huntington's Disease

HD is an autosomal dominant (chromosome 4) progressive neuropsychiatric disorder with peak onset in the fourth and fifth decades. Chorea—brief, random, nonstereotyped, purposeless movements—is often the first sign of the disease. However, the clinical presentation is variable, and cognitive and psychiatric manifestations may be the initial symptoms. Depression, irritability, and impulsive or erratic behavior are the most common psychiatric symptoms (Folstein 1989; Martin and Gusella 1986).

Epidemiology

Prevalence among Caucasians is 5–7 cases per 100,000, and prevalence in various European populations is relatively uniform (Harper 1992). Early onset is associated with paternal transmission and a more rapid course. In adult-onset cases, death usually occurs after 16–20 years. The rate of decline may be slower in patients with onset after the fifth decade of life.

Etiology

The HD gene locus is at the distal end of the short arm of chromosome 4. The mutant gene consists of an expanded trinucleotide cytosine-adenine-guanine (CAG) repeat sequence. Normal alleles have a range from 9 to 30 CAG repeats, whereas HD patients have from 40 to at least 121 repeats (Albin and Tagle 1995). Patients with repeat lengths between 36 and 39 may or may not become symptomatic. Although age at onset is related to the number of gene repeats, environmental factors contribute as much as 38% of the variability in age at onset (Wexler et al. 2004).

Diagnosis and Clinical Features

The key step in HD diagnosis is to consider it as a possibility, because laboratory diagnosis requires only confirmation of the expanded CAG repeats. The classic clinical syndrome of HD consists of chorea, dementia, and/or psychiatric disturbances in the setting of a positive family history consistent with autosomal dominant inheritance. Clinical diagnosis may be confounded by other movement disorders, atypical presentations, or a family history that is incomplete or misleading (e.g., mistaken paternity). In the 3%–9% of cases with adolescent onset (the so-called Westphal variant), parkinsonism, myoclonus, or dystonia may be the predominant movement conditions. The differential diagnosis of HD includes PD, Sydenham's chorea, ataxias, cerebrovascular disease, systemic lupus erythematosus, schizophrenia, mood disorder, thyroid disease, acanthocytosis, drug-induced chorea, and alcoholism.

Nearly half of HD patients initially present with emotional or cognitive symptoms, including depression, irritability, hallucinations, and apathy. Motor symptoms may be mild and attributed to another disorder. However, when the patient has a positive family history, HD is a very likely explanation of these symptoms. The clinical and ethical issues involved in preclinical genetic testing for HD have been widely discussed. These issues must be explored on an individual basis and may be aided by employing an experienced genetic counselor (Broadstock et al. 2000).

Neurobiology

The gross pathology in HD consistently affects the striatum, with degeneration beginning in the medial caudate nucleus and proceeding laterally to the putamen and occasionally to the globus pallidus.

The gene product of the HD gene is a protein called *huntingtin*. In unaffected individuals, it is a cytosolic protein, but in patients with HD, it is transported to the cell nucleus. The mechanism by which its abnormal transport and deposition in intraneuronal inclusions relate to molecular pathophysiology is currently unknown. The actual mechanisms of cell destruction in the caudate nucleus may include abnormal posttranslation cleavage products that disturb cellular metabolism (Albin and Tagle 1995) or N-methyl-D-aspartate (NMDA)–mediated excitotoxicity. Reductions occur in γ-aminobutyric acid (GABA), the main neurotransmitter of spiny output neurons, and acetylcholine, the main neurotransmitter of type I aspiny interneurons (Martin and Gusella 1986).

The degree of atrophy of the caudate nucleus correlates with cognitive dysfunction, including intelligence, memory, and visuospatial deficits. Atrophy of the caudate nucleus is generally more consistently correlated than measures of frontal atrophy, with impaired executive functions typically considered to be evidence of prefrontal cortical pathology. Similar associations between functional impairments and caudate nucleus pathology have been reported with positron emission tomography (PET) (Bamford et al. 1989; Morris 1995; Starkstein et al. 1988).

Motor Abnormalities

HD has also been called *Huntington's chorea,* emphasizing the prominence of chorea, which is characterized by involuntary sudden, jerky movements of the limbs, face, or trunk, unpredictable in timing or distribution. Patients can generally suppress chorea for only short periods. Parkinsonism or dystonia, in the absence of chorea, is common in juvenile-onset (Westphal variant) cases.

Early motor abnormalities include brief, irregular, jerky movements along with slower, writhing movements, often occurring in conjunction with the initiation of action. Irregular flexion-extension of individual fingers and ulnar deviation of the hands while walking are also common. Later, movements become almost constant, with severe grimacing, nodding, head bobbing, and a "dancing" gait. In late disease, chorea may decrease, and dystonia and an akinetic-rigid syndrome may supervene, especially in those with drug-induced parkinsonism.

Early in the course of the disease, chorea may be misdiagnosed as nervousness or intentional movements. Patients have abnormalities in initiation and inhibition of eye movements (saccades, fixation, and smooth pursuit), coordination of limb movements, and articulation. These abnormalities correlate better with intellectual impairment and capacity for activities of daily living than does chorea severity.

Cognitive Abnormalities

Cognitive deficits usually appear early in the course of HD and are progressive. Although cognitive deficits can occur very early, it is unclear whether neuropsychological deficits appear before other clinical signs of the disease (Giordani et al. 1995). When the deficits are severe, a brief mental status test is sufficient.

Memory deficits are the best-characterized neuropsychological feature of the disease. Early studies (Brandt and Butters 1986) suggested that HD was characterized by major deficits in the encoding or storage of new information. However, deficits in retrieval of memories and the acquisition of procedural memory appear to be even more pronounced (Folstein et al. 1990).

Mendez (1994) found that for any given level of dementia, the pattern of failure is different in HD and AD. At mild levels of dementia, patients with HD are more impaired in serial subtraction, whereas patients with AD are more likely to have errors in recall. HD patients also have difficulties in sustained concentration and visuospatial skills. Executive dysfunction also appears early in HD.

Language, with the exception of verbal fluency and prosody, is relatively preserved in HD (Mendez 1994). Patients, however, may have deficits in the ability to understand speech prosody.

Psychiatric Abnormalities

Psychiatric symptoms are common in HD and are often the first signs of the disorder. Estimates of the proportion of patients who first present with psychiatric symptoms range from 24% to 79% (Folstein 1989). The number of CAG repeats did not correlate with psychiatric symptoms (Vassos et al. 2008).

Studies suggest that affective disorders and intermittent explosive disorders are the most prevalent psychiatric conditions in HD (Folstein 1989; Folstein et al. 1990). Unipolar depression is common, but mania can also be seen in conjunction with HD. A markedly elevated risk of suicide is found in persons with HD, with the greatest risk for individuals in their 50s and 60s (Cummings 1995; Mendez 1994). Up to 85% of patients are reported to show altered sexual behavior (Mendez et al. 2011; Schmidt and Bonelli 2008). Later on in the disease, apathy and abulia are common psychiatric manifestations.

Treatment

Tetrabenazine, which has been approved in the United States for treatment of chorea, acts by depleting neurotransmitters. Tetrabenazine can increase the risk of depression and suicidal thoughts and behavior (suicidality) in patients with HD; given the frequency of depression in patients with HD, the drug's use must be carefully monitored.

Neuroleptics have long been used for suppressing chorea. Treatment is not always effective, and dopamine blockade increases the risk of tardive dyskinesia, worsening depression, and cognitive effects. Because the impairment of voluntary movement persists, reducing chorea generally does not improve disability.

Tricyclic antidepressants or lithium can be effective in the treatment of affective symptoms. Improvement may be greater for the somatic-vegetative aspects of the syndrome than for the subjective elements of depression. Manic symptoms may respond more to neuroleptics and carbamazepine than to lithium (Mendez 1994). Irritability and aggressive outbursts respond to both environmental changes and neuroleptics.

Social support along with case management can be very important in the adaptation of the family to the diagnosis of HD and the management of the illness within the family.

Parkinson's Disease

In 1817, James Parkinson described "the shaking palsy," now referred to as *Parkinson's disease*. The cardinal features include tremor, muscle rigidity, bradykinesia, and postural instability. When these features occur in another identified entity, the term *parkinsonism* or *secondary parkinsonism* is used.

Epidemiology and Etiology

PD shows dramatic age-related increases in prevalence. The prevalence of PD is approximately 150 per 100,000, increasing after age 65 to nearly 1,100 per 100,000. Genetic causes of PD are involved in 10%–20% of cases. Worldwide, the prevalence and incidence vary widely, possibly due to both genetic and environmental variability (Bekris et al. 2010; Muangpaisan et al. 2011).

Environmental risk factors are highlighted by the association of PD with use of a meperidine analogue (Langston et al. 1983). Positive associations have been found between PD risk and rural living and drinking of well water, and a negative association has been established between smoking and the risk for PD.

Dementia probably occurs in 20%–40% of patients with PD, and depression occurs in up to 50% of these patients. Family histories of dementia, depression, and severe motor disability increase dementia risk. The decline in mental status scores on the Mini-Mental State Examination is similar for patients with PD and patients with AD (Aarsland et al. 2004).

Neurobiology

PD is accompanied by the formation of Lewy bodies, which are hyaline inclusion bodies. Lewy bodies occur in brain stem nuclei, particularly the substantia nigra and locus coeruleus. Occurrence of Lewy bodies in the neocortex has led to the recognition of dementia with Lewy bodies (DLB). PD begins in lower brain stem structures (an asymptomatic stage), followed by the substantia nigra (onset of motor manifestations of PD) and ultimately other cerebral structures, including cortex (Braak et al. 2003). The loss of dopaminergic cells in the substantia nigra relates to akinesia and rigidity. Dementia in PD is most clearly associated with cortical Lewy bodies.

Motor Symptoms

The most disabling motor features of PD are asymmetric bradykinesia and rigidity. Poverty of associated movements (such as blinking or arm swing when walking) is characteristic. Rigidity can affect all muscle groups. Tremor is the presenting feature in most cases, is relatively slow (3–7 Hz), often occurs distally, and is prominent at rest. It increases with distraction and may increase during walking.

Postural changes are a late development in PD and take two forms. One is a characteristic flexion at the neck, waist, elbows, and knees. The other, postural instability or disequilibrium, can lead to falls and serious injury. Early occurrence of postural instability should raise suspicion of PSP, multiple system atrophy (MSA), or another akinetic-rigid syndrome. Treatment may improve tremor, rigidity, and akinesia but rarely has any effect on postural instability or dementia.

PD is frequently associated with development of restless legs syndrome, which responds to L-dopa, dopamine agonists, or benzodiazepines.

Cognitive Impairments

Cognitive impairment may complicate PD at any time during its course. Visuospatial impairment is common in PD. Constructional praxis is affected in PD, perhaps partly because of problems with spatial attention. The communication difficulties of PD are mostly due to hypophonia and dysarthria. Language impairments include reduced verbal fluency and naming difficulties. Executive and attentional abnormalities can be attributed to frontal lobe dysfunction. These deficits include difficulties in sequencing voluntary motor activities, difficulties in maintaining and switching set, and abnormalities in selective attention.

The relationships between the cognitive impairments and the motor symptoms in PD are complex. Poor performance on cognitive tests is not purely related to motor abnormalities. However, the presence of akinetic-rigid motor deficit makes comparisons with dementias such as AD or HD difficult to interpret.

Psychiatric Disturbances

Affective disorder is common in PD, with an estimated incidence of up to 90% (Mayeux et al. 1986). The frequency of depression is higher in early-onset cases (Kostic et al. 1994).

Anxiety such as fear of falling (a real risk in advanced PD) is common. Sleep is frequently problematic in PD, but this disturbance is frequently multifactorial, being affected by medications, motor and nonmotor symptoms, and age, as well as depression and anxiety.

Psychosis

Medications trigger the vast majority of episodes of psychosis in PD. Dementia is the most important risk factor for psychosis, and age and visual impairment contribute to risk. All of the antiparkinsonian medications can cause hallucinations, especially trihexyphenidyl.

Dementia

The occurrence of dementia in PD presents a diagnostic and therapeutic challenge, and the diagnosis may change over time as the patient's full clinical picture develops. In a study of rivastigmine, moderate improvements occurred, but treated patients had higher rates of nausea, vomiting, and tremor (Emre et al. 2004).

Nonmotor Impairments

Nonmotor impairments are common in PD and may precede motor symptoms by years. These include pain, chronic constipation, impaired olfactory function, impaired sleep, and cognitive disturbances.

Treatment

Treatment of Motor Dysfunction

Medication classes include L-dopa, which may be given with inhibitors of its breakdown, such as monoamine oxidase B (MAO-B) inhibitors and catechol O-methyltransferase (COMT) inhibitors; dopamine agonists; amantadine; and anticholinergic agents. As PD progresses, treatment with L-dopa is often complicated by dose-related fluctuations and dyskinesias, particularly in younger patients. Use of extended-release L-dopa and MAO-B and COMT inhibitors can help with this symptom. Other agents that can help in treating motor fluctuations are selegiline and subcutaneous apomorphine (Bowron 2004). Selegiline may cause the unusual side effect of transvestic fetishism, which in one case resolved when selegiline was discontinued (Riley 2002).

Dopamine agonists are associated with cognitive side effects, postural hypotension, and peripheral edema. Dopamine agonists may cause sedation, including sleep attacks while driving, and compulsive behaviors related to gambling, sexual activity, and eating.

Behavioral treatment begins with a careful assessment of the medical aspects and the functional effects of the illness on the patient and family. Nursing and social work assessments are important in providing a baseline for following the course of the illness, and follow-up care to modify the treatment plan is essential. Early planning, both financial and legal, is helpful to minimize the difficulty of gaining access to and financing home care, day care, or institutional care.

Interventions such as individual psychotherapy can help with depression early in the illness. Physical and occupational therapy may be very helpful, and a home safety evaluation may prevent falls.

Biological Treatment of Dementia

An important goal in treatment of patients with PD and dementia is prevention of so-called excess disability, which is frequently a result of intercurrent illnesses, psychological stress, or iatrogenic disease such as that due to overuse of medication.

Treatment of depression in PD parallels that of non-PD depression. Virtually all antidepressants may aggravate tremor, with the notable exception of mirtazapine. While helping motor disabilities, antidepressants or other medications with significant anticholinergic potential can aggravate dementia or orthostatic hypotension.

Antipsychotics may worsen motor symptoms, dementia, or both. Cholinesterase inhibitors may help with dementia and may minimally improve psychosis. The atypical neuroleptics that produce little if any exacerbation of parkinsonism are quetiapine and clozapine (Motsinger et al. 2003). Other atypical antipsychotics that were thought to cause few extrapyramidal side effects, such as risperidone, olanzapine, and aripiprazole, have been disappointments in this regard. Atypical antipsychotics have relatively high anticholinergic potential and can cause lethargy and conceivably affect cognition. Sleep disturbances are common with psychotic disorders, and a primary focus should be on teaching sleep hygiene techniques.

Although cholinesterase inhibitors occasionally lead to worsening of parkinsonism, they are usually well tolerated and may produce measurable levels of cognitive enhancement that equal or surpass their effectiveness in AD (Emre et al. 2004). The role of memantine in treating PD-related dementia is unclear, but no contraindication to its use is apparent.

Surgical Treatment

In some patients with PD, medication does not control motor manifestations or results in intolerable side effects. These patients may benefit from stereotactic surgery. The surgical treatment of choice is deep brain stimulation targeting the subthalamic nucleus. Deep brain stimulation often leads to more consistent control of PD symptoms and may allow for medication reduction, sometimes ameliorating cognitive dysfunction. Rarely, electrode implantation results in irreversible cognitive deterioration; worsened cognitive outcomes are more common in older patients and in those with preexisting dementia. A decrease in verbal fluency, particularly with left subthalamic nucleus stimulation, has been reported. Changes in personality and acute depression also have been reported (Hugdahl and Wester 2000; Schmand et al. 2000). Following surgery, some patients may experience improved cognitive scores, such as improvements in cognitive flexibility (Witt et al. 2004). In most patients, surgery is well tolerated from a cognitive standpoint, and cognitive complications are typically transient.

Dementia With Lewy Bodies

DLB is an increasingly recognized dementia. DLB occurs as the sole pathology but is often (approximately 50% of the time) mixed with AD pathology. Rest tremor was more common in patients with PD than in patients with DLB, whereas myoclonus was more common in those with DLB; the two groups did not differ in frequency of rigidity, bradykinesia, dystonia, or gaze palsies (Louis et al. 1997). Response to L-dopa is much more predictive of PD.

Clinical Diagnosis

Diagnostic criteria for DLB have long included the presence of two of three cardinal features: hallucinations (especially visual), spontaneous parkinsonism, and daily fluctuations in cognition. However, the clinical criteria have been criticized as being of low sensitivity (Hohl et al. 2000). False-negative DLB cases tended to lack hallucinations and spontaneous parkinsonism (McKeith et al. 2000). To improve diagnostic sensitivity, McKeith et al. (2005) created newer diagnostic criteria. Dementia is now obligatory for diagnosis of possible or probable DLB, with frequent occurrence of supportive features recognized, including rapid eye movement sleep behavior disorder, repeated falls and syncope, autonomic dysfunction, nonvisual hallucinations, delusions, depression, and reduced occipital regional cerebral blood flow.

Neurobiology

Genetic forms of DLB exist, including autosomal dominant forms, and patients with these forms of DLB may respond well to L-dopa therapy. Autopsy studies have shown that compared with patients with AD, about half of patients with DLB have similar numbers of neuritic plaques but fewer neurofibrillary tangles (Samuel et al. 1997). Sabbagh et al. (1999) found that reductions in synaptophysin and choline acetyltransferase did not correlate with dementia severity in DLB as they did in AD.

Neuroimaging

Neither structural nor functional neuroimaging is specifically helpful in diagnosing DLB.

Treatment

DLB patients may respond as well as or better than AD patients to cholinesterase inhibitors. No large controlled trials of memantine have been done to support a recommendation for its use in DLB. When taking nonselective neuroleptics, patients with DLB need to be observed for side effects such as neuroleptic malignant syndrome and extrapyramidal side effects.

Progressive Supranuclear Palsy

Progressive supranuclear palsy (also known as Steele-Richardson-Olszewski syndrome) is a progressive disorder with eye movement abnormalities, parkinsonism, and dementia. The prevalence is estimated at 1.4 per 100,000. Median age at onset of symptoms is approximately 63, and median survival is 6–10 years (Golbe et al. 1988).

Diagnosis

Patients with PSP often have parkinsonism without tremor, as well as early postural instability and eye movement abnormalities, especially decreased saccadic velocity (Leigh and Riley 2000). With disease progression, pursuit eye movements are also impaired. Testing of reflex eye movements with passive head turning shows relative preservation of vertical eye movements (hence the term *supranuclear*, because the oculocephalic reflexes determine the integrity of the lower motor neuron pathways for up and down gaze). Lack of vertical eye movement abnormalities is the largest obstacle to correct antemortem diagnosis of PSP (Litvan et al. 1999). Many patients with PSP have no noticeable dementia or it is often not severe early in the course, although patients may demonstrate slowing of thought processes, and emotional or personality changes. Other signs include axial dystonia, bradyphrenia, perseveration, forced grasping, and utilization behaviors. Pseudobulbar palsy may be observed in the later stages.

Neuropsychiatric Manifestations

Patients with PSP often have disturbances of sleep and depression and, rarely, a schizophreniform psychosis. They may experience memory loss, slowed thinking, personality changes, inappropriate crying or laughing, and obsessive-compulsive behaviors.

Levy et al. (1998) found that apathy correlated with lower cognitive function but not with depression. Patients with PSP have particular impairment in sequential movement tasks and in tasks requiring shifting of concepts, monitoring of the frequency of stimuli, or rapid retrieval of verbal information (Grafman et al. 1990). Apraxia may develop in cases with prominent cerebral cortical involvement (Bergeron et al. 1997).

Diagnostic Imaging

In patients with PSP, neuroimaging shows early atrophy of midbrain structures, with later atrophy of the pons and frontotemporal regions (Savoiardo et al. 1989). Fluorodeoxyglucose PET studies show marked frontal and temporal hypometabolism.

Neurobiology

Neuropathological findings in PSP include neuronal loss associated with gliosis and neurofibrillary tangles, most marked in the substantia nigra, basal forebrain, subthalamic nucleus, pallidum, and superior colliculus. Additional areas that might be involved include the locus coeruleus, the striatum, and a variety of upper brain stem and midbrain structures (Agid et al. 1987).

The tangles in PSP are straight filaments. Mutations in the tau gene on chromosome 17 are responsible for most clinical cases of PSP. In PSP, only the four-repeat tau isoform aggregating into straight filaments is found. Because of the presence of tau pathology and clinical overlapping syndromes, many experts now include PSP with the other FTD syndromes.

The neurochemistry of PSP is characterized by massive dopamine depletion in the striatum and reduced density of striatal dopamine type 2 receptors (Pierot et al. 1988). Additionally, widespread reduction occurs in choline acetyltransferase levels (Whitehouse et al. 1988).

Treatment

No treatment has been found to be effective in relieving the motor or cognitive deficiencies in PSP. L-Dopa treatment is generally not successful, correlating with the loss of postsynaptic striatal dopamine receptors, and may worsen cognitive function. Poor responses with frequent dose-limiting side effects often occur with dopamine agonists.

Corticobasal Ganglionic Degeneration

Corticobasal ganglionic degeneration (which we abbreviate as CBD) presents with asymmetric basal ganglia (akinesia, rigidity, dystonia) and cerebral cortical (apraxia, cortical sensory loss, alien limb) manifestations (Riley et al. 1990). The alien limb is seen with parietal lobe, medial frontal lobe, and corpus callosum pathology. Dementia is a variable but may be the presenting symptom (Lang 2003). The neuropsychological profile shows prominent executive dysfunction, explicit memory deficits without retention difficulties, and asymmetric apraxias (Pillon et al. 1995). Other neuropsychiatric abnormalities in CBD include depression, apathy or disinhibition, aberrant motor behaviors, and delusions (Litvan et al. 1998). Oculomotor involvement similar to that in PSP may occur. Survival ranges from 2.5 to 12 years, with a median of about 8 years.

CBD pathology shows abundant ballooned, achromatic neurons and focal cortical atrophy predominating in medial frontal and parietal lobes, plus degeneration of the substantia nigra. Astrocytic plaques are also seen in neocortex. CBD neuronal tau pathology shows wispy, fine-threaded tau inclusions (Dickson 1999).

Magnetic resonance imaging (MRI) may show asymmetric atrophy in the frontal and parietal lobes contralateral to the dominantly affected limbs (Soliveri et al. 1999).

Treatment of CBD is limited, with only a minority of patients responding to L-dopa preparations given for parkinsonism. Myoclonus may respond to benzodiazepines, particularly clonazepam. No specific treatment for the dementia is available, but it may not be cholinergic in nature, suggesting that cholinesterase inhibitors are of limited value. Depression is common in CBD, but few data exist on treatment response (Kampoliti et al. 1998; Litvan et al. 1998).

Frontotemporal Dementia

The FTDs constitute a heterogeneous group of conditions, often with prominent early behavioral disinhibitory symptoms. There are a confusing number of phenotypes, subsuming Pick's disease, semantic aphasia, hereditary dysphasic dementia (Morris et al. 1984), progressive aphasias (fluent and nonfluent), PSP, and CBD. Neuropsychiatric symptoms include Klüver-Bucy syndrome or social withdrawal, depression, and a schizophrenia-like illness in middle adulthood. Patients may develop parkinsonism and occasionally amyotrophy (Josephs et al. 2006).

Motor neuron disease presents as a form of FTD in about 20% of FTD cases, and amyotrophic lateral sclerosis may be admixed with dementia. A loss of neurons occurs in layers 2 and 3 of the cortical mantle, particularly in the frontal and temporal regions. Specific decreases in spindle-shaped cells called von Economo neurons have been linked to behavioral changes in FTD (Graham and Hodges 2008; Seeley et al. 2006).

The FTDs have been linked to mutations in the tau protein gene, progranulin gene, TAR DNA-binding protein 43 gene, and several rarer genes. The FTD phenotypes have been expanded in recent years to include tauopathies such as PSP and CBD (see sections earlier in this chapter).

Multiple System Atrophy

MSA is a disease concept that unifies striatonigral degeneration, Shy-Drager syndrome, and sporadic olivopontocerebellar atrophy. Diagnostic criteria require evidence of orthostatic hypotension or urinary incontinence in combination with either L-dopa–unresponsive parkinsonism or cerebellar dysfunction. Cognitive dysfunction is rare (Gilman et al. 1998); however, autopsy-proven cases of MSA have been associated with dementia (Schlossmacher et al. 2004).

Friedreich's Ataxia

Friedreich's ataxia is an autosomal recessive disorder presenting as slowly progressive ataxia, areflexia, pes cavus, and scoliosis. Mental changes are present in about a quarter of cases. Psychiatric disorders, including schizophrenia-like psychoses and depression, can occur. Personality abnormalities may be marked.

Spinocerebellar Ataxias

Spinocerebellar ataxia (SCA) classification has been revolutionized by the discovery of gene loci, with more than 25 loci described. The molecular pathogenesis may involve excess polyglutamine repeats, channelopathies, or gene expression disorders but remains unknown in most cases. The ataxic disorders may not be accompanied by intellectual changes until late in the illness, and frequency varies by SCA type. Patients may have apathy and psychomotor retardation and occasionally depression or schizophrenia-like psychosis. SCA-17 can have an HD-like phenotype (Bruni et al. 2004). Patients with SCA-2 or SCA-12 may develop dementia (Geschwind 1999; O'Hearn et al. 2001). Cerebellar ataxia itself is generally considered resistant to medications.

Wilson's Disease

Wilson's disease, also called *hepatolenticular degeneration,* affects the basal ganglia in association with abnormalities in liver function. It is the result of an autosomally recessive defect in copper metabolism, in a defective P-type adenosine triphosphatase (Cuthbert 1995), that leads to excessive copper deposition in the liver, corneas, and basal ganglia. Onset is usually in the second or third decade, with dystonia, parkinsonism, or cerebellar ataxia. Patients also may have dysarthria, dysphagia, hypophonia, or seizures. Chronic hepatitis or hemolytic anemia may be detected. Kayser-Fleischer rings consist of brown or green discolorations near the limbus of the cornea and are seen in nearly all patients with neurological signs. Imaging shows abnormal signal in the lenticular nuclei, caudate nuclei, thalamus, dentate nuclei, and brain stem. The diagnosis may be established by slit-lamp examination of the cornea, a serum ceruloplasmin level less than 20 mg/dL, a 24-hour copper excretion of more than 100 mg, or a liver biopsy showing increased hepatic copper concentration.

Wilson's disease may present with schizophrenia-like changes, depression, or manic-depressive states. Aggressive and self-destructive or antisocial acts may also occur. Intellectual deterioration is relatively mild in the early symptomatic stages (Akil and Brewer 1995).

Treatment of Wilson's disease consists of maintaining a negative copper balance and frequent administration of a copper-chelating agent (Brewer 2005). Patients with advanced disease may require liver transplantation. Neurological symptoms, including dementia, improve with long-term therapy. L-Dopa may be of some benefit in reversing neurological symptoms not improved by direct copper therapies.

Calcification of the Basal Ganglia (Fahr's Disease)

Calcification of the basal ganglia, or Fahr's disease, is a rare, occasionally autosomal dominant disorder (Geschwind et al. 1999). Computed tomography scans show extensive calcification of the basal ganglia and periventricular white matter. Dystrophic calcification occurs in pediatric acquired immunodeficiency syndrome, Aicardi-Goutières syndrome, trisomy 21, Kearns-Sayre syndrome, tumors (e.g., astrocytomas) or vascular lesions, and hypoparathyroidism. Patients may present in early adulthood with a schizophrenia-like psychosis or mood disorder or later in life with an extrapyramidal syndrome, dementia, and mood changes. Apathy, poor judgment, and impaired memory are usually prominent, and language function is often spared. Choreoathetosis, cerebellar ataxia, and dystonia also may be seen.

Normal-Pressure Hydrocephalus

Normal-pressure hydrocephalus (NPH) is a syndrome composed of the triad of dementia, gait disturbance, and urinary incontinence. It may be associated with a history of meningitis, intracranial bleeding, or head injury. A wide-based gait with slow steps and difficulty initiating locomotion are characteristic. Usually, no changes occur in motor strength or tone.

The diagnosis requires symptom recognition and neuroimaging showing an enlarged ventricle disproportionate to cerebral atrophy. MRI scanning may show transependymal fluid flux. Difficulties in diagnosis arise in determining whether hydrocephalus could be congenital or secondary to cerebral atrophy. It may be difficult to determine if dementia in suspected NPH is not due to other causes. In a series in which shunted patients also underwent brain biopsy, the prevalence of AD ranged from 31% to 50% (Savolainen et al. 1999).

Dementia of NPH presents primarily with attentional difficulties but can progress to include apathy, lethargy, mental slowing, perseveration, and memory dysfunction. Language is typically spared early in the course. Psychosis may occur, sometimes early in the course.

High-volume lumbar puncture (up to 50 mL) or external lumbar drainage and cerebrospinal fluid (CSF) pressure measurement and analysis are commonly recommended; sensitivity of specific tests may vary. Transient improvement in gait, urinary incontinence, or neuropsychological functioning may help predict surgical treatment response.

CSF shunting may help up to 70% of patients (Verrees and Selman 2004). The best cognitive results occur in patients whose cognitive disturbances are relatively mild and who have early onset of urinary incontinence and gait disturbance. After shunting, memory may improve more than frontostriatal dysfunction (Iddon et al. 1999). Use of programmable pressure valves reduces the rate of postshunting hematomas while ensuring optimal shunting in a given patient. Late shunt failure, as a result of mechanical failure or obstruction, may present as worsening clinical status (Williams et al. 1998).

Recommended Readings

Huntington's Disease

Hague SM, Klaffke S, Bandmann O: Neurodegenerative disorders: Parkinson's disease and Huntington's disease. J Neurol Neurosurg Psychiatry 76:1058–1063, 2005

Landles C, Bates GP: Huntingtin and the molecular pathogenesis of Huntington's disease. Fourth in molecular medicine review series. EMBO Rep 5:958–963, 2004

Parkinson's Disease

Jankovic J: An update on the treatment of Parkinson's disease. Mt Sinai J Med 73:682–689, 2006

Savitt JM, Dawson VL, Dawson TM: Diagnosis and treatment of Parkinson disease: molecules to medicine. J Clin Invest 116:1744–1754, 2006

Dementia With Lewy Bodies

Lippa CF, Duda JE, Grossman M, et al: DLB and PDD boundary issues: diagnosis, treatment, molecular pathology, and biomarkers. Neurology 68:812–819, 2007

McKeith IG, Rowan E, Askew K, et al: More severe functional impairment in dementia with Lewy bodies than Alzheimer disease is related to extrapyramidal motor dysfunction. Am J Geriatr Psychiatry 14:582–588, 2006

Mosimann UP, Rowan EN, Partington CE, et al: Characteristics of visual hallucinations in Parkinson disease dementia and dementia with Lewy bodies. Am J Geriatr Psychiatry 14:153–160, 2006

Weisman D, McKeith I: Dementia with Lewy bodies. Semin Neurol 27:42–47, 2007

Progressive Supranuclear Palsy

Rampello L, Butta V, Raffaele R, et al: Progressive supranuclear palsy: a systematic review. Neurobiol Dis 20:179–186, 2005

Corticobasal Ganglionic Degeneration

Sha S, Hou C, Viskontas IV, et al: Are frontotemporal lobar degeneration, progressive supranuclear palsy and corticobasal degeneration distinct diseases? Nat Clin Pract Neurol 2:658–665, 2006

Frontotemporal Dementia

Boxer AL, Miller BL: Clinical features of frontotemporal dementia. Alzheimer Dis Assoc Disord 19 (suppl 1):S3–S6, 2005

Multiple System Atrophy

Bak TH, Rogers TT, Crawford LM, et al: Cognitive bedside assessment in atypical parkinsonian syndromes. J Neurol Neurosurg Psychiatry 76:420–422, 2005

Singer W, Opfer-Gehrking TL, McPhee BR, et al: Acetylcholinesterase inhibition: a novel approach in the treatment of neurogenic orthostatic hypotension. J Neurol Neurosurg Psychiatry 74:1294–1298, 2003

Friedreich's Ataxia and Spinocerebellar Ataxias

Geschwind DH: Focusing attention on cognitive impairment in spinocerebellar ataxia. Arch Neurol 56:20–22, 1999

Motor Neuron Disease With Dementia

Ringholz GM, Greene SR: The relationship between amyotrophic lateral sclerosis and frontotemporal dementia. Curr Neurol Neurosci Rep 6:387–392, 2006

Wilson's Disease

Ala A, Walker AP, Ashkan K, et al: Wilson's disease. Lancet 369:397–408, 2007

Fahr's Disease
Schmidt U, Mursch K, Halatsch ME: Symmetrical intracerebral and intracerebellar calcification ("Fahr's disease"). Funct Neurol 20:15, 2005

Normal-Pressure Hydrocephalus
McGirt MJ, Woodworth G, Coon AL, et al: Diagnosis, treatment, and analysis of long-term outcomes in idiopathic normal-pressure hydrocephalus. Neurosurgery 57:699–705, 2005
Relkin N, Marmarou A, Klinge P, et al: Diagnosing idiopathic normal-pressure hydrocephalus. Neurosurgery 57 (suppl 3):S4–S16, 2005

References

Aarsland D, Andersen K, Larsen JP, et al: The rate of cognitive decline in Parkinson disease. Arch Neurol 61:1906–1911, 2004

Agid Y, Javoy-Agid F, Ruberg M, et al: Progressive supranuclear palsy: anatomoclinical and biochemical considerations, in Parkinson's Disease (Advances in Neurology Series, Vol 45). Edited by Yahr MD, Bergmann KJ. New York, Raven, 1987, pp 191–206

Akil M, Brewer GJ: Psychiatric and behavioral abnormalities in Wilson's disease, in Behavioral Neurology of Movement Disorders (Advances in Neurology Series, Vol 46). Edited by Weiner WJ, Lang AE. New York, Raven, 1995, pp 171–178

Albert ML, Feldman RG, Willis AL: The "subcortical dementia" of progressive supranuclear palsy. J Neurol Neurosurg Psychiatry 37:121–130, 1974

Albin RL, Tagle DA: Genetics and molecular biology of Huntington's disease. Trends Neurosci 18:11–14, 1995

Apaydin H, Ahlskog JE, Parisi JE, et al: Parkinson disease neuropathology: later-developing dementia and loss of the levodopa response. Arch Neurol 59:102–112, 2002

Bamford K, Caine E, Kido D, et al: Clinical-pathologic correlation in Huntington's disease: a neuropsychological and computed tomography study. Neurology 39:796–801, 1989

Bekris LM, Mata IF, Zabetian CP: The genetics of Parkinson disease. J Geriatr Psychiatry Neurol 23:228–242, 2010

Bergeron C, Pollanen MS, Weyer L, et al: Cortical degeneration in progressive supranuclear palsy: a comparison with cortical-basal ganglionic degeneration. J Neuropathol Exp Neurol 56:726–734, 1997

Bowron A: Practical considerations in the use of apomorphine injectable. Neurology 62 (suppl 4):S32–S36, 2004

Braak H, Del Tredici K, Rub U, et al: Staging of brain pathology related to sporadic Parkinson's disease. Neurobiol Aging 24:197–211, 2003

Brandt J, Butters N: The neuropsychology of Huntington's disease. Trends Neurosci 9:118–120, 1986

Brewer GJ: Neurologically presenting Wilson's disease: epidemiology, pathophysiology and treatment. CNS Drugs 19:185–192, 2005

Broadstock M, Michie S, Marteau T: Psychological consequences of predictive genetic testing: a systematic review. Eur J Hum Genet 8:731–738, 2000

Bruni AC, Takahashi-Fujigasaki J, Maltecca F, et al: Behavioral disorder, dementia, ataxia, and rigidity in a large family with TATA box-binding protein mutation. Arch Neurol 61:1314–1320, 2004

Cummings JL: Behavioral and psychiatric symptoms associated with Huntington's disease, in Behavioral Neurology of Movement Disorders (Advances in Neurology Series, Vol 65). Edited by Weiner WJ, Lang AE. New York, Raven, 1995, pp 179–186

Cuthbert JA: Wilson's disease: a new gene and an animal model for an old disease. J Investig Med 43:323–326, 1995

Dickson DW: Neuropathologic differentiation of progressive supranuclear palsy and corticobasal degeneration. J Neurol 246 (suppl 2):6–15, 1999

Emre M, Aarsland D, Albanese A, et al: Rivastigmine for dementia associated with Parkinson's disease. N Engl J Med 351:2509–2518, 2004

Folstein SE: Huntington's Disease: A Disorder of Families. Baltimore, MD, Johns Hopkins University Press, 1989

Folstein SE, Brandt J, Folstein MF: Huntington's disease, in Subcortical Dementia. Edited by Cummings JL. New York, Oxford University Press, 1990, pp 87–107

Geschwind DH: Focusing attention on cognitive impairment in spinocerebellar ataxia. Arch Neurol 56:20–22, 1999

Geschwind DH, Loginov M, Stern JM: Identification of a locus on chromosome 14Q for idiopathic basal ganglia calcification (Fahr disease). Am J Hum Genet 65:764–772, 1999

Gilman S, Low PA, Quinn N, et al: Consensus statement on the diagnosis of multiple system atrophy. J Auton Nerv Syst 74:189–192, 1998

Giordani B, Berent S, Boivin MJ, et al: Longitudinal neuropsychological and genetic linkage analysis of persons at risk for Huntington's disease. Arch Neurol 52:59–64, 1995

Golbe LI, Davis PH, Schoenberg BS, et al: Prevalence and natural history of progressive supranuclear palsy. Neurology 38:1031–1034, 1988

Grafman J, Litvan I, Gomez C, et al: Frontal lobe function in progressive supranuclear palsy. Arch Neurol 47:553–558, 1990

Graham A, Hodges JR: Frontotemporal dementia. Psychiatry 7(1):24–28, 2008

Harper PS: The epidemiology of Huntington's disease. Hum Genet 89:365–376, 1992

Hohl U, Tiraboschi P, Hansen LA, et al: Diagnostic accuracy of dementia with Lewy bodies. Arch Neurol 57:347–351, 2000

Hugdahl K, Wester K: Neurocognitive correlates of stereotactic thalamotomy and thalamic stimulation in parkinsonian patients. Brain Cogn 42:231–252, 2000

Iddon JL, Pickard JD, Cross JJ, et al: Specific patterns of cognitive impairment in patients with idiopathic normal pressure hydrocephalus and Alzheimer's disease: a pilot study. J Neurol Neurosurg Psychiatry 67:723–732, 1999

Josephs KA, Parisi JE, Knopman DS, et al: Clinically undetected motor neuron disease in pathologically proven frontotemporal lobar degeneration with motor neuron disease. Arch Neurol 63:506–512, 2006

Kampoliti K, Goetz CG, Boeve BF, et al: Clinical presentation and pharmacological therapy in corticobasal degeneration. Arch Neurol 55:957–961, 1998

Kostic VS, Filipovic SR, Lecic D, et al: Effect of age at onset on frequency of depression in Parkinson's disease. J Neurol Neurosurg Psychiatry 57:1265–1267, 1994

Lang AE: Corticobasal degeneration: selected developments. Mov Disord 18 (suppl 6): S51–S56, 2003

Langston JW, Ballard P, Tetrud JW, et al: Chronic parkinsonism in humans due to a product of meperidine-analog synthesis. Science 219:979–980, 1983

Leigh RJ, Riley DE: Eye movements in parkinsonism: it's saccadic speed that counts. Neurology 54:1018–1019, 2000

Levy ML, Cummings JL, Fairbanks LA, et al: Apathy is not depression. J Neuropsychiatry Clin Neurosci 10:314–319, 1998

Litvan I, Cummings JL, Mega M: Neuropsychiatric features of corticobasal degeneration. J Neurol Neurosurg Psychiatry 65:717–721, 1998

Litvan I, Grimes DA, Lang AE, et al: Clinical features differentiating patients with postmortem confirmed progressive supranuclear palsy and corticobasal degeneration. J Neurol 246 (suppl 2):1–5, 1999

Louis ED, Klatka LA, Liu Y, et al: Comparison of extrapyramidal features in 31 pathologically confirmed cases of diffuse Lewy body disease and 34 pathologically confirmed cases of Parkinson's disease. Neurology 48:376–380, 1997

Martin JB, Gusella JF: Huntington's disease: pathogenesis and management. N Engl J Med 20:1267–1276, 1986

Mayeux R, Stern Y, Rosen J, et al: Is "subcortical dementia" a recognizable clinical entity? Ann Neurol 14:278–283, 1983

Mayeux R, Stern Y, Williams JBW, et al: Clinical and biochemical features of depression in Parkinson's disease. Am J Psychiatry 143:756–759, 1986

McKeith IG, Ballard CG, Perry RH, et al: Prospective validation of consensus criteria for the diagnosis of dementia with Lewy bodies. Neurology 54:1050–1058, 2000

McKeith IG, Dickson DW, Lowe J, et al: Diagnosis and management of dementia with Lewy bodies: third report of the DLB Consortium. Neurology 65:1863–1872, 2005

Mendez MF: Huntington's disease: update and review of neuropsychiatric aspects. Int J Psychiatry Med 24:189–208, 1994

Mendez MF, Shapira JS, Saul RE: The spectrum of sociopathy in dementia. J Neuropsychiatry Clin Neurosci 23:132–140, 2011

Morris JC, Cole M, Banker BQ, et al: Hereditary dysphasic dementia and the Pick-Alzheimer spectrum. Ann Neurol 16:455–466, 1984

Morris M: Dementia and cognitive changes in Huntington's disease, in Behavioral Neurology of Movement Disorders (Advances in Neurology Series, Vol 65). Edited by Weiner WJ, Lang AE. New York, Raven, 1995, pp 187–200

Motsinger CD, Perron GA, Lacy TJ: Use of atypical antipsychotic drugs in patients with dementia. Am Fam Physician 67:2335–2340, 2003

Muangpaisan W, Mathews A, Hori H, et al: A systematic review of the worldwide prevalence and incidence of Parkinson's disease. J Med Assoc Thai 94:749–755, 2011

O'Hearn E, Holmes SE, Calvert PC, et al: SCA-12: tremor with cerebellar and cortical atrophy is associated with a CAG repeat expansion. Neurology 56:299–303, 2001

Pierot L, Desnos C, Blin J, et al: D1 and D2-type dopamine receptors in patients with Parkinson's disease and progressive supranuclear palsy. J Neurol Sci 86:291–306, 1988

Pillon B, Blin J, Vidailhet M, et al: The neuropsychological pattern of corticobasal degeneration: comparison with progressive supranuclear palsy and Alzheimer's disease. Neurology 45:1477–1483, 1995

Riley DE: Reversible transvestic fetishism in a man with Parkinson's disease treated with selegiline. Clin Neuropharmacol 25:234–237, 2002

Riley DE, Lang AE, Lewis A, et al: Cortical-basal ganglionic degeneration. Neurology 40:1203–1212, 1990

Sabbagh MN, Corey-Bloom J, Tiraboschi P, et al: Neurochemical markers do not correlate with cognitive decline in the Lewy body variant of Alzheimer disease. Arch Neurol 45:1458–1461, 1999

Samuel W, Alford M, Hofstetter CR, et al: Dementia with Lewy bodies versus pure Alzheimer disease: differences in cognition, neuropathology, cholinergic dysfunction, and synapse density. J Neuropathol Exp Neurol 56:499–508, 1997

Savoiardo M, Strada L, Girotti F, et al: MR imaging in progressive supranuclear palsy and Shy-Drager syndrome. J Comput Assist Tomogr 13:555–560, 1989

Savolainen S, Paljärvi L, Vapalahti M: Prevalence of Alzheimer's disease in patients investigated for presumed normal pressure hydrocephalus: a clinical and neuropathological study. Acta Neurochir (Wien) 141:849–853, 1999

Schlossmacher MG, Hamann C, Cole AG, et al: Case records of the Massachusetts General Hospital: weekly clinicopathological exercises. Case 27–2004: a 79-year-old woman with disturbances in gait, cognition, and autonomic function. N Engl J Med 351:912–922, 2004

Schmand B, de Bie RM, Koning-Haanstra M, et al: Unilateral pallidotomy in PD: a controlled study of cognitive and behavioral effects. The Netherlands Pallidotomy Study (NEPAS) group. Neurology 54:1058–1064, 2000

Schmidt EZ, Bonelli RM: Sexuality in Huntington's disease. Wien Med Wochenschr 158:78–83, 2008

Seeley WW, Carlin DA, Allman JM, et al: Early frontotemporal dementia targets neurons unique to apes and humans. Ann Neurol 60:660–667, 2006

Soliveri P, Monza D, Paridi D, et al: Cognitive and magnetic resonance imaging aspects of corticobasal degeneration and progressive supranuclear palsy. Neurology 53:502–507, 1999

Starkstein SE, Brandt J, Folstein S, et al: Neuropsychologic and neuropathologic correlates in Huntington's disease. J Neurol Neurosurg Psychiatry 51:1259–1263, 1988

Vassos E, Panas M, Kladi A, et al: Effect of CAG repeat length on psychiatric disorders in Huntington's disease. J Psychiatr Res 42:544–549, 2007

Verrees M, Selman WR: Management of normal pressure hydrocephalus. Am Fam Physician 70:1071–1078, 2004

Wexler NS, Lorimer J, Porter J, et al: Venezuelan kindreds reveal that genetic and environmental factors modulate Huntington's disease age of onset. Proc Natl Acad Sci U S A 101:3498–3503, 2004

Whitehouse PJ: The concept of subcortical and cortical dementia: another look. Ann Neurol 19:1–6, 1986

Whitehouse PJ, Martino AM, Marcus KA, et al: Reductions in acetylcholine and nicotine binding in several degenerative diseases. Arch Neurol 45:722–724, 1988

Williams MA, Razumovsky AY, Hanley DF: Evaluation of shunt function in patients who are never better, or better than worse after shunt surgery for NPH. Acta Neurochir (Wien) 71:368–370, 1998

Witt K, Pulkowski U, Herzog J, et al: Deep brain stimulation of the subthalamic nucleus improves cognitive flexibility but impairs response inhibition in Parkinson disease. Arch Neurol 61:697–700, 2004

10

Alzheimer's Disease and Other Dementing Illnesses

Liana G. Apostolova, M.D., M.S.

Jeffrey L. Cummings, M.D.

The dementias are a large group of neuropsychiatric disorders that preferentially affect elderly people. The socioeconomic significance of these disorders is on a steady rise as the number of elderly persons continues to increase. The most common dementia, Alzheimer's disease (AD), accounts for 60%–70% of all dementias in older individuals. More than 90% of patients with AD are age 65 years or older. The second most common dementia, dementia with Lewy bodies (DLB), accounts for 15%–20% of newly diagnosed dementia cases, and vascular dementia (VaD) accounts for another 5%–10% (Corey-Bloom 2004). DLB and VaD also occur in seniors. In patients younger than 65 years, frontotemporal dementia (FTD) is as common as AD; it accounts for 5%–9% of all newly diagnosed dementia cases (Graff-Radford and Woodruff 2004).

Diagnostic and Research Criteria

DSM-IV-TR (American Psychiatric Association 2000) defines *dementia* as an acquired cognitive syndrome of sufficient severity to result in functional decline. The diagnosis requires that the following two conditions be met: 1) impairments of memory and in at least one additional cognitive domain and 2) functional decline resulting in impaired activities of daily living, vocational abilities, or social interactions. Because these criteria are broad and nonspecific, dementia experts have developed more refined research criteria for each of the major dementia syndromes (see Tables 10–1, 10–2, 10–3, and 10–4, later in chapter) (Dubois et al. 2007; McKeith et al. 2005; Neary et al. 1998; Roman et al. 1993).

Alzheimer's Disease

AD (Table 10–1) is the most common cause of cognitive decline among elderly people. It frequently follows a prodromal stage during which amyloid pathology is already accumulating but has not reached the threshold for interfering with activities of daily living (Dubois et al. 2007). As the disease progresses, the initially isolated memory deficits evolve into more multidimensional cognitive decline, with disturbance in language, visuospatial skills, and executive and social functioning.

Early in the disease course, the patients have deficient verbal and visual encoding, impaired delayed recall, concrete thinking, and mild anomia (Pasquier 1999). They may have trouble operating a vehicle and managing their finances. Patients may have deficient emotional processing manifested in difficulty with interpretation of facial expression and speech prosody (Cummings 2003). As the disease progresses, they develop transcortical sensory aphasia, with relatively preserved syntax and phonological abilities (Pasquier 1999). Their judgment and ability to perform instrumental activities of daily living decline. Neurovegetative disturbances such as appetite loss and sleep-wake cycle disruption are common (Cummings 2003). As patients continue to deteriorate, they progressively lose the ability to perform the more basic activities of daily living, such as dressing, eating, toileting, and finally communicating and ambulating. They typically succumb to the complications of immobilization (Kukull et al. 1994).

Table 10–1. Diagnostic criteria for Alzheimer's disease (AD)

Definite AD	Probable AD
Sporadic late-onset AD: Both a diagnosis of probable AD and histopathologic evidence of AD should be present Autosomal dominant AD: Both clinical and genetic evidence for autosomal dominant AD should be present	*Core criterion:* Early significant episodic memory impairment • With gradual and progressive course over more than 6 months • With objective evidence of impaired episodic memory on neuropsychological testing that does not normalize with cueing or recognition testing • Concomitant impairments in other cognitive domains are possible *Supportive features (one or more required)* • Evidence of medial temporal lobe atrophy (hippocampus, amygdala, entorhinal atrophy) • Positive cerebrospinal fluid biomarkers such as low Aβ (amyloid-beta protein), increased total tau or phosphorylated tau individually or in combination • Functional neuroimaging suggestive of AD pathology (bilateral temporoparietal hypometabolism/hypoperfusion or positive amyloid ligand imaging [using PIB (Pittsburgh Compound B) or FDDNP]) • Proven AD autosomal dominant mutation in the immediate family *Exclusion criteria* • Sudden onset of cognitive decline or early occurrence of gait or behavioral disturbances or seizures • Clinical features: focal neurological signs or early extrapyramidal signs • Other disorders severe enough to account for the clinical manifestation such as non-AD dementia, major depression, cerebrovascular disease, toxic/metabolic abnormalities

Source. Dubois et al. 2007.

Neuropsychiatric Features

Patients with AD display a host of personality and behavior changes in addition to cognitive decline. Some behaviors are more stage specific than others. Early in the disease course, patients show apathy, depressed mood, anxiety, and irritability (Lyketsos et al. 2000; Mega et al. 1996). Depression in AD is associated with decreased quality of life, functional impairment, increased aggression, and increased institutionalization, as well as caregiver burden and caregiver depression (Cummings 2003; Lyketsos and Olin 2002). Depression in AD has been linked to more precipitous cognitive decline (Heun et al. 2003).

Apathy in AD is a complex syndrome, consisting of loss of interest, motivation, volition, enjoyment, spontaneity, and emotional behavior. It is the most common neuropsychiatric symptom in AD, affecting 42% of the patients with mild, 80% with moderate, and 92% with advanced AD (Mega et al. 1996). Apathy may occur up to 3 years prior to diagnosis (Jost and Grossberg 1996). Apathy and the associated executive dysfunction (Boyle et al. 2003; McPherson et al. 2002) result in inefficient social and environmental interaction, decreased engagement in day-to-day activities and personal care, and worse quality of life (Boyle et al. 2003; Freels et al. 1992). Apathy most likely results from disruption of the anterior cingulate and dorsolateral prefrontal circuits (Apostolova et al. 2007a; Mega and Cummings 1994).

Anxiety is another early feature of AD. It can present with apprehension and inner feelings of nervousness and autonomic signs such as tachycardia, perspiration, dry mouth, or chest tightness. Relative to elderly persons without dementia, in whom the prevalence of anxiety is 5.8% (Lyketsos et al. 2002), and to persons with mild cognitive impairment (MCI), in whom the prevalence is 11%–39% (Apostolova and Cummings 2008), the frequency of anxiety in persons with AD dementia averages 48% (Mega et al. 1996).

Irritability is seen in 4.6% of cognitively normal elderly people, 29% of patients with MCI, and 42% of patients with AD (Lyketsos et al. 2002).

As AD progresses, its behavioral profile expands. Some behaviors that are only rarely encountered in the premorbid amnestic MCI or in the mild AD stages, such as disinhibition, abnormal motor behaviors, hallucinations, and delusions, ensue (Piccininni et al. 2005). In advanced AD, agitation, aggression, irritability, and violent behaviors are prominent and may prompt nursing home placement.

Disinhibition may manifest with impulsivity, tactlessness, loss of empathy, and violation of social boundaries. It results from dysfunction in the fronto-subcortical circuits (Cummings 1993).

Aberrant motor behaviors include a variety of manifestations, such as fidgetiness, pacing, and inability to stay still. The prevalence of these behaviors exponentially increases with disease progression (Lyketsos et al. 2000; Mega et al. 1996).

Psychotic symptoms such as delusions and hallucinations are common features of AD and several other neurodegenerative disorders. They can result in patient distress, caregiver dissatisfaction, and early residential placement (Steele et al. 1990). The delusions are rarely as bizarre as in some primary psychiatric disorders such as schizophrenia. Common delusional themes are paranoia, theft, and infidelity. Content-specific delusions and misidentification syndromes occur mostly later in the disease course (Devanand et al. 1997).

Hallucinations in AD are typically in the visual modality and tend to resolve with time (Marin et al. 1997). Both hallucinations and delusions correlate with poor insight (Migliorelli et al. 1995) and faster cognitive and functional decline (Rosen and Zubenko 1991). Other disturbing behaviors are wandering, occurring in up to 43% of AD patients, and disturbed diurnal sleep, occurring in 56% (Jost and Grossberg 1996).

Pathology

AD is a neurodegenerative disorder that results from accumulation of amyloid-β (Aβ) and tau protein. Aβ is a segment of the amyloid precursor protein (APP) that is liberated by the joint action of two proteases: β-secretase and γ-secretase. In healthy individuals, these two enzymes are responsible for only a small fraction of the APP cleavage, while the majority is accomplished by a third protease, α-secretase, which splits the large APP molecule in the midst of the Aβ sequence and prevents the formation of the potentially toxic 39- to 43-amino acid Aβ protein (Mesulam 2000). Aβ polymerizes, producing first oligomeres and later polymers that clump together and form several types of amyloid inclusions. The diffuse and neuritic plaques deposit extracellularly. *Vascular amyloid* is the term for Aβ accumulation within the walls of cortical blood vessels (Duyckaerts and Dickson 2003).

Tau, a structural protein of the microtubular transport system, plays a role in microtubule stabilization. Tau's affinity for microtubules is closely regulated by phosphorylation/dephosphorylation. AD tau is hyperphosphorylated, whereby its function is severely compromised. Tau forms intracellular neurofibrillary tangles and dendritic inclusions in the form of neuropil threads and dystrophic neurites (Duyckaerts and Dickson 2003).

Genetics

Sporadic AD (e.g., late-onset AD) generally occurs after age 65. Its mode of inheritance is governed by the synergistic action of a constellation of genes further modified by epigenetic influences. The risk for and the age at onset of AD are modified by the apolipoprotein E gene (*APOE*) on chromosome 19. *APOE* encodes a 299–amino acid glycoprotein functioning as cholesterol transporter. *APOE*E4*, one of the gene's three alleles, promotes Aβ aggregation (Esler et al. 2002) and suppresses neural plasticity (Nathan et al. 2002). It has been shown to accelerate disease onset in a dose-dependent fashion (Khachaturian et al. 2004). The *APOE*E4* effect is modified by race, being stronger in Caucasians than African Americans (Evans et al. 2003), and inversely by advancing age (Blacker et al. 1997). Epigenetic influences, such as mental and physical exercise, high educational level, and a healthy diet rich in polyunsaturated as opposed to saturated fats (Luchsinger et al. 2007), offer protection from AD.

When AD presents before age 65 years (early-onset AD), consideration should be given to three autosomal dominant mutations: the APP gene mutation on chromosome 21, the presenilin-1 gene mutation on chromosome 14, and the presenilin-2 gene mutation on chromosome 1. Autosomal dominant early-onset AD is known for its atypical clinical features, which may include aphasia, dysarthria, myoclonus, seizures, paraplegia, and dystonia (Binetti et al. 2003; Miklossy et al. 2003; Rippon et al. 2003).

Some of the atypical neuropsychiatric symptoms of early-onset AD are emotional lability, obsessive-compulsive behavior (Rippon et al. 2003), an FTD type of presentation, and hyperoral, hyperphagic, and hypersexual behavior resembling Klüver-Bucy syndrome (Tang-Wai et al. 2002).

Neuroimaging

The American Academy of Neurology (2001) currently recommends a noncontrast structural image—either computed tomography or magnetic resonance imaging (MRI)—as part of the initial evaluation for cognitive impairment. MRI has several advantages—most notably, better resolution. The classic structural changes of AD are global cerebral atrophy with mesial temporal and parietal predilection. Hippocampal volume loss is evident not only in the predementia stage of MCI (Apostolova et al. 2006) but also in the presymptomatic (i.e., pre-MCI) stages of AD (Apostolova et al. 2010a). Gray matter atrophy can be visualized easily with computational anatomy techniques. It is most pronounced in the association cortices, while primary cortices are relatively spared (Apostolova and Thompson 2008; Apostolova et al. 2007b).

Functional neuroimaging techniques such as single-photon emission computed tomography and positron emission tomography add another dimension to the workup. They provide an estimate of neuronal function rather than cerebral structure and reveal early hypoperfusion/hypometabolic changes in lateral temporal and parietal distribution and in the posterior cingulate (Apostolova et al. 2010b). Later in the disease, global hypoperfusion/hypometabolism is the rule, with relative sparing of the basal ganglia and the primary sensorimotor and visual cortices (Silverman 2004).

Therapy

The acetylcholinesterase inhibitors donepezil (Doody 2003), galantamine (Raskind 2003), and rivastigmine (Farlow 2003) were the first class of pharmaceuticals approved by the U.S. Food and Drug Administration (FDA) for treatment of AD. Their effect is mediated by increased availability of acetylcholine in the synaptic cleft. These three agents have modest cognitive, functional, and behavioral effects and a safe side-effect profile.

Memantine is approved for treatment of moderate to severe AD. Memantine is a weak N-methyl-D-aspartate (NMDA) receptor blocker and as such prevents the deleterious effects of continuous toxic low levels of glutamate while allowing the physiologically advantageous large glutamate surge to exert its required cognitive effect. Memantine has also been shown to stimulate long-term potentiation and ameliorate tau hyperphosphorylation (Li et al. 2004; Voisin et al. 2004).

Management of Neuropsychiatric Disturbances

Treatment of the neuropsychiatric manifestations of AD remains rather empirical to date. No agents for the behavioral aspects of AD have been approved by the FDA. Depressive mood may respond to selective serotonin reuptake inhibitors (SSRIs) such as citalopram, sertraline, or escitalopram. In depression with psychotic symptoms or for treatment of psychosis in AD, the newer-generation antipsychotics, such as risperidone, quetiapine, olanzapine, aripiprazole, or ziprasidone, are typically helpful. Anxiety is best approached with SSRIs rather than benzodiazepines. The atypical antipsychotics may be useful in refractory cases. Agitation, irritability, and aggression, when mild, are best treated with behavioral modifications such as structure, gentle reassurance, and redirection. The educational and emotional support of caregivers in the management of these challenging behaviors is of utmost importance. When absolutely necessary, one should once again consider the use of atypical antipsychotics or the SSRIs.

When prescribing atypical antipsychotics, physicians should take into consideration the FDA warning of the associated increased risk for stroke in elderly persons with dementia—which emerged after post hoc data analyses of randomized placebo-controlled trials of risperidone and olanzapine—and the increased risk of death associated with all antipsychotics, typical and atypical. This risk is highest for patients with risk factors for stroke, such as hypertension, diabetes, or atrial fibrillation (Bullock 2005; Sink et al. 2005).

Dementia With Lewy Bodies

DLB accounts for 15%–20% of all late-onset dementias and is the second most prevalent dementing disorder of the elderly population (Corey-Bloom 2004). The most recent diagnostic criteria (McKeith et al. 2005) are listed in Table 10–2.

Cognitive decline in DLB is somewhat different from that observed in AD. Memory impairment is less severe in DLB, but attention and visuospatial and visuoperceptual functions can be severely affected early in the disease course. Cognitive fluctuations in AD are minor; however, in DLB they are profound, resulting in significant variability in cognitive performance, fluctuating alertness, and frank episodes of delirium. Cognitive fluctuations can be short lived, lasting a few minutes, or persist for several days. Fluctuations are described in as many as 50%–75% of patients with DLB (McKeith et al. 2004).

DLB is closely related to Parkinson's disease dementia; it is arbitrarily accepted to diagnose Parkinson's disease dementia if motor symptoms precede cognitive decline by more than 12 months and DLB if they occur within 12 months of each other. The extrapyramidal symptoms observed in DLB—bradykinesia, rigidity, resting tremor, and gait disturbance—are typically symmetric. Extrapy-

Table 10-2.   Diagnostic criteria for dementia with Lewy bodies (DLB)

Central feature

Progressive cognitive decline interfering with activities of daily living (with prominent decline in attention, executive function, or visuospatial performance)

Core features

Cognitive fluctuations

Recurrent visual hallucinations

Spontaneous features of parkinsonism (bradykinesia, rigidity, gait disturbance)

Suggestive features

Repeated falls

Severe autonomic dysfunction (orthostatic hypotension, urinary incontinence)

Transient loss of consciousness

Neuroleptic sensitivity

Systematized delusions

Hallucinations in other modalities

Depression

Relative preservation of medial temporal lobe structures on computed tomography/magnetic resonance imaging

Generalized hypometabolism/hypoperfusion with reduced occipital activity

Low uptake on myocardial scintigraphy

Prominent slow-wave activity on electroencephalographic examination, with transient sharp waves in the temporal lobes

Source.   McKeith et al. 2005.

ramidal symptoms are one of the initial presenting symptoms of DLB in 25%–50% of patients and develop later in the disease course in up to 100% of the patients (McKeith et al. 2004).

Distinguishing DLB from AD and VaD may be challenging. Early falls and presyncopal/syncopal episodes are characteristic of DLB. DLB features prominent sleep disorders, most notably rapid eye movement sleep behavior disorder. This sleep disorder bears a positive predictive value of 92% for DLB (Boeve et al. 2001) and can precede the onset of extrapyramidal symptoms, cognitive decline, and fluctuations and visual hallucinations in up to 80% of patients with DLB (Ferman et al. 2002).

A characteristic but ominous clinical symptom is the unusual sensitivity of patients with DLB to neuroleptic medications. Adverse extrapyramidal symptoms were reported in 81% of DLB patients versus 19% of AD patients. The reactions included sedation, confusion, severe parkinsonism with extreme rigidity and immobility, and neuroleptic malignant syndrome. The mortality hazard ratio is 2.3 (McKeith et al. 1992). Thus, neuroleptic use is contraindicated in patients with DLB.

Neuropsychiatric Features

Up to 98% of patients with DLB experience at least one psychiatric symptom during the course of their illness. Multiple simultaneous psychiatric symptoms are almost universal (Ballard et al. 1996). At disease onset, neuropsychiatric features are much more common in DLB than in AD (Simard et al. 2000).

Delusions are common in DLB, with a prevalence of 50% compared with 30% in AD (Simard et al. 2000). The most common theme is delusional misidentification (see Table 10–2), followed by paranoid beliefs (theft, conspiracy, harassment, abandonment, infidelity) and phantom boarder syndrome. Of the delusional misidentifications, mistaking TV images for real occurs in 19% of patients, followed by Capgras syndrome in 10%, mistaking one's mirror image for another person in 9.5%, and reduplicative paramnesia in 2.4% (Ballard et al. 1996).

Depression is more common in DLB than in AD (Ballard et al. 1999), although the symptomatology seems not to differ (Samuels et al. 2004). A depressed cognitively impaired patient has a 16 times higher likelihood to harbor DLB than of having AD pathology (Papka et al. 1998). Major depression per DSM-III-R criteria (American Psychiatric Association 1987) was observed in 33% of the patients with DLB (McKeith et al. 1992).

Anxiety disorder per DSM-IV-TR criteria is rare in DLB, whereas feeling anxious is very common (Ballard et al. 1996). Up to 84% of DLB patients appear or feel anxious (Rockwell et al. 2000). Of three studies that used the Neuropsychiatric Inventory, two found anxiety to be one of the most prominent neuropsychiatric features of DLB (Del Ser et al. 2000; Hirono et al. 1999; McKeith 2000).

Very few studies have assessed the full neuropsychiatric spectrum in DLB. Among the three Neuropsychiatric Inventory studies, apathy emerged as the most common psychopathology. Agitation, aberrant motor behavior, and aggression were also significant in DLB, whereas euphoria and disinhibition were rarely reported (Del Ser et al. 2000; Hirono et al. 1999; McKeith 2000).

Neuropsychiatric remission occurs less frequently in DLB than in AD or VaD patients (28%, 63%, and 33%, respectively), largely because of persistent visual hallucinations.

Pathology

The major pathological finding in DLB is the *Lewy body*. The major component of the Lewy body—α-synuclein—is a natively unfolded 140–amino acid polypeptide. α-Synuclein functions as a modulator of synaptic transmission and synaptic vesicle transport. It also plays a role in neuronal plasticity (Jellinger 2003; Spillantini 2003).

Lewy bodies are frequently seen in the amygdala and brain stem nuclei of patients with DLB, Parkinson's disease, or AD, and occasionally in cognitively intact elderly persons. Cortical Lewy bodies, however, are seen in temporal, insular, and cingulate cortices in dementia patients with DLB, Parkinson's disease dementia, and sometimes AD (Jellinger 2003).

Neuroimaging

On structural imaging, patients with DLB manifest brain atrophy in a pattern similar to that observed in patients with AD but with lesser severity (Burton et al. 2002; Harvey et al. 1999; Hashimoto et al. 1998).

Functional imaging has demonstrated temporoparietal and occipital involvement in DLB. Occipital involvement helps differentiate DLB from AD (Lobotesis et al. 2001; Minoshima et al. 2001).

The most distinctive and useful imaging modality to date is dopamine transporter imaging, which shows impaired dopamine transporter function in DLB and normal function in AD (O'Brien et al. 2004).

Therapy

Similar to AD, DLB is characterized by cholinergic deficits. Two randomized placebo-controlled rivastigmine trials showed cognitive improvement specifically in vigilance, working memory, episodic memory, attention, and executive function (McKeith et al. 2000; Wesnes et al. 2002). The noncognitive symptoms in DLB also tend to respond favorably to therapy with acetylcholinesterase inhibitors. Most responsive to this therapy are hallucinations, paranoid delusions, daytime somnolence, apathy, aggression, and agitation (Simard and van Reekum 2004). Most important, neuroleptic use is contraindicated in DLB because of the extreme risk of severe side effects such as neuroleptic malignant syndrome and death. Neuroleptic malignant syndrome is only rarely reported with atypical antipsychotics (McKeith et al. 1995). Extreme caution in instituting atypical antipsychotic therapy in DLB is advised. Treatment should begin with very low dosages under close supervision for cognitive or extrapyramidal side effects (Swanberg and Cummings 2002).

Frontotemporal Dementia

FTD is a group of disorders that, as the name implies, result from focal atrophy of the frontal and/or temporal lobes, with characteristic behavioral and neuropsychological features. The three subtypes of FTD are frontal variant FTD, primary progressive aphasia, and semantic dementia (Table 10–3). Onset around age 70 is typical for semantic dementia, whereas primary progressive aphasia and frontal variant FTD tend to occur in younger persons.

Neuropsychiatric Features

Relative to patients with AD, patients with FTD have significantly more apathy, euphoria, disinhibition, and abnormal motor behavior. In addition, patients with frontal variant FTD show other behavioral features such as emotional lability, profound emotional coldness, loss of social comportment, and loss of empathy.

Obsessive-compulsive behavior, in either its simple form (lip smacking, hand clapping, counting) or its complex form (hoarding, repeating a fixed route, having a strict routine, hyperorality, food craving, eating the same food item every day, complex ritualistic behaviors), is present in 24% of patients with FTD at presentation and in 47% two years after diagnosis (Bathgate et al. 2001; Mendez and Perryman 2002).

Table 10–3.   Diagnostic criteria for frontotemporal dementia (FTD)

Frontal variant FTD

Insidious onset and gradual progression

Early decline in interpersonal conduct

Early decline in personal conduct

Emotional blunting

Loss of insight

Decline in personal hygiene and grooming

Mental rigidity and inflexibility

Distractibility and impersistence

Hyperorality and dietary changes

Preparations and/or stereotyped behavior

Utilization behavior

Neuroimaging evidence of predominant frontal and temporal lobe involvement

Primary progressive aphasia

Insidious onset and gradual progression

Dysfluent speech output with at least one of the following: agrammatism, phonemic paraphasias, anomia

Supportive features: stuttering, apraxia of speech, impaired repetition, alexia, agraphia, early preservation of single word comprehension, late mutism, early preservation of social skills, late behavioral changes similar to frontal variant FTD

Neuroimaging evidence of predominant superior temporal, inferior frontal, and insular involvement

Semantic dementia

Insidious onset and gradual progression

Progressive fluent empty spontaneous speech

Loss of semantic word knowledge with impaired naming and single word comprehension

Semantic paraphasias

Supportive features: pressured speech, idiosyncratic word substitution, surface dyslexia and dysgraphia

Neuroimaging evidence of predominant anterior temporal lobe involvement

Source.   Modified from Neary et al. 1998.

Pathology

Pathologically, FTD is divided into tau-positive and tau-negative forms. Pick's disease is characterized by striking frontotemporal atrophy, with underlying intraneuronal argyrophil spherical tau inclusions (i.e., Pick bodies), striking neuronal loss, and swollen neurons (i.e., Pick cells) (Lantos and Cairns 2001). Some hereditary FTD forms show tau inclusions in neurons and glia, neuronal loss, and vacuolation of the superficial cortical layers (Ghetti et al. 2003; Lantos and Cairns 2001).

Several tau-negative forms of FTD have been described. One is pathologically defined as dementia lacking distinctive histopathology (DLDH), in which neuronal loss, gliosis, and microvacuolation are the sole pathological features. Nevertheless, when biochemical analyses were conducted, substantial reductions in the soluble brain tau content in both gray and white matter were found (Zhukareva et al. 2003). The tau-negative ubiquitin-positive FTD is frequently a familial disorder and may present as FTD, as amyotrophic lateral sclerosis (ALS), or as a combination of the two (Lantos and Cairns 2001).

Genetics

Forty percent of FTD patients have a positive family history. Such kinships have allowed the identification of multiple pathogenic mutations of the tau gene on chromosome 17. These mutations are all autosomal dominant and have high penetrance but also significant phenotypic variability (Ghetti et al. 2003; Hodges and Miller 2001). FTD with DLDH pathology has been linked to chromosome 3, and the ubiquitin positive–tau negative FTD-ALS forms have revealed causative mutations on chromosomes 9 and 17 (Lowe and Rossor 2003). The responsible gene on chromosome 17 has been recognized as the progranulin gene (Gijselinck et al. 2008).

Neuroimaging

The neuroimaging profiles of the three subtypes of FTD are distinct (Gorno-Tempini et al. 2004; Rosen et al. 2002). The behavioral variant of FTD has predominant frontal and to a lesser extent temporal atrophy, usually more significant on the right. Primary progressive aphasia is associated with left inferior frontal, left insular, and left superior temporal involvement. Semantic dementia is associated with atrophy of the left anterior temporal pole and gray matter loss in temporal, parietal, and frontal lobes. Functional imaging shows frontotemporal hypometabolism.

Therapy

Presently, no effective therapy for FTD is available. SSRIs have been tested in open-label fashion. They provide symptomatic relief from compulsive behaviors, depression, disinhibition, and carbohydrate craving, and reduce caregiver burden (Moretti et al. 2003; Swartz et al. 1997). Selegiline, a monoamine oxidase B inhibitor, may influence behavior and improve executive performance (Moretti et al. 2002).

Vascular Dementia

VaD (Table 10–4) is the third leading cause of dementia in the elderly population, with an incidence of 6–12 per 1,000 persons over age 70 years (Corey-Bloom 2004). VaD is a highly heterogeneous dementia syndrome that can result from small or large vessel arteriosclerotic disease, cardiac embolism, vasospasm, hypoperfusion, hematological/rheological disturbances, or hypoxic ischemic injury. Currently, the following VaD syndromes are recognized: multi-infarct dementia, single strategically placed infarct, lacunar state, and poststroke cognitive deterioration (Bowler 2002; Korczyn 2002). Common risk factors for VaD are cerebrovascular atherosclerosis, hypertension, hyperlipidemia, hyperhomocysteinemia, diabetes mellitus, and smoking (Bowler 2002; Korczyn 2002).

The cognitive deficits in VaD are frequently those of psychomotor slowing and executive dysfunction. Difficulty with spontaneous retrieval of previously learned information is readily observed, as are declines in attention, processing speed, and set shifting (Schmidtke and Hull 2002). Cortical (aphasia) and subcortical (dysarthria) language deficits may be present. Confrontation naming is frequently impaired. Visuospatial difficulties may result from either parietal or frontal lobe involvement, and these impairments are associated with deficiencies in planning and executive functioning (McPherson and Cummings 1996).

The neurological examination is an important step in the evaluation of patients with VaD, because it frequently reveals abnormalities. Focal or generalized upper motor neuron signs (weakness, spasticity, hyperreflexia, exten-

Table 10–4.   Diagnostic criteria for vascular dementia (VaD)

Probable VaD

Cognitive decline in two or more cognitive domains that interferes with activities of daily living

Absence of delirium, aphasia, or sensorimotor impairment that would preclude administration of neuropsychological tests

Absence of another medical or psychiatric disorder that can cause cognitive decline

Focal neurological signs consistent with stroke

Neuroimaging evidence of extensive cerebrovascular disease

Onset of dementia within 3 months of a documented stroke

Abrupt onset, stepwise deterioration, and/or fluctuating course

Supporting features

Early gait disturbance

History of unsteadiness and frequent falls

Early urinary problems not explained by genitourinary condition

Pseudobulbar palsy

Neuropsychiatric manifestations such as mood changes, abulia, depression, emotional incontinence

Psychomotor retardation or executive dysfunction

Possible VaD

Dementia otherwise meeting criteria for probable VaD but without neuroimaging confirmation of definite cerebrovascular disease

Dementia otherwise meeting criteria for probable VaD but without a clear temporal relationship with a stroke event

Dementia otherwise meeting criteria for probable VaD but with subtle onset and gradual course of cognitive decline

Source.   Adapted from Roman et al. 1993.

sor plantar reflex), extrapyramidal findings (bradykinesia, rigidity, lower-body parkinsonism), and gait apraxia are common (Chui 2001).

Neuropsychiatric Features

In a large epidemiological study of community-dwelling elderly persons with VaD, Lyketsos et al. (2000) used the Neuropsychiatric Inventory to assess the frequency and severity of individual neuropsychiatric symptoms. The most common were depression and aggressive behaviors, followed by apathy, irritability, and anxiety. Less frequent were delusions, hallucinations, disinhibition, and abnormal motor behaviors, and the least common was euphoria. Relative to AD, VaD has more severe depression, agitation, and apathy (Aharon-Peretz et al. 2000).

Pathology

The pathological findings in VaD are heterogeneous (Jellinger 2002). Multi-infarct dementia typically has underlying infarcts in the territory of the middle cerebral artery and the watershed regions. Microangiopathic changes and lacunar infarcts are commonly seen in the basal ganglia, periventricular white matter, or cortical and subcortical areas. They can lead to strategic infarct dementia in the case of thalamic, mesial temporal lobe, posterior cerebral artery territory, or basal forebrain strokes; to Binswanger's disease in the case of confluent lacunes and/or cystic infarcts in periventricular or hemispheric white matter; or to multilacunar state in the case of basal ganglia and brain stem lacunar infarcts. Hypoperfusion VaD is characterized by multiple watershed cortical and subcortical microinfarcts and is most commonly due to tight stenosis of the internal carotid or middle cerebral arteries. Postischemic encephalopathy is characterized by cortical laminar necrosis and hippocampal and cerebellar ischemia and is most commonly due to cardiorespiratory collapse.

Neuroimaging

Chronic VaD lesions are best visualized on T2 and fluid-attenuated inverse recovery (FLAIR) MRI sequences as hyperintense lesions. Acutely, infarcts are most easily appreciated on diffusion-weighted imaging as hyperintense and on apparent diffusion coefficient maps as hypointense lesions. Functional imaging shows deficits in the areas corresponding with the stroke location.

Therapy

The most important therapy in VaD is stroke prevention. Smoking cessation and tight control of hypertension, hyperlipidemia, and diabetes mellitus are imperative. Aspirin should be used for routine prophylaxis. Physical, occupational, and speech therapy may be beneficial for the functional recovery of many patients.

In acetylcholinesterase inhibitor trials, patients with VaD showed improvement on cognitive, behavioral, and functional scales (Erkinjuntti et al. 2004). Depression may respond to antidepressant therapy (Alexopoulos et al. 1997a, 1997b; Starkstein and Robinson 1994). Pseudobulbar palsy may improve with antidepressant therapy or a combination of dextromethorphan and quinidine. Atypical antipsychotics are best avoided or used only with greatest caution in this patient population, because they have been shown to increase the risk of stroke and death in elderly dementia patients with vascular risk factors (Bullock 2005; Sink et al. 2005).

Creutzfeldt-Jakob Disease

Prion disorders are a rare subgroup of the neurodegenerative diseases caused by infectious agents with proteinlike properties. Creutzfeldt-Jakob disease (CJD), the most common prion disorder, characteristically presents with rapid cognitive decline. In its sporadic form, CJD presents mostly in the seventh decade of life (range= 45–75 years) (Collinge and Palmer 1996), whereas the familial forms and new variant CJD (nvCJD) tend to present at a younger age.

The classic CJD presentation is that of rapidly progressing cognitive decline, with ataxia, multifocal myoclonic jerks, and startle myoclonus. Other features may include weakness, neuropathy, chorea, hallucinations, visual field cuts, language disturbance, and seizures. One-third of the patients have prodromal fatigue, headache, insomnia, malaise, or depression. Once myoclonus appears, electroencephalographic recording typically shows periodic paroxysmal triphasic or sharp wave discharges against a slow background. Cerebrospinal fluid (CSF) exam may show nonspecific abnormalities such as increased protein (Collinge and Palmer 1996). A sensitive but not specific CSF laboratory finding is the presence of protein 14-3-3 (Collinge and Palmer 1996; Mastrianni and Roos 2000). To date, the only definitive means for establishing the diagnosis of CJD is brain biopsy or postmortem examination of the brain. Several promising diagnostic techniques under development rely on immunostaining for the causative variant of the prion protein (PrP^{sc}) in tonsillar, olfactory mucosal, or muscle tissue (Collinge and Palmer 1996; Glatzel et al. 2005; Mastrianni and Roos 2000).

Iatrogenic CJD has been reported from inoculation of prion protein via blood transfusions, inadequately sterilized surgical equipment or depth electrodes, dural grafts, corneal implants, and human pituitary–derived growth hormone. In these cases, ataxia may be the predominant presentation following severe cerebellar involvement (Collinge and Palmer 1996; Mastrianni and Roos 2000).

The first reports of nvCJD occurred in 1995 in the United Kingdom. These cases represented interspecies (cow to human) transmission of bovine spongiform encephalopathy via alimentary intake of beef or beef products. Most commonly affected were children and adolescents (average age at onset=26.3 years). nvCJD manifests with early prominent anxiety, depression and apathy, rapidly progressive ataxia, dementia, chorea, or myoclonus. Dysesthesias may be present. Average survival time is 14 months (Collinge and Palmer 1996; Ironside and Bell 1996).

Familial CJD accounts for about 15% of the CJD cases and is caused by point mutations, insertions, or deletions in the prion gene on chromosome 20. It tends to present a decade earlier than the sporadic variant and has a longer course (Collinge and Palmer 1996; Mastrianni and Roos 2000).

Neuropsychiatric Features

Apathy, depression, sleep disorders, anorexia (Ajax and Rodnitzky 1998), and/or voracious appetite (personal observation) can occur. Some patients have hallucinations (Mastrianni and Roos 2000). Prominent early neuropsychiatric changes are a classic feature in nvCJD (Collinge and Palmer 1996).

Pathology

PrP^{sc} is a protease-resistant, β-pleated isoform of the normal nonpathogenic membrane-bound PrP protein. Disease progression is thought to occur by template-directed refolding, whereas PrP^{sc} serves as a template for misfolding of the nonpathogenic PrP protein to PrP^{sc} within the cells. The most striking microscopic abnormality in sporadic CJD is the pancortical vacuolation commonly referred to as *spongiosis*. The vacuoles are axonal and dendritic swellings with accumulation of membranous material. Neuronal vacuolation may occasionally be present. Vacuoles can be seen in the cerebellum, white matter, basal ganglia, and brain stem. Reactive gliosis is present, but inflammatory cells are characteristically absent. Spongiosis is commonly found in the occipital, inferior temporal, and parietal cortex. Prion amyloid plaques rarely seen in sporadic and familial CJD are typical of nvCJD and iatrogenic CJD (Ajax and Rodnitzky 1998; Ironside and Bell 1996). Immunostaining of PrP^{sc} is a sensitive technique allowing for definitive diagnosis of CJD and is extremely useful for questionable cases with very mild spongiform change; even the normal-appearing tissue without vacuolation stains positive in affected cases (Ironside and Bell 1996).

Neuroimaging

MRI in CJD can show very specific abnormalities and aid the correct diagnosis. Increased T2, FLAIR, and diffusion signal intensity in the basal ganglia or the cortical ribbon are thought to be pathognomonic in patients with rapidly progressive cognitive decline (Hirose et al. 1998; Matoba et al. 2001; Milton et al. 1991; Yee et al. 1999; Zeidler et al. 2000).

Therapy

Because definitive therapy for CJD is not yet available, only secondary prevention through transmission interception is possible.

Conclusion

The dementias are a prominent group of neurological disorders occurring mainly in elderly people. The full assessment of the patient with cognitive decline includes a thorough history of the current illness, with particular attention to activities of daily living, as well as social, family, and medication history. Alcohol and drug abuse and sexually transmitted diseases (e.g., syphilis, AIDS) need to be excluded in the appropriate patients. A detailed neuropsychiatric assessment of personality changes, mood disorders, and psychotic symptoms can help in the differential diagnosis. Such changes are sometimes present years before the onset of the cognitive decline. Genetic tests may be considered in young patients with a family history of dementia.

Recommended Readings

Apostolova LG, Cummings JL: Neuropsychiatric features of dementia with Lewy bodies, in Dementia With Lewy Bodies and Parkinson's Disease. Edited by O'Brien J, McKeith I, Ames D, et al. Oxford, UK, Taylor & Francis, 2006, pp 73–94

Ballard CG, Waite J, Birks J: Atypical antipsychotics for aggression and psychosis in Alzheimer's disease. Cochrane Database of Systematic Reviews 2006, Issue 1. Art. No.: CD003476. DOI: 10.1002/14651858.CD003476.pub2.

Craig D, Mirakhur A, Hart DJ, et al: A cross-sectional study of neuropsychiatric symptoms in 435 patients with Alzheimer's disease. Am J Geriatr Psychiatry 13:460–468, 2005

Lyketsos CG, Lopez O, Jones B, et al: Prevalence of neuropsychiatric symptoms in dementia and mild cognitive impairment: results from the Cardiovascular Health Study. JAMA 288:1475–1483, 2002

McKeith IG, Dickson DW, Lowe J, et al: Diagnosis and management of dementia with Lewy bodies: third report of the DLB Consortium. Neurology 65:1863–1872, 2005

Sink KM, Holden KF, Yaffe K: Pharmacological treatment of neuropsychiatric symptoms of dementia: a review of the evidence. JAMA 293:596–608, 2005

References

Aharon-Peretz J, Kliot D, Tomer R: Behavioral differences between white matter lacunar dementia and Alzheimer's disease: a comparison on the Neuropsychiatric Inventory. Dement Geriatr Cogn Disord 11:294–298, 2000

Ajax T, Rodnitzky R: Creutzfeldt-Jacob disease. Home Healthcare Consultant 5:8–16, 1998

Alexopoulos GS, Meyers BS, Young RC, et al: Clinically defined vascular depression. Am J Psychiatry 154:562–565, 1997a

Alexopoulos GS, Meyers BS, Young RC, et al: "Vascular depression" hypothesis. Arch Gen Psychiatry 54:915–922, 1997b

American Psychiatric Association: Diagnostic and Statistical Manual of Mental Disorders, 3rd Edition, Revised. Washington, DC, American Psychiatric Association, 1987

American Psychiatric Association: Diagnostic and Statistical Manual of Mental Disorders, 4th Edition, Text Revision. Washington, DC, American Psychiatric Association, 2000

Apostolova LG, Cummings JL: Neuropsychiatric manifestations in mild cognitive impairment: a systematic review of the literature. Dement Geriatr Cogn Disord 25:115–126, 2008

Apostolova LG, Thompson PM: Mapping progressive brain structural changes in early Alzheimer's disease and mild cognitive impairment. Neuropsychologia 46:1597–1612, 2008

Apostolova LG, Dutton RA, Dinov ID, et al: Conversion of mild cognitive impairment to Alzheimer disease predicted by hippocampal atrophy maps. Arch Neurol 63:693–699, 2006

Apostolova LG, Akopyan GG, Partiali N, et al: Structural correlates of apathy in Alzheimer's disease. Dement Geriatr Cogn Disord 24:91–97, 2007a

Apostolova LG, Steiner CA, Akopyan GG, et al: Three-dimensional gray matter atrophy mapping in mild cognitive impairment and mild Alzheimer disease. Arch Neurol 64:1489–1495, 2007b

Apostolova LG, Mosconi L, Thompson PM, et al: Subregional hippocampal atrophy predicts future decline to Alzheimer's dementia in cognitively normal subjects. Neurobiol Aging 31:1077–1088, 2010a

Apostolova LG, Thompson PM, Rogers SA, et al: Surface feature–guided mapping of cerebral metabolic changes in cognitively normal and mildly impaired elderly. Mol Imaging Biol 12:218–224, 2010b

Ballard C, Lowery K, Harrison R, et al: Noncognitive symptoms in Lewy body dementia, in Dementia With Lewy Bodies. Edited by Perry R, McKeith I, Perry E. Cambridge, UK, Cambridge University Press, 1996, pp 67–84

Ballard C, Holmes C, McKeith I, et al: Psychiatric morbidity in dementia with Lewy bodies: a prospective clinical and neuropathological comparative study with Alzheimer's disease. Am J Psychiatry 156:1039–1045, 1999

Bathgate D, Snowden JS, Varma A, et al: Behaviour in frontotemporal dementia, Alzheimer's disease and vascular dementia. Acta Neurol Scand 103:367–378, 2001

Binetti G, Signorini S, Squitti R, et al: Atypical dementia associated with a novel presenilin-2 mutation. Ann Neurol 54:832–836, 2003

Blacker D, Haines JL, Rodes L, et al: ApoE-4 and age at onset of Alzheimer's disease: the NIMH genetics initiative. Neurology 48:139–147, 1997

Boeve BF, Silber MH, Ferman TJ, et al: Association of REM sleep behavior disorder and neurodegenerative disease may reflect an underlying synucleinopathy. Mov Disord 16:622–630, 2001

Bowler JV: The concept of vascular cognitive impairment. J Neurol Sci 203–204:11–15, 2002

Boyle PA, Malloy PF, Salloway S, et al: Executive dysfunction and apathy predict functional impairment in Alzheimer disease. Am J Geriatr Psychiatry 11:214–221, 2003

Bullock R: Treatment of behavioural and psychiatric symptoms in dementia: implications of recent safety warnings. Curr Med Res Opin 21:1–10, 2005

Burton EJ, Karas G, Paling SM, et al: Patterns of cerebral atrophy in dementia with Lewy bodies using voxel-based morphometry. Neuroimage 17:618–630, 2002

Chui H: Dementia attributable to subcortical ischemic vascular disease. Neurologist 7:208–219, 2001

Collinge J, Palmer M: Human prion diseases, in Prion Diseases. Edited by Collinge J, Palmer M. New York, Oxford University Press, 1996, pp 18–56

Corey-Bloom J: Alzheimer's disease. Continuum: Lifelong Learning in Neurology 10:29–57, 2004

Cummings JL: Frontal-subcortical circuits and human behavior. Arch Neurol 50:873–880, 1993

Cummings JL: Alzheimer's disease, in The Neuropsychiatry of Alzheimer's Disease and Related Dementias. Edited by Cummings JL. London, Martin Dunitz, 2003, pp 57–116

Del Ser T, McKeith I, Anand R, et al: Dementia with Lewy bodies: findings from an international multicentre study. Int J Geriatr Psychiatry 15:1034–1045, 2000

Devanand DP, Jacobs DM, Tang MX, et al: The course of psychopathologic features in mild to moderate Alzheimer disease. Arch Gen Psychiatry 54:257–263, 1997

Doody RS: Update on Alzheimer drugs: donepezil. Neurologist 9:225–229, 2003

Dubois B, Feldman HH, Jacova C, et al: Research criteria for the diagnosis of Alzheimer's disease: revising the NINCDS-ADRDA criteria. Lancet Neurol 6:734–746, 2007

Duyckaerts C, Dickson DW: Neuropathology of Alzheimer's disease, in Neurodegeneration: The Molecular Pathology of Dementia and Movement Disorders. Edited by Dickson DW. Basel, Switzerland, ISN Neuropath Press, 2003, pp 47–65

Erkinjuntti T, Roman G, Gauthier S: Treatment of vascular dementia: evidence from clinical trials with cholinesterase inhibitors. J Neurol Sci 226:63–66, 2004

Esler WP, Marshall JR, Stimson ER, et al: Apolipoprotein E affects amyloid formation but not amyloid growth in vitro: mechanistic implications for apoE4 enhanced amyloid burden and risk for Alzheimer's disease. Amyloid 9:1–12, 2002

Evans DA, Bennett DA, Wilson RS, et al: Incidence of Alzheimer disease in a biracial urban community: relation to apolipoprotein E allele status. Arch Neurol 60:185–189, 2003

Farlow M: Update on rivastigmine. Neurologist 9:230–234, 2003

Ferman TJ, Boeve BF, Smith GE, et al: Dementia with Lewy bodies may present as dementia and REM sleep behavior disorder without parkinsonism or hallucinations. J Int Neuropsychol Soc 8:907–914, 2002

Freels S, Cohen D, Eisdorfer C, et al: Functional status and clinical findings in patients with Alzheimer's disease. J Gerontol 47:M177–M182, 1992

Ghetti B, Hutton ML, Wszolek ZK: Frontotemporal dementia and parkinsonism linked to chromosome 17 associated with tau gene mutations, in Neurodegeneration: The Molecular Pathology of Dementia and Movement Disorders. Edited by Dickson DW. Basel, Switzerland, ISN Neuropath Press, 2003, pp 86–102

Gijselinck I, Van Broeckhoven C, Cruts M: Granulin mutations associated with frontotemporal lobar degeneration and related disorders: an update. Hum Mutat 29:1373–1386, 2008

Glatzel M, Stoeck K, Seeger H, et al: Human prion diseases: molecular and clinical aspects. Arch Neurol 62:545–552, 2005

Gorno-Tempini ML, Dronkers NF, Rankin KP, et al: Cognition and anatomy in three variants of primary progressive aphasia. Ann Neurol 55:335–346, 2004

Graff-Radford N, Woodruff B: Frontotemporal dementia. Continuum: Lifetime Learning in Neurology 10:58–80, 2004

Harvey GT, Hughes J, McKeith IG, et al: Magnetic resonance imaging differences between dementia with Lewy bodies and Alzheimer's disease: a pilot study. Psychol Med 29:181–187, 1999

Hashimoto M, Kitagaki H, Imamura T, et al: Medial temporal and whole-brain atrophy in dementia with Lewy bodies: a volumetric MRI study. Neurology 51:357–362, 1998

Heun R, Kockler M, Ptok U: Lifetime symptoms of depression in Alzheimer's disease. Eur Psychiatry 18:63–69, 2003

Hirono N, Mori E, Tanimukai S, et al: Distinctive neurobehavioral features among neurodegenerative dementias. J Neuropsychiatry Clin Neurosci 11:498–503, 1999

Hirose Y, Mokuno K, Abe Y, et al: [A case of clinically diagnosed Creutzfeldt-Jakob disease with serial MRI diffusion weighted images] (in Japanese). Rinsho Shinkeigaku 38:779–782, 1998

Hodges JR, Miller B: The neuropsychology of frontal variant frontotemporal dementia and semantic dementia: introduction to the special topic papers, part II. Neurocase 7:113–121, 2001

Ironside J, Bell J: Pathology of prion diseases, in Prion Diseases. Edited by Collinge J, Palmer M. New York, Oxford University Press, 1996, pp 57–88

Jellinger KA: The pathology of ischemic-vascular dementia: an update. J Neurol Sci 203–204:153–157, 2002

Jellinger KA: Neuropathological spectrum of synucleinopathies. Mov Disord 18 (suppl 6): S2–S12, 2003

Jost BC, Grossberg GT: The evolution of psychiatric symptoms in Alzheimer's disease: a natural history study [see comment]. J Am Geriatr Soc 44:1078–1081, 1996

Khachaturian AS, Corcoran CD, Mayer LS, et al: Apolipoprotein E epsilon4 count affects age at onset of Alzheimer disease, but not lifetime susceptibility: the Cache County Study. Arch Gen Psychiatry 61:518–524, 2004

Knopman DS, DeKosky ST, Cummings JL, et al: Practice parameter: diagnosis of dementia (an evidence-based review). Report of the Quality Standards Subcommittee of the American Academy of Neurology. Neurology 56:1143–1153, 2001

Korczyn AD: The complex nosological concept of vascular dementia. J Neurol Sci 203–204:3–6, 2002

Kukull WA, Brenner DE, Speck CE, et al: Causes of death associated with Alzheimer disease: variation by level of cognitive impairment before death. J Am Geriatr Soc 42:723–726, 1994

Lantos PL, Cairns NJ: Neuropathology, in Early Onset Dementia. Edited by Hodges JR. New York, Oxford University Press, 2001, pp 227–262

Li L, Sengupta A, Haque N, et al: Memantine inhibits and reverses the Alzheimer type abnormal hyperphosphorylation of tau and associated neurodegeneration. FEBS Lett 566:261–269, 2004

Lobotesis K, Fenwick JD, Phipps A, et al: Occipital hypoperfusion on SPECT in dementia with Lewy bodies but not AD. Neurology 56:643–649, 2001

Lowe J, Rossor M: Frontotemporal lobar degeneration, in Neurodegeneration: The Molecular Pathology of Dementia and Movement Disorders. Edited by Dickson DW. Basel, Switzerland, ISN Neuropath Press, 2003, pp 342–348

Luchsinger JA, Noble JM, Scarmeas N: Diet and Alzheimer's disease. Curr Neurol Neurosci Rep 7:366–372, 2007

Lyketsos CG, Olin J: Depression in Alzheimer's disease: overview and treatment. Biol Psychiatry 52:243–252, 2002

Lyketsos CG, Steinberg M, Tschanz JT, et al: Mental and behavioral disturbances in dementia: findings from the Cache County Study on Memory in Aging. Am J Psychiatry 157:708–714, 2000

Lyketsos CG, Lopez O, Jones B, et al: Prevalence of neuropsychiatric symptoms in dementia and mild cognitive impairment: results from the Cardiovascular Health Study. JAMA 288:1475–1483, 2002

Marin DB, Green CR, Schmeidler J, et al: Noncognitive disturbances in Alzheimer's disease: frequency, longitudinal course, and relationship to cognitive symptoms. J Am Geriatr Soc 45:1331–1338, 1997

Mastrianni JA, Roos RP: The prion diseases. Semin Neurol 20:337–352, 2000

Matoba M, Tonami H, Miyaji H, et al: Creutzfeldt-Jakob disease: serial changes on diffusion-weighted MRI. J Comput Assist Tomogr 25:274–277, 2001

McKeith IG: Spectrum of Parkinson's disease, Parkinson's dementia, and Lewy body dementia. Neurol Clin 18:865–902, 2000

McKeith IG, Perry RH, Fairbairn AF, et al: Operational criteria for senile dementia of Lewy body type (SDLT). Psychol Med 22:911–922, 1992

McKeith IG, Ballard CG, Harrison RW: Neuroleptic sensitivity to risperidone in Lewy body dementia (letter). Lancet 346:699, 1995

McKeith I, Del Ser T, Spano P, et al: Efficacy of rivastigmine in dementia with Lewy bodies: a randomised, double-blind, placebo-controlled international study [see comment]. Lancet 356:2031–2036, 2000

McKeith I, Mintzer J, Aarsland D, et al: Dementia with Lewy bodies. Lancet Neurol 3:19–28, 2004

McKeith IG, Dickson DW, Lowe J, et al: Diagnosis and management of dementia with Lewy bodies: third report of the DLB Consortium. Neurology 65:1863–1872, 2005

McPherson SE, Cummings JL: Neuropsychological aspects of vascular dementia. Brain Cogn 31:269–282, 1996

McPherson S, Fairbanks L, Tiken S, et al: Apathy and executive function in Alzheimer's disease. J Int Neuropsychol Soc 8:373–381, 2002

Mega MS, Cummings JL: Frontal-subcortical circuits and neuropsychiatric disorders. J Neuropsychiatry Clin Neurosci 6:358–370, 1994

Mega MS, Cummings JL, Fiorello T, et al: The spectrum of behavioral changes in Alzheimer's disease. Neurology 46:130–135, 1996

Mendez MF, Perryman KM: Neuropsychiatric features of frontotemporal dementia: evaluation of consensus criteria and review. J Neuropsychiatry Clin Neurosci 14:424–429, 2002

Mesulam MM: Aging, Alzheimer's disease and dementia, in Principles of Behavioral and Cognitive Neurology. Edited by Mesulam MM. Oxford, UK, Oxford University Press, 2000, pp 439–510

Migliorelli R, Teson A, Sabe L, et al: Prevalence and correlates of dysthymia and major depression among patients with Alzheimer's disease [see comment]. Am J Psychiatry 152:37–44, 1995

Miklossy J, Taddei K, Suva D, et al: Two novel presenilin-1 mutations (Y256S and Q222H) are associated with early onset Alzheimer's disease. Neurobiol Aging 24:655–662, 2003

Milton WJ, Atlas SW, Lavi E, et al: Magnetic resonance imaging of Creutzfeldt-Jacob disease. Ann Neurol 29:438–440, 1991

Minoshima S, Foster NL, Sima AA, et al: Alzheimer's disease versus dementia with Lewy bodies: cerebral metabolic distinction with autopsy confirmation. Ann Neurol 50:358–365, 2001

Moretti R, Torre P, Antonello RM, et al: Effects of selegiline on fronto-temporal dementia: a neuropsychological evaluation. Int J Geriatr Psychiatry 17:391–392, 2002

Moretti R, Torre P, Antonello RM, et al: Frontotemporal dementia: paroxetine as a possible treatment of behavior symptoms: a randomized, controlled, open 14-month study. Eur Neurol 49:13–19, 2003

Nathan BP, Jiang Y, Wong GK, et al: Apolipoprotein E4 inhibits, and apolipoprotein E3 promotes neurite outgrowth in cultured adult mouse cortical neurons through the low-density lipoprotein receptor-related protein. Brain Res 928:96–105, 2002

Neary D, Snowden JS, Gustafson L, et al: Frontotemporal lobar degeneration: a consensus on clinical diagnostic criteria. Neurology 51:1546–1554, 1998

O'Brien JT, Colloby S, Fenwick J, et al: Dopamine transporter loss visualized with FP-CIT SPECT in the differential diagnosis of dementia with Lewy bodies. Arch Neurol 61:919–925, 2004

Papka M, Rubio A, Schiffer RB, et al: Lewy body disease: can we diagnose it? J Neuropsychiatry Clin Neurosci 10:405–412, 1998

Pasquier F: Early diagnosis of dementia: neuropsychology. J Neurol 246:6–15, 1999

Piccininni M, Di Carlo A, Baldereschi M, et al: Behavioral and psychological symptoms in Alzheimer's disease: frequency and relationship with duration and severity of the disease. Dement Geriatr Cogn Disord 19:276–281, 2005

Raskind MA: Update on Alzheimer drugs: galantamine. Neurologist 9:225–229, 2003

Rippon GA, Crook R, Baker M, et al: Presenilin 1 mutation in an African American family presenting with atypical Alzheimer dementia. Arch Neurol 60:884–888, 2003

Rockwell E, Choure J, Galasko D, et al: Psychopathology at initial diagnosis in dementia with Lewy bodies versus Alzheimer disease: comparison of matched groups with autopsy-confirmed diagnoses. Int J Geriatr Psychiatry 15:819–823, 2000

Roman GC, Tatemichi TK, Erkinjuntti T, et al: Vascular dementia: diagnostic criteria for research studies. Report of the NINDS-AIREN International Workshop. Neurology 43:250–260, 1993

Rosen HJ, Gorno-Tempini ML, Goldman WP, et al: Patterns of brain atrophy in frontotemporal dementia and semantic dementia. Neurology 58:198–208, 2002

Rosen J, Zubenko GS: Emergence of psychosis and depression in the longitudinal evaluation of Alzheimer's disease. Biol Psychiatry 29:224–232, 1991

Samuels SC, Brickman AM, Burd JA, et al: Depression in autopsy-confirmed dementia with Lewy bodies and Alzheimer's disease. Mt Sinai J Med 71:55–62, 2004

Schmidtke K, Hull M: Neuropsychological differentiation of small vessel disease, Alzheimer's disease and mixed dementia. J Neurol Sci 203–204:17–22, 2002

Silverman DH: Brain 18F-FDG PET in the diagnosis of neurodegenerative dementias: comparison with perfusion SPECT and with clinical evaluations lacking nuclear imaging. J Nucl Med 45:594–607, 2004

Simard M, van Reekum R: The acetylcholinesterase inhibitors for treatment of cognitive and behavioral symptoms in dementia with Lewy bodies. J Neuropsychiatry Clin Neurosci 16:409–425, 2004

Simard M, van Reekum R, Cohen T: A review of the cognitive and behavioral symptoms in dementia with Lewy bodies. J Neuropsychiatry Clin Neurosci 12:425–450, 2000

Sink KM, Holden KF, Yaffe K: Pharmacological treatment of neuropsychiatric symptoms of dementia: a review of the evidence. JAMA 293:596–608, 2005

Spillantini MG: Introduction to synucleinopathies, in Neurodegeneration: The Molecular Pathology of Dementia and Movement Disorders. Edited by Dickson DW. Basel, Switzerland, ISN Neuropath Press, 2003, pp 156–158

Starkstein S, Robinson R: Neuropsychiatric aspects of stroke, in The American Psychiatric Press Textbook of Geriatric Neuropsychiatry. Edited by Coffey C, Cummings J. Washington, DC, American Psychiatric Press, 1994, pp 457–475

Steele C, Rovner B, Chase GA, et al: Psychiatric symptoms and nursing home placement of patients with Alzheimer's disease. Am J Psychiatry 147:1049–1051, 1990

Swanberg MM, Cummings JL: Benefit-risk considerations in the treatment of dementia with Lewy bodies. Drug Saf 25:511–523, 2002

Swartz JR, Miller BL, Lesser IM, et al: Frontotemporal dementia: treatment response to serotonin selective reuptake inhibitors. J Clin Psychiatry 58:212–216, 1997

Tang-Wai D, Lewis P, Boeve B, et al: Familial frontotemporal dementia associated with a novel presenilin-1 mutation. Dement Geriatr Cogn Disord 14:13–21, 2002

Voisin T, Reynish E, Portet F, et al: What are the treatment options for patients with severe Alzheimer's disease? CNS Drugs 18:575–583, 2004

Wesnes K, McKeith I, Ferrara R, et al: Effects of rivastigmine on cognitive function in dementia with Lewy bodies: a randomised placebo-controlled international study using the Cognitive Drug Research computerised assessment system. Dement Geriatr Cogn Disord 13:183–192, 2002

Yee AS, Simon JH, Anderson CA, et al: Diffusion-weighted MRI of right-hemisphere dysfunction in Creutzfeldt-Jakob disease. Neurology 52:1514–1515, 1999

Zeidler M, Sellar RJ, Collie DA, et al: The pulvinar sign on magnetic resonance imaging in variant Creutzfeldt-Jakob disease. Lancet 355:1412–1418, 2000

Zhukareva V, Sundarraj S, Mann D, et al: Selective reduction of soluble tau proteins in sporadic and familial frontotemporal dementias: an international follow-up study. Acta Neuropathol (Berl) 105:469–476, 2003

11

Psychopharmacological Treatments for Patients With Neuropsychiatric Disorders

Paul E. Holtzheimer III, M.D.

Mark Snowden, M.D., M.P.H.

Peter P. Roy-Byrne, M.D.

Modern neuropsychiatry is concerned with the understanding and treatment of cognitive, emotional, and behavioral syndromes in patients with known neurological illness or central nervous system (CNS) dysfunction. Although some psychiatric syndromes in patients with neurological disease are clinically similar to those in patients experiencing the syndromes without neurological illness, treatment response may be quite different.

Despite dissimilarities in the pathophysiology, clinical presentation, and treatment response of neuropsychiatric and "idiopathic" psychiatric syndromes, the treatment of neuropsychiatric illness has largely been modeled on known treatments of idiopathic psychiatric disorders. In addition to identifying efficacious treatments, attention to altered side-effect sensitivity and pertinent interactions with commonly used neurological drugs is an especially important aspect of the treatment of neuropsychiatric patients.

Approach to the Neuropsychiatric Patient

The psychiatrist who is asked to assess a neuropsychiatric patient for pharmacological treatment must first have familiarity with the pathophysiology and treatment of the underlying neurological illness. The psychiatrist must consider other medical conditions and treatments, recent surgeries, and health habits. Importantly, a patient's history of alcohol and drug use must be explored because substance abuse, intoxication, and withdrawal can lead to a vast array of psychiatric symptoms (Rosse et al. 1997).

Establishing good rapport with a patient will increase the integrity of data obtained via the patient and history, as well as improve adherence to recommendations. Presenting the pharmacological intervention as a way to optimize treatment of the primary neurological disease can be helpful. However, realistic expectations, including the possibility of incomplete remission of symptoms, should be conveyed from the outset.

The neuropsychiatrist must also be aware of his or her own desire to help—even in the absence of data to guide treatment. The psychiatrist must resist the frequent urge to "do something…anything." Some symptoms may be long-standing and unlikely to resolve quickly, whereas others may result from an adjustment disorder that may dissipate without pharmacological treatment; also, the treatments themselves may not be benign.

When assessing the patient, the clinician must look beyond DSM-IV-TR (American Psychiatric Association 2000) criteria when appropriate. A careful, detailed focus on identifying problematic symptoms may establish clear symptom clusters (e.g., anhedonia, apathy, poor energy) that may respond to pharmacological intervention, even when specific diagnostic criteria for a particular disorder (e.g., major depression) are not fully met.

Optimal treatment must also take into account whether the psychiatric symptoms appeared before the neurological disorder or arose as a neurologically or psychologically mediated result of the neurological disease. Because CNS insults, particularly in the frontal lobe, can amplify underlying character traits (Prigatano 1992), complete eradication of behaviors that at first appear to be a direct result of the neurological insult may not be possible. In addition, certain premorbid traits, such as IQ, may have important implications for course of illness (Palsson et al. 1999).

During the patient interview, the clinician must remember that the neurological disorder may dampen (or heighten) the patient's emotional expressivity. Importantly, patients and their caregivers may disagree about which symptoms are most troubling; for example, a patient often reports cognitive difficulties as more disabling, whereas family members may view the patient's emotional or behavior changes as more problematic (Hendryx 1989). Careful prospective documentation of symptoms will help in tracking what are often slow improvements that seem subjectively inconsequential to the patient and caregiver but that lead to noticeable improvements in overall functioning. Although documenting all symptoms completely may be impractical, specific target symptoms and functional goals should be measured in as much detail as possible.

A basic tenet of treating psychiatric symptoms in patients with neurological disorders is to limit polypharmacy. Patients with CNS pathology are more susceptible to CNS side effects. Treatment of symptoms secondary to the primary neurological disorder, such as pain and sleep disturbance, may decrease psychiatric symptoms sufficiently to allow avoidance of further psychopharmacotherapy. For example, analgesia has been shown to alleviate agitation, irritability, and anger in both patients and caregivers (Perry et al. 1991). Similarly, appropriate treatment of psychiatric symptoms early in presentation may prevent exacerbation of the underlying neurological disorder. For example, emotional distress has been shown to precipitate and/or worsen multiple sclerosis exacerbations (Grant et al. 1989).

Detailed knowledge of the patient's stage in rehabilitation, as well as the patient's current social, occupational, and interpersonal status, is required in order to tailor the pharmacological regimen to specific practical needs and limitations. For example, starting a potentially sedating medication when rigorous physical therapy is being initiated or during reentry into the workplace would be ill advised. Social and interpersonal status can affect access to treatment (Ferrando et al. 1999), the ability of caregivers to participate in treatment (Donaldson et al. 1998), vulnerability of patients to domestic violence (Diaz-Olavarrieta et al. 1999), and psychiatric outcome (Max et al. 1998).

Because of the neurological patient's susceptibility to medication side effects, the clinician should typically start the medication at a lower dosage and titrate more slowly, although the patient may ultimately require the same dosage as the non-neurological patient (i.e., "Start low and go slow...but go!"). Side effects should be well documented, and standardized measures should be used whenever possible. Because neurological patients may have cognitive deficits, the anticipated benefit of the medication, the dosing regimen, and any potential side effects must be thoroughly explained to the patient and caregiver, as well as to all other physicians caring for the patient.

Once medication has been initiated, all available tools to subjectively monitor pharmacokinetics and pharmacological efficacy must be considered. Objective rating scales for symptoms and side effects should be considered. Additionally, monitoring medication blood levels and physiological response (such as vital signs), as well as other laboratory monitoring when appropriate, can be helpful. Medication blood levels do not always correlate with medication efficacy but can still provide information about compliance, drug metabolism, and potential toxicity. Because some neuropsychiatric patients with impaired cognition or communication ability may not be able to convey information adequately about efficacy and side effects, more objective monitoring is required.

Depression, Apathy, and "Deficit" States

Major depression and dysthymia are among the most common psychiatric disorders, including in neurological patients. Untreated depression can have a significant negative impact on quality of life and management of the underlying neurological disease; therefore, timely identification and treatment are essential. Because the symptoms of depression overlap significantly with symptoms of many neurological conditions, confirming the presence or absence of depression in the neuropsychiatric patient can be quite difficult.

In neuropsychiatric patients, selective serotonin reuptake inhibitors (SSRIs) may have more favorable side-effect profiles than tricyclic antidepressants (TCAs). Sedation, postural hypotension, modest hypertension, and seizure threshold–

lowering effects are common with TCAs and may be more pronounced in medically ill, especially neuropsychiatric, patients. SSRIs also have been shown to improve "emotional incontinence" in neuropsychiatric patients (Iannaccone and Ferini-Strambi 1996; Müller et al. 1999; Nahas et al. 1998; Tan and Dorevitch 1996).

A growing database suggests that various brain stimulation techniques may have efficacy in treating depression, although they have not been extensively studied in neuropsychiatric patients. Electroconvulsive therapy (ECT) is an effective treatment for depression in Parkinson's disease patients that can also transiently improve core motor symptoms (Fall et al. 1995; Moellentine et al. 1998). Five of six patients with Huntington's disease also improved with ECT, although two patients developed notable side effects (Ranen et al. 1994). Reports of a high rate of ECT-induced delirium in patients with Parkinson's disease have been interpreted as being due to denervation supersensitivity of dopamine receptors; therefore, reduction of dopaminergic drugs before ECT has been advised (Rudorfer et al. 1992).

Repetitive transcranial magnetic stimulation (rTMS) has shown antidepressant efficacy (Burt et al. 2002; Holtzheimer et al. 2001; O'Reardon et al. 2007), and some data suggest efficacy in depressed patients with Parkinson's disease (Fregni et al. 2004) and patients with poststroke depression (Jorge et al. 2004). Vagus nerve stimulation (VNS) has led to mood improvements in patients with epilepsy (Elger et al. 2000) and was recently approved by the U.S. Food and Drug Administration for treatment-resistant depression (George et al. 2005; Rush et al. 2005). Deep brain stimulation (DBS) of the subthalamic nucleus or internal globus pallidus has shown efficacy in treating motor symptoms associated with Parkinson's disease (Deep-Brain Stimulation for Parkinson's Disease Study Group 2001), essential tremor (Schuurman et al. 2000), and dystonia (Lozano and Abosch 2004) but has also been associated with negative mood changes (Bejjani et al. 1999; Berney et al. 2002). Studies of DBS of the white matter adjacent to the subgenual cingulate region or the ventral striatum/anterior internal capsule have shown antidepressant efficacy in patients without neurological disease (Lozano et al. 2008; Malone et al. 2009; Mayberg et al. 2005).

In summary, SSRIs are generally considered the treatment of choice in neuropsychiatric patients with depression. SSRIs with relatively shorter half-lives (paroxetine, fluvoxamine) or absence of inhibition of select microsomal enzyme systems (citalopram, sertraline, paroxetine, fluvoxamine) may be advantageous in some cases. Because of the potentially activating properties of the SSRIs, they should be started at about half the usual starting dosage and titrated up to standard antidepressant dosages in the first 1–3 weeks. Venlafaxine at lower dosages is less likely to cause hypertension but also acts more like a pure SSRI, with noradrenergic properties requiring higher dosages (≥ 225 mg). Mirtazapine's effect of increased appetite could be advantageous in patients with wasting, although sedative side effects may limit its use. Apathetic states could be treated with dopaminergic strategies, including bupropion, bromocriptine, amantadine, and stimulants. TCAs, if used, should probably be limited to desipramine (lowest anticholinergic effects) and nortriptyline (lowest hypotensive effects, low anticholinergic effects). Nonselective monoamine oxidase inhibitors should probably be avoided in neuropsychiatric patients. Table 11–1 lists characteristic antidepressants recommended in this section, dose ranges, side effects, and relevant drug interactions.

In severely ill patients who do not respond to or cannot tolerate pharmacological treatments, ECT is a reasonable treatment option. Other brain stimulation techniques (rTMS, VNS, DBS) have shown promising results in treating depression but require further study before their utility in neuropsychiatric patients can be determined.

Psychosis

Psychotic states—for example, hallucinations, delusions, and formal thought disorder—occur principally in schizophrenia and less commonly in mania and depression. In neurological patients, psychosis generally occurs less frequently than does depression, agitation, or cognitive impairment and often may be associated with and result from cognitive impairment. Psychosis can have a serious effect on patient care, such that rapid, definitive, and independent treatment is warranted.

Neuroleptic (antipsychotic) medications remain the mainstay in the pharmacological treatment of psychosis. Although typical neuroleptics (e.g., haloperidol, perphenazine, chlorpromazine) have proven efficacy in the treatment of psychosis, side effects that include the risk of severe adverse reactions (e.g., tardive dyskinesia, neuroleptic malignant syndrome) can limit their usefulness. Alternatively, the atypical neuroleptics (clozapine, risperidone, olanza-

Table 11–1. Antidepressants

Drug	Starting daily dose (mg)	Target daily dose (mg)	Neuropsychiatric side effects	Neuropsychiatric drug interactions	Comments
Tricyclic antidepressants (TCAs)					
Nortriptyline	10	30–100	Dizziness, fatigue, drowsiness, tremor, nervousness, confusion, insomnia, headache, seizures, anticholinergic effects Other: orthostatic hypotension, ECG alterations, cardiac conduction delay, tachycardia, sexual dysfunction, weight gain	Increased blood levels with SSRIs, neuroleptics, methylphenidate, VPA, opioids	Low, but present, anticholinergic and hypotensive potential
Desipramine	25	75–200			Blood level monitoring available
Amitriptyline	10	50–150			Antiarrhythmic properties
Imipramine	10	50–200		Decreased blood levels with CBZ, phenytoin, barbiturates	Analgesic effects, even at low doses, for neuropathic pain
Clomipramine	25	75–200		Increased blood levels of neuroleptics, CBZ, opioids	
Doxepin	10	50–200		Decreased blood levels of levodopa	
Protriptyline	2.5	10–30		Additive anticholinerg.c effects with neuroleptics, antiparkinsonian agents, antihistamines	

Table 11–1. Antidepressants (continued)

Drug	Starting daily dose (mg)	Target daily dose (mg)	Neuropsychiatric side effects	Neuropsychiatric drug interactions	Comments
SSRIs and SNRIs					
Fluoxetine	5	10–80	Drowsiness (especially with paroxetine, fluvoxamine), nervousness or agitation (especially with fluoxetine), fatigue (especially with paroxetine), insomnia, tremor, dizziness, headache, confusion, paresthesia Other: nausea, diarrhea, sexual dysfunction, weight loss, hyponatremia, blood pressure changes (especially with venlafaxine)	Increased sedation with hypnotics, chloral hydrate, antihistamines Lethargy, impaired consciousness with metoprolol, propranolol Excitation and hallucinations with narcotics EPS with neuroleptics Neurotoxicity with lithium Serotonergic effects with lithium, buspirone, sumatriptan Serotonin syndrome with other serotonergic drugs (e.g., TCAs, MAOIs, atypical neuroleptics, opioids)	Fluoxetine: may require up to 8 weeks to reach steady state; most inhibition of hepatic cytochrome P450 2D6 enzymes; also inhibits 2C and 3A4; potential use in cataplexy; antimyoclonic adjunct with oxitriptan Sertraline: increased blood level with food; most likely to cause diarrhea; least inhibition of cytochrome P450 2D6 but does inhibit 2C and 3A4 Paroxetine: more sedating, less stimulating, and shorter half-life than fluoxetine, sertraline; withdrawal syndrome more likely/severe; inhibition of cytochrome P450 2D6 but not 2C or 3A4; can inhibit trazodone metabolism
Sertraline	25	50–200			
Paroxetine	10	20–50			
Fluvoxamine	25	50–300			
Citalopram	10	20–60			
Escitalopram	5–10	10–20			
Venlafaxine	37.5	150–300			
Duloxetine	20–30	60			

Table 11–1. Antidepressants *(continued)*

Drug	Starting daily dose (mg)	Target daily dose (mg)	Neuropsychiatric side effects	Neuropsychiatric drug interactions	Comments
SSRIs and SNRIs (continued)					
				Contraindicated with MAOIs (hypertensive crisis)	Fluvoxamine: use twice-daily administration; most sedating and shortest half-life of SSRIs; withdrawal syndrome most likely; least bound to plasma proteins and no inhibition of hepatic cytochrome P450 2D6 enzymes; does inhibit 1A2, 2C, and 3A4 enzymes; less ejaculatory delay compared with fluoxetine, sertraline, paroxetine
				Increased blood levels with valproate	
				Decreased blood levels with CBZ	
				Increased blood levels of TCAs, neuroleptics, BZDs, CBZ, valproate, phenytoin, propranolol (especially with fluoxetine, paroxetine)	Citalopram: Minimal to no cytochrome inhibition; most purely serotonergic in vitro
					Venlafaxine: hypertensive exacerbation likely dose related; extended-release formulation much better tolerated than immediate release
					Duloxetine: cytochrome P450 inhibition similar to fluoxetine; less hypertensive exacerbation than venlafaxine

Table 11–1. Antidepressants *(continued)*

Drug	Starting daily dose (mg)	Target daily dose (mg)	Neuropsychiatric side effects	Neuropsychiatric drug interactions	Comments
Other antidepressants					
Bupropion	75–150	200–450	Nervousness, tremor, dizziness, insomnia, headache, confusion, paresthesia, drowsiness, seizures	Contraindicated with MAOIs Decreased blood level with CBZ	Risk of seizures, especially with dosages >450 mg/day, >150 mg/dose Contraindicated in seizure disorders, bulimia, anorexia nervosa Fewer drug interactions than SSRIs
Mirtazapine	15	30–60	Sedation (less with higher doses); weight gain, agranulocytosis (very rare)	Contraindicated with MAOIs	No in vitro cytochrome enzyme inhibition May be more effective at higher doses (>60 mg/day) but few controlled data

Table 11–1. Antidepressants *(continued)*

Drug	Starting daily dose (mg)	Target daily dose (mg)	Neuropsychiatric side effects	Neuropsychiatric drug interactions	Comments
Psychostimulants					
Methyl-phenidate	5–30	10–90	Nervousness, insomnia, dizziness, headache, dyskinesia, drowsiness, confusion, delusions, rebound depression, hallucinations, Tourette's, tics Other: anorexia, palpitations, blood pressure and pulse changes, cardiac arrhythmia, weight loss	Hypertension with MAOIs	Contraindicated in marked anxiety, tension, agitation Fast onset of action
Dextroam-phetamine	2.5–20	5–60		Increased blood levels of TCAs, phenytoin, phenobarbital, primidone Antagonistic effect by neuroleptics, phenobarbital	Give early in day, divided doses (methylphenidate three times daily, dextroamphetamine twice daily) Dependence rare in medically ill May precipitate or worsen Tourette's or dyskinesia

Note. BZD=benzodiazepine; CBZ=carbamazepine; ECG=electrocardiogram; EPS=extrapyramidal side effects; MAOI=monoamine oxidase inhibitor; SNRI=serotonin-norepinephrine reuptake inhibitor; SSRI=selective serotonin reuptake inhibitor; TCA=tricyclic antidepressant; VPA=valproic acid.

Source. Reprinted from Holtzheimer PE III, Snowden M, Roy-Byrne PP: "Psychopharmacological Treatments for Patients With Neuropsychiatric Disorders," in *Essentials of Neuropsychiatry and Behavioral Neurosciences*, 2nd Edition. Edited by Yudofsky SC, Hales RE. Washington, DC, American Psychiatric Publishing, 2010, pp. 495–530. Used with permission. Copyright © 2010 American Psychiatric Association.

pine, quetiapine, ziprasidone, aripiprazole) have been shown to be as effective as typical neuroleptics in the treatment of psychosis and are generally associated with different, somewhat more tolerable side effects. These advantages are even more relevant in neuropsychiatric patients, who are more prone to neurological side effects. However, the association of atypical neuroleptics with metabolic alterations (hyperglycemia, hyperlipidemia) may present difficulties for long-term use. These medications have also been associated with tardive dyskinesia and neuroleptic malignant syndrome, though at much lower rates than typical neuroleptics.

Neuroleptic medications should be considered first-line agents for the treatment of psychosis across the full range of neuropsychiatric conditions. Many neuropsychiatric patients will show exaggerated sensitivity to motor side effects, making atypical antipsychotics the treatment of choice. Clozapine is least likely to have motor side effects, although seizure threshold–lowering and other side effects may be problematic. It may be preferred in patients who are unusually sensitive to extrapyramidal side effects, such as those with Parkinson's disease, Huntington's disease, or other conditions with basal ganglia involvement. Table 11–2 lists characteristic antipsychotics recommended in this section, dose ranges, side effects, and relevant drug interactions.

Agitated States, Including Anxiety and Mania

Agitation and anxiety occur in a wide spectrum of psychiatric illness, including mood disorders, anxiety disorders, psychosis, dementia, and impulse-control disorders. The differential diagnosis of prominent agitation remains broad and may include agitated depression, mixed bipolar states, severe anxiety, delirium, medication side effects (e.g., akathisia), and pain.

An important step in treating agitated states in neuropsychiatric patients is identifying and addressing both medical factors (e.g., infection, electrolyte imbalance, metabolic abnormalities) and pharmacological factors (e.g., corticosteroids, thyroid hormone replacements, antiemetics, anticholinergics) that may be causing or contributing to symptoms. Although specific pharmacological management of the agitated state still may be required, equally if not more important actions are to treat associated medical conditions and stop offending medications if possible.

Table 11–2. Antipsychotics/neuroleptics

Drug	Starting daily dose (mg)	Target daily dose (mg)	Neuropsychiatric side effects	Neuropsychiatric drug interactions	Comments
Typical neuroleptics					
Haloperidol	1–5	2–20	Parkinsonism, dystonia, akathisia, perioral (rabbit) tremor, anticholinergic effects, sedation, confusion, impaired psychomotor performance, TD, NMS, orthostatic hypotension, ejaculatory inhibition, priapism, dysphagia, urinary incontinence, temperature dysregulation, sudden death (possibly due to cardiac arrhythmia) Other: slowed cardiac repolarization, photosensitivity, hyperthermia, hyperprolactinemia, weight gain	Additive CNS depressant effects with other CNS depressants Additive anticholinergic effects with other anticholinergic drugs Increased EPS with SSRIs, lithium, buspirone Neurotoxicity with lithium Increased blood level of TCAs, valproate, phenytoin, β-adrenergic blockers Decreased blood level with lithium, CBZ, phenytoin, phenobarbital, antiparkinsonian agents Increased blood level with TCAs, SSRIs, MAOIs, alprazolam, buspirone, β-adrenergic blockers	Haloperidol: most EPS potential, especially with low calcium, akathisia with low iron; intravenous route provides rapid onset of action with potentially lower risk of EPS; available in decanoate form; useful in Huntington's, Tourette's Perphenazine: available in decanoate form
Perphenazine	4–16	8–40			

Table 11–2. Antipsychotics/neuroleptics (*continued*)

Drug	Starting daily dose (mg)	Target daily dose (mg)	Neuropsychiatric side effects	Neuropsychiatric drug interactions	Comments
Atypical antipsychotics					
Risperidone	0.25–1	2–6	Sedation, insomnia, agitation, EPS, headache, anxiety, dizziness, aggressive reaction, NMS Other: anticholinergic side effects, weight gain, possible glucose control and cholesterol abnormalities	May antagonize effects of levodopa and dopamine agonists Increased blood level with clozapine, inhibitor of cytochrome P450 2D6 Decreased blood level with CBZ	Maximum efficacy for most patients at 4–6 mg/day Less EPS potential than haloperidol but more than other atypical agents Typically use two divided daily doses

Table 11–2. Antipsychotics/neuroleptics *(continued)*

Drug	Starting daily dose (mg)	Target daily dose (mg)	Neuropsychiatric side effects	Neuropsychiatric drug interactions	Comments
Atypical antipsychotics (continued)					
Clozapine	15–50	200–600	Drowsiness, dizziness, headache, tremor, syncope, insomnia, restlessness, hypokinesia/akinesia, agitation, seizures, rigidity, akathisia, confusion, fatigue, hyperkinesia, weakness, lethargy, ataxia, slurred speech, depression, abnormal movements, anxiety, EPS, NMS, obsessive-compulsive symptoms Other: salivation, weight gain, glucose intolerance, hypercholesterolemia, agranulocytosis	Additive CNS depressant effects with other CNS depressants Occasional collapse (hypotension, respiratory depression, loss of consciousness) with BZDs Increased risk of bone marrow suppression with CBZ, possibly lithium Increased risk of NMS with other antipsychotics, lithium, CBZ Decreased blood level with CBZ, phenytoin Serotonin syndrome with other serotonergic drugs	Initially monitor WBC count weekly; may increase interval if stable for several months; lower risk of EPS, TD, NMS, and higher risk of lowering seizure threshold than typical neuroleptics have May improve motor function in Tourette's, Huntington's, drug-induced persistent dyskinesia, spasmodic torticollis, essential tremor

Table 11–2.   Antipsychotics/neuroleptics *(continued)*

Drug	Starting daily dose (mg)	Target daily dose (mg)	Neuropsychiatric side effects	Neuropsychiatric drug interactions	Comments
Atypical antipsychotics (continued)					
Olanzapine	5	10–20	Somnolence, headache, dizziness, NMS Other: dry mouth, weight gain, glucose control abnormalities, hypercholesterolemia, nausea, constipation, elevated transaminase	Additive CNS depressant effects with other CNS depressants Increased blood level with fluoxetine, duloxetine Decreased blood level with smoking and CBZ	Once-daily dosing
Quetiapine	12.5–25	300–450	Sedation, EPS, dizziness, agitation Other: moderate weight gain, postural hypotension, dry mouth, elevated transaminase, glucose control abnormalities, lipid abnormalities	Additive CNS depressant effects with other CNS depressants	Very sedating; often used in low doses for treating insomnia

Table 11–2. Antipsychotics/neuroleptics *(continued)*

Drug	Starting daily dose (mg)	Target daily dose (mg)	Neuropsychiatric side effects	Neuropsychiatric drug interactions	Comments
Atypical antipsychotics (continued)					
Ziprasidone	20–40	120–160	Agitation, akathisia, insomnia, NMS. Other: QT prolongation possible, may affect lipid and glucose metabolism	Serotonin syndrome with other serotonergic drugs. Increased cardiac rhythm effects with other medications that affect conduction	Use divided daily doses. Appears to cause little weight gain and few effects on glucose and lipid metabolism
Aripiprazole	5–15	20–30	Agitation, akathisia, insomnia, NMS	Decreased blood level with barbiturates, CBZ	Appears to cause little weight gain and few effects on glucose and lipid metabolism. Long half-life

Note. BZD=benzodiazepine; CBZ=carbamazepine; CNS=central nervous system; EPS=extrapyramidal side effects; MAOI=monoamine oxidase inhibitor; NMS=neuroleptic malignant syndrome; SSRI=selective serotonin reuptake inhibitor; TCA=tricyclic antidepressant; TD=tardive dyskinesia; WBC=white blood cell.

Source. Reprinted from Holtzheimer PE III, Snowden M, Roy-Byrne PP: "Psychopharmacological Treatments for Patients With Neuropsychiatric Disorders," in *Essentials of Neuropsychiatry and Behavioral Neurosciences*, 2nd Edition. Edited by Yudofsky SC, Hales RE. Washington, DC, American Psychiatric Publishing, 2010, pp. 495–530. Used with permission. Copyright © 2010 American Psychiatric Association.

Some data support the efficacy of several pharmacological agents in the treatment of agitation and anxiety in neuropsychiatric patients, although well-designed clinical trials are needed to better guide treatment. The anticonvulsants carbamazepine and valproate have a reasonably strong database supporting their use in treating agitation and anxiety across a range of neuropsychiatric conditions and generally would be considered first-line agents; however, the side effects and risks associated with these medications are not inconsequential. In the presence of prominent anxiety or an underlying depressive syndrome, antidepressant medications should be considered. Benzodiazepines should be reserved for severe or treatment-resistant cases; when benzodiazepines are used, agents with shorter half-lives and no active metabolites should be chosen, and dosages should be started very low and titrated carefully. In the absence of clear mania, lithium is not supported as a first- or second-line agent. Neuroleptics, a mainstay in the treatment of agitated neuropsychiatric patients, are coming under closer scrutiny given concerns about increased mortality risk when they are used in agitated patients with dementia. However, these agents, especially the atypical antipsychotics, have shown efficacy in treating agitation across a range of conditions. Before using these agents, a careful risk-benefit analysis should be performed, and informed consent should be carefully documented. Tables 11–3 and 11–4, respectively, list characteristic mood stabilizers and anxiolytics recommended in this section, including dose ranges, side effects, and relevant drug interactions.

Aggression, Impulsivity, and Behavioral Dyscontrol

Behavioral dyscontrol is a common complication in neuropsychiatric patients and includes aggressive acts, paraphilias, compulsions, rituals, self-mutilation, and other socially inappropriate behaviors. Such symptoms can be associated with psychosis, agitation, mania, depression, or cognitive impairment. They may also be part of acute delirium or chronic severe brain dysfunction. Less often, behavioral dyscontrol (e.g., aggression, hypersexuality) may result from specific neurological lesions.

Treatment for behavioral dyscontrol should target primarily the clinical syndrome associated with the maladaptive behavior. Thus, the irritable, depressed patient should first be given an antidepressant; the agitated, paranoid patient

Table 11–3.   Mood stabilizers

Drug	Starting daily dose (mg)	Target daily dose (mg)	Neuropsychiatric side effects	Neuropsychiatric drug interactions	Comments
Lithium	300–900	600–2,400	Lethargy, fatigue, muscle weakness, tremor, headache, confusion, dulled senses, ataxia, dysarthria, aphasia, muscle hyperirritability, hyperactive deep tendon reflexes, hypertonia, choreoathetoid movements, cogwheel rigidity, dizziness, drowsiness, disturbed accommodation, dystonia, seizures, EPS Other: nausea, diarrhea, polyuria, nephrogenic diabetes insipidus, hypothyroidism, hyperparathyroidism, T-wave depression, acne, leukocytosis	EPS and NMS with neuroleptics Neurotoxicity with SSRIs, neuroleptics. CBZ, valproate, phenytoin, calcium channel blockers Increased blood level with SSRIs, NSAIDs, dehydration Increased or decreased blood levels with diuretics Increased or decreased blood level of neuroleptics	Lowers seizure threshold Predominantly renally excreted Once-daily dosing more tolerable with less renal toxicity Blood levels correlate with therapeutic response and toxicity Used in Huntington's, cluster headaches, torticollis, Tourette's, SIADH, leukopenia

Table 11–3.   Mood stabilizers (continued)

Drug	Starting daily dose (mg)	Target daily dose (mg)	Neuropsychiatric side effects	Neuropsychiatric drug interactions	Comments
Carbamazepine	200–600	400–2,000	Dizziness, drowsiness, incoordination, confusion, headache, fatigue, blurred vision, hallucinations, diplopia, oculomotor disturbance, nystagmus, speech disturbance, abnormal involuntary movement, peripheral neuritis, paresthesia, depression, agitation, talkativeness, tinnitus, hyperacusis Other: nausea, bone marrow suppression, hepatotoxicity, SIADH	Additive CNS depressant effects with other CNS depressants Contraindicated with MAOIs Neurotoxicity with lithium, neuroleptics Bone marrow suppression with clozapine Increased blood level with SSRIs, verapamil Decreased blood level with TCAs, haloperidol, valproate, phenytoin, phenobarbital Decreased blood levels of TCAs, BZDs, neuroleptics, valproate, phenytoin, phenobarbital, methadone, propranolol	Induces own hepatic metabolism (2–5 weeks) Monitor CBC, LFTs, electrolytes Blood level of approximately 4–12 μg/mL Useful in trigeminal neuralgia, neuropathic pain, sedative-hypnotic withdrawal

Table 11–3. Mood stabilizers (continued)

Drug	Starting daily dose (mg)	Target daily dose (mg)	Neuropsychiatric side effects	Neuropsychiatric drug interactions	Comments
Valproate	250–750	500–3,000	Sedation, tremor, paresthesia, headache, lethargy, dizziness, diplopia, confusion, incoordination, ataxia, dysarthria, psychosis, nystagmus, asterixis, "spots before eyes" Other: nausea, hair loss, thrombocytopenia, impaired platelet aggregation, elevated liver transaminases, hepatotoxicity, pancreatitis	Additive CNS depressant effects with other CNS depressants Increased blood level with chlorpromazine Decreased blood level with SSRIs, CBZ, phenytoin, phenobarbital Increased blood level of TCAs, chlorpromazine, CBZ, phenytoin, pheno-barbital, primidone, BZDs	Monitor CBC with platelets, LFTs Blood level of approximately 50–150 µg/mL Useful in neuropathic pain

Note. BZD=benzodiazepine; CBC=complete blood count; CBZ=carbamazepine; CNS=central nervous system; EPS=extrapyramidal side effects; LFT=liver function test; MAOI=monoamine oxidase inhibitor; NMS=neuroleptic malignant syndrome; NSAID=nonsteroidal anti-inflammatory drug; SIADH=syndrome of inappropriate antidiuretic hormone; SSRI=selective serotonin reuptake inhibitor; TCA=tricyclic antidepressant.
Source. Reprinted from Holtzheimer PE III, Snowden M, Roy-Byrne PP: "Psychopharmacological Treatments for Patients With Neuropsychiatric Disorders," in *Essentials of Neuropsychiatry and Behavioral Neurosciences*, 2nd Edition. Edited by Yudofsky SC, Hales RE. Washington, DC, American Psychiatric Publishing, 2010, pp. 495–530. Used with permission. Copyright © 2010 American Psychiatric Association.

Table 11–4. Anxiolytics and sedative-hypnotics

Drug	Starting daily dose (mg)	Target daily dose (mg)	Neuropsychiatric side effects	Neuropsychiatric drug interactions	Comments
Benzodiazepines					
Alprazolam	0.25–0.50	0.75–6.00	Drowsiness, incoordination, confusion, dysarthria, fatigue, agitation, dizziness, akathisia, anterograde amnesia (especially alprazolam, lorazepam) Other: sexual dysfunction	Augments respiratory depression with opioids Neurotoxicity and sexual dysfunction with lithium Additive CNS depressant effects with other CNS depressants Increased blood level with SSRIs, phenytoin Decreased blood level with CBZ Decreased blood level of levodopa, phenytoin	May develop tolerance to psychotropic and anticonvulsant effects Do not induce own metabolism Addictive potential May cause withdrawal syndrome May cause EEG changes May worsen delirium and dementia May be useful in treating akathisia Clonazepam may accumulate in bloodstream May have utility in pain syndromes, movement disorders
Lorazepam	0.5–1.0	1.5–12.0			
Clonazepam	0.25–0.50	1–5			

Table 11–4. Anxiolytics and sedative-hypnotics *(continued)*

Drug	Starting daily dose (mg)	Target daily dose (mg)	Neuropsychiatric side effects	Neuropsychiatric drug interactions	Comments
Others					
Buspirone	10–15	15–60	Nervousness, headache, confusion, weakness, numbness, drowsiness, tremor, paresthesia, incoordination	EPS with neuroleptics Hypertension with MAOIs Increased ALT with trazodone Increased blood level of BZDs, haloperidol	Has antidepressant effects as adjunct to SSRI but may produce dysphoria at higher doses Slow onset of action Nonaddictive Usually does not impair psychomotor performance
Diphenhydramine	25–50	25–200	Drowsiness, fatigue, dizziness, confusion, anticholinergic effects, incoordination, tremor, nervousness, insomnia, euphoria, paresthesia	Additive CNS depressant effects with other CNS depressants Increased anticholinergic effects with MAOIs, TCAs	Minimal effects on EEG Anticholinergic effects may decrease EPS but may exacerbate delirium May help with insomnia; tolerance may develop Unpredictable anxiolytic properties

Table 11–4. Anxiolytics and sedative-hypnotics *(continued)*

Drug	Starting daily dose (mg)	Target daily dose (mg)	Neuropsychiatric side effects	Neuropsychiatric drug interactions	Comments
Others *(continued)*					
Clonidine	0.05–0.20	0.15–0.80	Nervousness, agitation, depression, headache, insomnia, vivid dreams or nightmares, behavior changes, restlessness, anxiety, hallucinations, delirium, sedation, weakness, fatigue	Additive CNS depressant effects with other CNS depressants Impaired blood pressure control with neuroleptics Decreased blood level with TCAs	Useful in opiate withdrawal, Tourette's, and possibly mania, anxiety, akathisia, ADHD, aggression Available in transdermal form

Note. ADHD=attention-deficit/hyperactivity disorder; ALT=alanine transaminase; BZD=benzodiazepine; CBZ=carbamazepine; CNS=central nervous system; EEG=electroencephalogram; EPS=extrapyramidal side effects; MAOI=monoamine oxidase inhibitor; SSRI=selective serotonin reuptake inhibitor; TCA=tricyclic antidepressant.

Source. Reprinted from Holtzheimer PE III, Snowden M, Roy-Byrne PP: "Psychopharmacological Treatments for Patients With Neuropsychiatric Disorders," in *Essentials of Neuropsychiatry and Behavioral Neurosciences,* 2nd Edition. Edited by Yudofsky SC, Hales RE. Washington, DC, American Psychiatric Publishing, 2010, pp. 495–530. Used with permission. Copyright © 2010 American Psychiatric Association.

should receive a trial of a neuroleptic; and the agitated, angry patient may benefit from an anticonvulsant. However, common side effects of medications used to treat anger and aggression can themselves exacerbate the symptoms (e.g., benzodiazepine-induced disinhibition), and anticholinergic agents can aggravate cognitive deficits, lower seizure threshold, and promote delirium, particularly when combined with other delirium-promoting agents.

β-Adrenergic blockers have been studied in a wide range of neuropsychiatric disorders and been shown to be efficacious (Alpert et al. 1990; Connor et al. 1997; Greendyke and Kanter 1986; Ratey et al. 1992b); however, not all data are consistent (Silver et al. 1999). β-Blockers are effective in reducing anger and aggression in patients with acute traumatic brain injury (TBI) (Fleminger et al. 2006) and patients with developmental disability (Connor et al. 1997). Secondary depression resulting from β-blockers appears to be a rare occurrence, but these medications are contraindicated in patients with certain medical conditions (e.g., chronic obstructive pulmonary disease, type 1 diabetes). Yudofsky et al. (1987) proposed titrating the dose of propranolol to as high as 12 mg/kg or up to 800 mg/day and maintaining maximum tolerable dosages for up to 8 weeks to achieve the desired clinical response, although dosages between 160 and 320 mg/day have also been effective.

Parenteral benzodiazepines are often used to manage both acute aggression and behavioral dyscontrol and can be as effective as neuroleptics (Dorevitch et al. 1999). However, they can also produce disinhibition, which worsens agitation and arousal (Yudofsky et al. 1987). Benzodiazepines with rapid onset of action and relatively short half-lives that can be given intramuscularly or intravenously, such as lorazepam, are most useful in the acute situation. Diazepam and chlordiazepoxide are less reliably and rapidly absorbed intramuscularly (Garza-Trevino et al. 1989). Although longer-acting benzodiazepines, such as clonazepam (Freinhar and Alvarez 1986), can be useful in patients with more chronic agitation and aggression, particularly when symptoms of anxiety coexist, their use in treating or preventing more chronic aggression is not supported (Salzman 1988). Impairment of cognitive function by benzodiazepines could potentially aggravate aggression by increasing confusion.

Buspirone can reduce anxiety-associated agitation and has a benign side-effect profile. It has been reported to be effective in treating aggression in patients with head injury (Gualtieri 1991), developmental disability (Verhoeven and Tuinier 1996), dementia (Colenda 1988; Tiller et al. 1988), or Huntington's

disease (Byrne et al. 1994). Although the effect of buspirone on anxiety can reduce agitation, its effect on aggression is probably independent of anxiolysis.
The usual dose is between 30 and 60 mg (total daily dose) (Verhoeven and Tuinier
1996), but lower doses (5–15 mg) have been useful in some reports (Ratey et al.
1992a). Buspirone is typically given in divided doses two to three times per day.

Serotonergic antidepressants also have been effective in the treatment of
aggression and behavioral dyscontrol. Open trials support efficacy for SSRIs
(typically at standard dosages) in patients with TBI (Sobin et al. 1989), Huntington's disease (Ranen et al. 1996), dementia (Pollock et al. 1997; Swartz et
al. 1997), and mental retardation/developmental disability (Cook et al. 1992;
Davanzo et al. 1998; Hellings et al. 1996; McDougle et al. 1996). Trazodone
may be effective in reducing aggression secondary to organic mental disorders
or dementia (Greenwald et al. 1986; Pinner and Rich 1988).

Although anticonvulsants are particularly effective in treating mood lability,
impulsivity, and aggression in patients with seizure disorders, lack of electroencephalographic abnormalities does not preclude potential benefit (Mattes
1990). Carbamazepine has been effective in managing aggression and irritability
in a variety of neuropsychiatric patients (Chatham-Showalter 1996; Mattes
1990; McAllister 1985); however, a placebo-controlled trial in children with
conduct disorder showed no benefit (Cueva et al. 1996). Valproate has been found
to be effective for aggression in patients with mental retardation (Ruedrich et al.
1999), TBI (Wroblewski et al. 1997), or dementia (Haas et al. 1997); however,
placebo-controlled data are generally lacking (Lindenmayer and Kotsaftis 2000).
Blood levels below 50 µg/mL have been effective in some reports (Mazure et al.
1992) but not others (Sival et al. 2002). A review of 17 reports showed a 77% response rate with normal blood level range (Lindenmayer and Kotsaftis 2000).
Phenytoin has been effective for impulsive aggression in inmates (Barratt 1993;
Stanford et al. 2005). Limited data are available for other anticonvulsants.

Lithium was effective in treating aggressive behavior and affective instability in brain-injured patients (Glenn et al. 1989) and in a double-blind, placebo-controlled trial with 42 adult patients with mental retardation (Craft et
al. 1987). Open trials in aggressive children with mental retardation and patients chronically hospitalized for severe aggression also support its use (Bellus
et al. 1996; Campbell et al. 1995). Although higher plasma levels are more
likely to result in clinical improvement, the potential for lower serum levels of
lithium to cause neurotoxicity in neuropsychiatric patients may limit its use.

Neuroleptics are effective in treating aggression in neuropsychiatric patients (Rao et al. 1985). Their use, however, should generally be reserved for patients who have psychotic symptoms or who require rapid behavioral control. Although typical neuroleptics may decrease arousal and agitation in the acute setting, the extrapyramidal and anticholinergic properties of these medications can further increase agitation, particularly when the agents are combined with other drugs that have anticholinergic properties (Tune et al. 1992). Akathisia can be confused with worsening aggression, thus prompting a detrimental increase in neuroleptic dosage. Neuroleptics can also, in some cases, impair executive cognitive functioning (Medalia et al. 1988). In the chronically aggressive psychotic patient, clozapine at dosages of 300–500 mg/day may be the most effective antipsychotic (Cohen and Underwood 1994). Open studies showed good effects for risperidone in patients with autism (Horrigan and Barnhill 1997) or mental retardation (Cohen et al. 1998). Overall, data support the use of risperidone, olanzapine, and quetiapine in patients with dementia, although side effects can still limit their use (Kindermann et al. 2002; Lawlor 2004; Tariot et al. 2004); also, the potentially increased mortality of patients with dementia taking atypical antipsychotics raises serious questions about the use of these agents. Various atypical antipsychotics have also shown efficacy in treating aggression in patients with developmental disability and mental retardation (Barnard et al. 2002; McCracken et al. 2002; Posey and McDougle 2000); again, side effects and potential long-term risks should be considered.

Other medications, such as amantadine, a dopamine agonist, and clonidine, an α-adrenergic agonist, have been used to treat aggression. Gualtieri et al. (1989) used amantadine successfully at dosages of 50–400 mg/day in agitated patients recovering from coma. Clonidine at a dosage of 0.6 mg/day reduced violent outbursts in an autistic adult (Koshes and Rock 1994), but its depressogenic and hypotensive risks may be problematic in the neurological patient.

Cognitive Disturbance

Cognitive disturbance is almost always the result of etiologically identifiable brain dysfunction. However, difficulties with concentration, memory, and more complicated executive cognitive functions occur not just as primary components of neurological disease but also as epiphenomena in the course of major mood disturbance (i.e., pseudodementia) and as a core feature of schizophrenia and chronic bipolar disorder; cognitive disturbance can also be secondary to medications used to treat neurological and other medical illnesses. Treating cognitive disturbance can lead to improvements in quality of life, and even minor improvements in cognition can produce substantial savings in health care costs (Ernst and Hay 1997).

Only a few approved treatments for cognitive impairment, principally in Alzheimer's disease, are available. Donepezil, rivastigmine, and galantamine are generally well tolerated, with modest efficacy at slowing cognitive decline. Memantine may have benefit in patients with moderate to severe dementia and as a combination therapy. It is actively being studied as a potential neuroprotective agent. Other agents have been investigated, but data are too limited to provide strong recommendations. Table 11–5 lists characteristic cognitive agents recommended in this section and the dose ranges, side effects, and relevant drug interactions for each.

Recommended Readings

Charney D, Nestler E (eds): Neurobiology of Mental Illness, 2nd Edition. New York, Oxford University Press, 2005

Davis KL, Charney D, Coyle JT, et al (eds): Neuropsychopharmacology: The Fifth Generation of Progress: An Official Publication of the American College of Neuropsychopharmacology. Philadelphia, PA, Lippincott Williams & Wilkins, 2002

Nestler EJ, Hyman SE, Malenka RC (eds): Molecular Basis of Neuropharmacology: A Foundation for Clinical Neuroscience. New York, McGraw-Hill, 2001

References

Alpert M, Allan ER, Citrome L, et al: A double-blind, placebo-controlled study of adjunctive nadolol in the management of violent psychiatric patients. Psychopharmacol Bull 26:367–371, 1990

American Psychiatric Association: Diagnostic and Statistical Manual of Mental Disorders, 4th Edition, Text Revision. Washington, DC, American Psychiatric Association, 2000

Barnard L, Young AH, Pearson J, et al: A systematic review of the use of atypical antipsychotics in autism. J Psychopharmacol 16:93–101, 2002

Table 11–5. Cognitive agents

Drug	Starting daily dose (mg)	Target daily dose (mg)	Neuropsychiatric side effects	Neuropsychiatric drug interactions	Comments
Acetylcholinesterase inhibitors					
Donepezil	5	10	Headache, fatigue, dizziness, insomnia Other: nausea, diarrhea, weight loss, muscle cramps, joint pain	Effects antagonized by anticholinergic drugs	Donepezil has once-daily dosing Rivastigmine and galantamine have twice-daily dosing; once-daily formulation for galantamine also available
Rivastigmine	3	12			
Galantamine	8	24			
NMDA antagonist					
Memantine	5	20	Fatigue, headache, dizziness, psychosis, confusion Other: nausea, diarrhea, pain, increased blood pressure	Carbonic anhydrase inhibitors (such as acetazolamide) may increase blood levels Possible interactions with other NMDA antagonists (such as amantadine) are unknown	Twice-daily dosing

Note. NMDA=*N*-methyl-D-aspartate.
Source. Reprinted from Holtzheimer PE III, Snowden M, Roy-Byrne PP: "Psychopharmacological Treatments for Patients With Neuropsychiatric Disorders," in *Essentials of Neuropsychiatry and Behavioral Neurosciences*, 2nd Edition. Edited by Yudofsky SC, Hales RE. Washington, DC, American Psychiatric Publishing, 2010, pp. 495–530. Used with permission. Copyright © 2010 American Psychiatric Association

Barratt ES: The use of anticonvulsants in aggression and violence. Psychopharmacol Bull 29:75–81, 1993

Bejjani BP, Damier P, Arnulf I, et al: Transient acute depression induced by high-frequency deep-brain stimulation. N Engl J Med 340:1476–1480, 1999

Bellus SB, Stewart D, Vergo JG, et al: The use of lithium in the treatment of aggressive behaviours with two brain-injured individuals in a state psychiatric hospital. Brain Inj 10:849–860, 1996

Berney A, Vingerhoets F, Perrin A, et al: Effect on mood of subthalamic DBS for Parkinson's disease: a consecutive series of 24 patients. Neurology 59:1427–1429, 2002

Burt T, Lisanby SH, Sackeim HA: Neuropsychiatric applications of transcranial magnetic stimulation: a meta-analysis. Int J Neuropsychopharmacol 5:73–103, 2002

Byrne A, Martin W, Hnatko G: Beneficial effects of buspirone therapy in Huntington's disease (letter). Am J Psychiatry 151:1097, 1994

Campbell M, Kafantaris V, Cueva JE: An update on the use of lithium carbonate in aggressive children and adolescents with conduct disorder. Psychopharmacol Bull 31:93–102, 1995

Chatham-Showalter PE: Carbamazepine for combativeness in acute traumatic brain injury. J Neuropsychiatry Clin Neurosci 8:96–99, 1996

Cohen SA, Underwood MT: The use of clozapine in a mentally retarded and aggressive population. J Clin Psychiatry 55:440–444, 1994

Cohen SA, Ihrig K, Lott RS, et al: Risperidone for aggression and self-injurious behavior in adults with mental retardation. J Autism Dev Disord 28:229–233, 1998

Colenda CC III: Buspirone in treatment of agitated demented patient (letter). Lancet 1:1169, 1988

Connor DF, Ozbayrak KR, Benjamin S, et al: A pilot study of nadolol for overt aggression in developmentally delayed individuals. J Am Acad Child Adolesc Psychiatry 36:826–834, 1997

Cook EH Jr, Rowlett R, Jaselskis C, et al: Fluoxetine treatment of children and adults with autistic disorder and mental retardation. J Am Acad Child Adolesc Psychiatry 31:739–745, 1992

Craft M, Ismail IA, Krishnamurti D, et al: Lithium in the treatment of aggression in mentally handicapped patients: a double-blind trial. Br J Psychiatry 150:685–689, 1987

Cueva JE, Overall JE, Small AM, et al: Carbamazepine in aggressive children with conduct disorder: a double-blind and placebo-controlled study. J Am Acad Child Adolesc Psychiatry 35:480–490, 1996

Davanzo PA, Belin TR, Widawski MH, et al: Paroxetine treatment of aggression and self-injury in persons with mental retardation. Am J Ment Retard 102:427–437, 1998

Deep-Brain Stimulation for Parkinson's Disease Study Group: Deep-brain stimulation of the subthalamic nucleus or the pars interna of the globus pallidus in Parkinson's disease. N Engl J Med 345:956–963, 2001

Diaz-Olavarrieta C, Campbell J, Garcia de la Cadena C, et al: Domestic violence against patients with chronic neurologic disorders. Arch Neurol 56:681–685, 1999

Donaldson C, Tarrier N, Burns A: Determinants of carer stress in Alzheimer's disease. Int J Geriatr Psychiatry 13:248–256, 1998

Dorevitch A, Katz N, Zemishlany Z, et al: Intramuscular flunitrazepam versus intramuscular haloperidol in the emergency treatment of aggressive psychotic behavior. Am J Psychiatry 156:142–144, 1999

Elger G, Hoppe C, Falkai P, et al: Vagus nerve stimulation is associated with mood improvements in epilepsy patients. Epilepsy Res 42:203–210, 2000

Ernst RL, Hay JW: Economic research on Alzheimer disease: a review of the literature. Alzheimer Dis Assoc Disord 11 (suppl 6):135–145, 1997

Fall PA, Ekman R, Granérus AK, et al: ECT in Parkinson's disease: changes in motor symptoms, monoamine metabolites and neuropeptides. J Neural Transm Park Dis Dement Sect 10:129–140, 1995

Ferrando SJ, Rabkin JG, de Moore GM, et al: Antidepressant treatment of depression in HIV-seropositive women. J Clin Psychiatry 60:741–746, 1999

Fleminger S, Greenwood RRJ, Oliver DL: Pharmacological management for agitation and aggression in people with acquired brain injury. Cochrane Database of Systematic Reviews 2006, Issue 4. Art. No.: CD003299. DOI: 10.1002/14651858. CD003299.pub2.

Fregni F, Santos CM, Myczkowski ML, et al: Repetitive transcranial magnetic stimulation is as effective as fluoxetine in the treatment of depression in patients with Parkinson's disease. J Neurol Neurosurg Psychiatry 75:1171–1174, 2004

Freinhar JP, Alvarez WA: Clonazepam treatment of organic brain syndromes in three elderly patients. J Clin Psychiatry 47:525–526, 1986

Garza-Trevino ES, Hollister LE, Overall JE, et al: Efficacy of combinations of intramuscular antipsychotics and sedative-hypnotics for control of psychotic agitation. Am J Psychiatry 146:1598–1601, 1989

George MS, Rush AJ, Marangell LB, et al: A one-year comparison of vagus nerve stimulation with treatment as usual for treatment-resistant depression. Biol Psychiatry 58:364–373, 2005

Glenn MB, Wroblewski B, Parziale J, et al: Lithium carbonate for aggressive behavior or affective instability in ten brain-injured patients. Am J Phys Med Rehabil 68:221–226, 1989

Grant I, Brown GW, Harris T, et al: Severely threatening events and marked life difficulties preceding onset or exacerbation of multiple sclerosis. J Neurol Neurosurg Psychiatry 52:8–13, 1989

Greendyke RM, Kanter DR: Therapeutic effects of pindolol on behavioral disturbances associated with organic brain disease: a double-blind study. J Clin Psychiatry 47:423–426, 1986

Greenwald BS, Marin DB, Silverman SM: Serotoninergic treatment of screaming and banging in dementia. Lancet 2:1464–1465, 1986

Gualtieri CT: Buspirone for the behavior problems of patients with organic brain disorders. J Clin Psychopharmacol 11:280–281, 1991

Gualtieri T, Chandler M, Coons TB, et al: Amantadine: a new clinical profile for traumatic brain injury. Clin Neuropharmacol 12:258–270, 1989

Haas S, Vincent K, Holt J, et al: Divalproex: a possible treatment alternative for demented, elderly aggressive patients. Ann Clin Psychiatry 9:145–147, 1997

Hellings JA, Kelley LA, Gabrielli WF, et al: Sertraline response in adults with mental retardation and autistic disorder. J Clin Psychiatry 57:333–336, 1996

Hendryx PM: Psychosocial changes perceived by closed-head-injured adults and their families. Arch Phys Med Rehabil 70:526–530, 1989

Holtzheimer PE III, Russo J, Avery DH: A meta-analysis of repetitive transcranial magnetic stimulation in the treatment of depression [erratum in Psychopharmacol Bull 37:5, 2003]. Psychopharmacol Bull 35:149–169, 2001

Horrigan JP, Barnhill LJ: Risperidone and explosive aggressive autism. J Autism Dev Disord 27:313–323, 1997

Iannaccone S, Ferini-Strambi L: Pharmacologic treatment of emotional lability. Clin Neuropharmacol 19:532–535, 1996

Jorge RE, Robinson RG, Tateno A, et al: Repetitive transcranial magnetic stimulation as treatment of poststroke depression: a preliminary study. Biol Psychiatry 55:398–405, 2004

Kindermann SS, Dolder CR, Bailey A, et al: Pharmacological treatment of psychosis and agitation in elderly patients with dementia: four decades of experience. Drugs Aging 19:257–276, 2002

Koshes RJ, Rock NL: Use of clonidine for behavioral control in an adult patient with autism (letter). Am J Psychiatry 151:1714, 1994

Lawlor BA: Behavioral and psychological symptoms in dementia: the role of atypical antipsychotics. J Clin Psychiatry 65 (suppl 11):5–10, 2004

Lindenmayer JP, Kotsaftis A: Use of sodium valproate in violent and aggressive behaviors: a critical review. J Clin Psychiatry 61:123–128, 2000

Lozano AM, Abosch A: Pallidal stimulation for dystonia. Adv Neurol 94:301–308, 2004

Lozano AM, Mayberg HS, Giacobbe P, et al: Subcallosal cingulate gyrus deep brain stimulation for treatment-resistant depression. Biol Psychiatry 64:461–467, 2008

Malone DA Jr, Dougherty DD, Rezai AR, et al: Deep brain stimulation of the ventral capsule/ventral striatum for treatment-resistant depression. Biol Psychiatry 65:267–275, 2009

Mattes JA: Comparative effectiveness of carbamazepine and propranolol for rage outbursts. J Neuropsychiatry Clin Neurosci 2:159–164, 1990

Max JE, Robin DA, Lindgren SD, et al: Traumatic brain injury in children and adolescents: psychiatric disorders at one year. J Neuropsychiatry Clin Neurosci 10:290–297, 1998

Mayberg HS, Lozano AM, Voon V, et al: Deep brain stimulation for treatment-resistant depression. Neuron 45:651–660, 2005

Mazure CM, Druss BG, Cellar JS: Valproate treatment of older psychotic patients with organic mental syndromes and behavioral dyscontrol. J Am Geriatr Soc 40:914–916, 1992

McAllister TW: Carbamazepine in mixed frontal lobe and psychiatric disorders. J Clin Psychiatry 46:393–394, 1985

McCracken JT, McGough J, Shah B, et al: Risperidone in children with autism and serious behavioral problems. N Engl J Med 347:314–321, 2002

McDougle CJ, Naylor ST, Cohen DJ, et al: A double-blind, placebo-controlled study of fluvoxamine in adults with autistic disorder. Arch Gen Psychiatry 53:1001–1008, 1996

Medalia A, Gold J, Merriam A: The effects of neuroleptics on neuropsychological test results of schizophrenics. Arch Clin Neuropsychol 3:249–271, 1988

Moellentine C, Rummans T, Ahlskog JE, et al: Effectiveness of ECT in patients with parkinsonism. J Neuropsychiatry Clin Neurosci 10:187–193, 1998

Müller U, Murai T, Bauer-Wittmund T, et al: Paroxetine versus citalopram treatment of pathological crying after brain injury. Brain Inj 13:805–811, 1999

Nahas Z, Arlinghaus KA, Kotrla KJ, et al: Rapid response of emotional incontinence to selective serotonin reuptake inhibitors. J Neuropsychiatry Clin Neurosci 10:453–455, 1998

O'Reardon JP, Solvason HB, Janicak PG, et al: Efficacy and safety of transcranial magnetic stimulation in the acute treatment of major depression: a multisite randomized controlled trial. Biol Psychiatry 62:1208–1216, 2007

Palsson S, Aevarsson O, Skoog I: Depression, cerebral atrophy, cognitive performance and incidence of dementia: population study of 85-year-olds. Br J Psychiatry 174:249–253, 1999

Perry EK, McKeith I, Thompson P, et al: Topography, extent, and clinical relevance of neurochemical deficits in dementia of Lewy body type, Parkinson's disease, and Alzheimer's disease. Ann N Y Acad Sci 640:197–202, 1991

Pinner E, Rich CL: Effects of trazodone on aggressive behavior in seven patients with organic mental disorders. Am J Psychiatry 145:1295–1296, 1988

Pollock BG, Mulsant BH, Sweet R, et al: An open pilot study of citalopram for behavioral disturbances of dementia: plasma levels and real-time observations. Am J Geriatr Psychiatry 5:70–78, 1997

Posey DJ, McDougle CJ: The pharmacotherapy of target symptoms associated with autistic disorder and other pervasive developmental disorders. Harv Rev Psychiatry 8:45–63, 2000

Prigatano GP: Personality disturbances associated with traumatic brain injury. J Consult Clin Psychol 60:360–368, 1992

Ranen NG, Peyser CE, Folstein SE: ECT as a treatment for depression in Huntington's disease. J Neuropsychiatry Clin Neurosci 6:154–159, 1994

Ranen NG, Lipsey JR, Treisman G, et al: Sertraline in the treatment of severe aggressiveness in Huntington's disease. J Neuropsychiatry Clin Neurosci 8:338–340, 1996

Rao N, Jellinek HM, Woolston DC: Agitation in closed head injury: haloperidol effects on rehabilitation outcome. Arch Phys Med Rehabil 66:30–34, 1985

Ratey JJ, Leveroni CL, Miller AC, et al: Low-dose buspirone to treat agitation and maladaptive behavior in brain-injured patients: two case reports. J Clin Psychopharmacol 12:362–364, 1992a

Ratey JJ, Sorgi P, O'Driscoll GA, et al: Nadolol to treat aggression and psychiatric symptomatology in chronic psychiatric inpatients: a double-blind, placebo-controlled study. J Clin Psychiatry 53:41–46, 1992b

Rosse RB, Riggs RL, Dietrich AM, et al: Frontal cortical atrophy and negative symptoms in patients with chronic alcohol dependence. J Neuropsychiatry Clin Neurosci 9:280–282, 1997

Rudorfer MV, Manji HK, Potter WZ: ECT and delirium in Parkinson's disease. Am J Psychiatry 149:1758–1759; author reply 1759–1760, 1992

Ruedrich S, Swales TP, Fossaceca C, et al: Effect of divalproex sodium on aggression and self-injurious behaviour in adults with intellectual disability: a retrospective review. J Intellect Disabil Res 43:105–111, 1999

Rush AJ, Marangell LB, Sackeim HA, et al: Vagus nerve stimulation for treatment-resistant depression: a randomized, controlled acute phase trial. Biol Psychiatry 58:347–354, 2005

Salzman C: Treatment of agitation, anxiety, and depression in dementia. Psychopharmacol Bull 24:39–42, 1988

Schuurman PR, Bosch DA, Bossuyt PM, et al: A comparison of continuous thalamic stimulation and thalamotomy for suppression of severe tremor. N Engl J Med 342:461–468, 2000

Silver JM, Yudofsky SC, Slater JA, et al: Propranolol treatment of chronically hospitalized aggressive patients. J Neuropsychiatry Clin Neurosci 11:328–335, 1999

Sival RC, Haffmans PM, Jansen PA, et al: Sodium valproate in the treatment of aggressive behavior in patients with dementia—a randomized placebo controlled clinical trial. Int J Geriatr Psychiatry 17:579–585, 2002

Sobin P, Schneider L, McDermott H: Fluoxetine in the treatment of agitated dementia (letter). Am J Psychiatry 146:1636, 1989

Stanford MS, Helfritz LE, Conklin SM, et al: A comparison of anticonvulsants in the treatment of impulsive aggression. Exp Clin Psychopharmacol 13:72–77, 2005

Swartz JR, Miller BL, Lesser IM, et al: Frontotemporal dementia: treatment response to serotonin selective reuptake inhibitors. J Clin Psychiatry 58:212–216, 1997

Tan I, Dorevitch M: Emotional incontinence: a dramatic response to paroxetine (letter). Aust N Z J Med 26:844, 1996

Tariot PN, Profenno LA, Ismail MS: Efficacy of atypical antipsychotics in elderly patients with dementia. J Clin Psychiatry 65 (suppl 11):11–15, 2004

Tiller JW, Dakis JA, Shaw JM: Short-term buspirone treatment in disinhibition with dementia (letter). Lancet 2:510, 1988

Tune L, Carr S, Hoag E, et al: Anticholinergic effects of drugs commonly prescribed for the elderly: potential means for assessing risk of delirium. Am J Psychiatry 149:1393–1394, 1992

Verhoeven WM, Tuinier S: The effect of buspirone on challenging behaviour in mentally retarded patients: an open prospective multiple-case study. J Intellect Disabil Res 40:502–508, 1996

Wroblewski BA, Joseph AB, Kupfer J, et al: Effectiveness of valproic acid on destructive and aggressive behaviours in patients with acquired brain injury. Brain Inj 11:37–47, 1997

Yudofsky SC, Silver JM, Schneider SE: Pharmacologic treatment of aggression. Psychiatr Ann 17:397–407, 1987

12

Cognitive Rehabilitation and Behavior Therapy for Patients With Neuropsychiatric Disorders

Michael D. Franzen, Ph.D.

Mark R. Lovell, Ph.D.

Increasing evidence indicates that the treatment of central nervous system (CNS) disorders is a viable and productive endeavor even for traumatic brain injury (TBI) (Cicerone et al. 2000; NIH Consensus Statement 1998). Psychiatry plays a central role in the assessment and treatment of individuals with neurological impairment. The role of the psychiatrist in diagnosis and treatment has become a crucial one with the continued development of sophisticated neuropharmacological treatments for both the cognitive and the psychosocial components of brain impairment (Gualtieri 1988).

The use of selective serotonin reuptake inhibitors appears to hold some promise in the treatment of patients with brain injury. The psychiatrist can greatly enhance the patient's recovery by combining a pharmacological approach with nonpharmacological, behavioral methods of assessment. Additionally, the psychiatrist should be aware of the potential neuropsychological effects of disorders of other somatic systems that have some effect on CNS operations, such as cancer (Anderson-Hanley et al. 2003) and hypertension (Muldoon et al. 2002), as well as potential neuropsychological side effects of the treatment for those disorders.

Neuroanatomical and Neurophysiological Determinants of Recovery

Recovery from brain injury or disease involves a number of separate but interacting processes. After an acute brain injury, some degree of improvement is likely because of a lessening of the temporary or treatable consequences of the injury. Factors such as degree of cerebral edema and extent of increased intracranial pressure are well known to temporarily affect brain function after a closed head injury or stroke (Lezak 1995). Extracellular changes after injury to the cell also have been shown to affect neural functioning. In addition, the regrowth of neural tissue to compensate for an injured area has been shown to occur to some minimal extent in animal studies on both anatomical (Kolata 1983) and physiological (Wall and Egger 1971) levels and may have some limited relevance for humans.

The differences in prognosis among various neurological disorders obviously affect the structure of the rehabilitation program. The goals will vary as a function of the severity of memory impairment in patients with closed head injury. A program designed for patients with head injury and consequent moderate memory impairment is likely to focus on teaching alternative strategies for remembering new information. A program designed for a patient with Alzheimer's disease would probably focus on improving the patient's functioning with regard to activities of daily living. Some intriguing data suggest that at least for stroke, brain reorganization for motor skills may be possible even a decade past the time of the stroke (Liepert et al. 2000).

Cognitive Rehabilitation of Patients With Neuropsychiatric Disorders

The terms *cognitive rehabilitation* and *cognitive retraining* have been used to describe treatments designed to maximize recovery of an individual's abilities. Ideally, treatment should be tailored to each patient's particular needs based on a thorough neuropsychological assessment of cognitive and behavioral deficits, as well as an estimation of how these deficits affect daily life. Sinforiani et al. (2004) reported that a cognitive rehabilitation program was effective in reversing the cognitive deficits associated with the early stages of Parkinson's disease. Such a program, however, may not be effective in later stages.

The use of pharmacological agents in the treatment of affective and behavior changes following TBI has been reported in case studies (Khouzam and Donnelly 1998; Mendez et al. 1999). Carbamazepine has been used in the treatment of behavioral agitation following severe TBI (Azouvi et al. 1999).

Systematic research concerning the effectiveness of cognitive and behavioral treatment strategies in patients with TBI is increasing. Medd and Tate (2000) reported the effects of anger management training in individuals with TBI. Pharmacological methods have been used to treat the physical and emotional symptoms (Holzer 1998; McIntosh 1997; Wroblewski et al. 1997). Although amantadine was at first promising, it has not provided robust effects in improving cognitive and behavioral functioning in subjects with brain injuries (Schneider et al. 1999). The treatment of frontal lobe injury with dopaminergic agents may beneficially affect other rehabilitation efforts (Kraus and Maki 1997). Furthermore, the use of psychostimulants in facilitating treatment effects has been reported for pediatric subjects with TBI (Williams et al. 1998) as well as for adults (Glen 1998).

The results of psychological treatment methods for the cognitive deficits associated with TBI generally show larger effects for skills as measured by standardized tests than as measured by ecologically relevant behaviors (Ho and Bennett 1997).

Flesher (1990) presented an intriguing discussion of an approach to using this type of intervention with schizophrenic patients, although reports of applications have been limited. An exception is Benedict et al.'s (1994) study of computer vigilance training to treat the attentional deficits shown by a group of patients with schizophrenia. Early criticisms regarding a need for empirical evaluation of the efficacy of this approach (Bellack and Mueser 1993) still hold. A more recent study evaluated the use of computerized methods in treating executive dysfunction in brain-impaired teenagers (Wade et al. 2010). In contrast, the use of behavioral methods for training in social skills in patients with schizophrenia is well documented (Corrigan and Penn 2001).

Attentional Processes

Recognition and treatment of attentional disorders are extremely important, because an inability to focus and sustain attention may directly limit the patient's ability to actively participate in the rehabilitation program. Progress on these tasks is a prerequisite for further training on higher-level tasks. Modafinil has been found to improve performance on measures of attention, reaction time, and executive function in healthy subjects who have been sleep deprived (Walsh et al. 2004), but the generalizability of these findings to individuals with CNS injury has yet to be demonstrated.

Memory

Within the field of cognitive rehabilitation, much emphasis has been placed on the development of treatment approaches to improve memory. Franzen and Haut (1991) divided the strategies into three basic categories: 1) the use of spared skills in the form of mnemonic devices or alternative functional systems, 2) the use of direct retraining with repetitive practice and drills, and 3) the use of behavioral prosthetics or external devices or strategies to improve memory.

Use of Spared Skills

Mnemonic strategies are approaches to memory rehabilitation that are specifically designed to promote the encoding and remembering of a specific type of information, depending on the patient's particular memory impairment, by capitalizing on the spared skills. Visual imagery (Glisky and Schacter 1986) involves the use of visual images to assist in the learning and retention of verbal information. Probably the oldest and best-known visual imagery strategy is the method of loci, which involves the association of verbal information to be remembered with locations that are familiar to the patient (e.g., the room in a house or the location on a street).

Peg mnemonics requires the patient to learn a list of peg words and to associate these words with a given visual image, such as "one bun," "two shoe," and so on. After the learned association of the numbers with the visual image, sequential information can be remembered in order by association with the visual image (Gouvier et al. 1986). Research, however, has suggested that this approach may not be highly effective because patients with brain injuries are unable to generate visual images (Crovitz et al. 1979) and have difficulty maintaining this information over time.

Face-name association has been used by patients with brain injuries to promote the remembering of people's names based on visual cues. A series of single-subject experiments reported by Wilson (1987) indicated that the strategy of visual imagery to learn people's names may be differentially effective for various individuals, even when the etiology of memory impairment is similar.

In addition to the extensive use of visual imagery strategies for improving memory in patients with brain injuries, the use of verbally based mnemonic strategies also has become quite popular, particularly with patients who have difficulty using visual imagery. One such procedure, semantic elaboration, involves constructing a story out of new information to be remembered. Rhyming strategies involve remembering verbal information by incorporating the information into a rhyme. This procedure was originally demonstrated by Gardner (1977) with a globally amnesic patient who was able to recall pertinent personal information by learning and subsequently singing a rhyme.

Repetitive Practice

Cognitive rehabilitation strategies that emphasize repetitive practice of information are extremely popular in rehabilitation settings, despite little experimental evidence of lasting improvement in memory. Glisky and Schacter (1986) suggested that attempts to remedy memory disorders should be focused on the acquisition of domain-specific knowledge that is likely to be relevant to everyday functioning. Initial research has established that even patients with severe brain injuries are indeed capable of acquiring discrete pieces of information that are important to their ability to function on a daily basis (Glasgow et al. 1977; Wilson 1982). Chiaravalloti et al. (2003) found that repetition was not helpful in remediating the memory deficits of individuals with multiple sclerosis, who instead may benefit from other rehabilitation strategies in addition to the repetition.

External Memory Aids

External aids to memory generally fall into two categories: memory storage devices and memory-cuing strategies (Harris 1984). The study by Schmitter-Edgecombe et al. (1995) supported the efficacy of memory notebook training to improve memory for everyday activities, although no improvement was evident in laboratory-based memory tasks, and the gains were not maintained at a 6-month follow-up evaluation. Handheld electronic storage devices allow for the storage of large amounts of information, but their often complicated operation requirements may obviate their use in all but the mildest cases of brain injury or disease.

Memory cuing involves the use of prompts designed to remind the patient to engage in a specific behavioral sequence at a given time. To be maximally effective, the cue should be given as close as possible to the time that the behavior is required, must be active rather than passive, and should provide a reminder of the specific behavior that is desired (Harris 1984). One particularly useful cuing device is the alarm wristwatch.

Visual-Perceptual Disorders

Deficits in visual perception are most common in patients who have undergone right hemisphere cerebrovascular accidents (Gouvier et al. 1986). Given the importance of visual-perceptual processing to many occupational tasks and to the safe operation of an automobile (Sivak et al. 1985), the rehabilitation of deficits in this area could have important implications for the recovery of neuropsychiatric patients.

Hemispatial neglect syndrome, common in stroke patients, is an inability to recognize stimuli in the contralateral visual field and has been treated with visual scanning training (Diller and Weinberg 1977; Gianutsos et al. 1983). A light board with 20 colored lights and a target that can be moved around the board at different speeds is used to train the patient to attend to the neglected visual field. This procedure, with the addition of other tasks (e.g., a size estimation and body awareness task), was found to be effective (Gordon et al. 1985). Other researchers have produced similar therapeutic gains in scanning and other aspects of visual-perceptual functioning through rehabilitation strategies. (For a more complete review of this area, see Gianutsos and Matheson 1987 and Gordon et al. 1985.)

Problem Solving and Executive Functions

Neuropsychiatric patients often experience a breakdown in their ability to reason, to form concepts, to solve problems, to execute and terminate behavioral sequences, and to engage in other complex cognitive activities (Goldstein and Levin 1987). Executive dysfunction correlates with white matter changes seen in diffusion tensor magnetic resonance imaging of patients with vascular dementia (O'Sullivan et al. 2004). These deficits are debilitating because they often underlie changes in the basic abilities to function interpersonally, socially, and vocationally. Executive function appears to have a relationship to other, simpler tasks—for example, lower-extremity coordination and walking speed in older healthy individuals (Ble et al. 2005).

Injury to the parieto-occipital area is likely to result in a problem-solving deficit secondary to difficulty with comprehension of logico-grammatical structure, whereas a frontal lobe injury may impede problem solving by disrupting the individual's ability to plan and to carry out the series of steps necessary to process the grammatical material (Luria and Tsvetkova 1990). Executive dysfunction may also affect the capacity to give consent to medical treatment in patients with Alzheimer's disease (Marson and Harrell 1999). An apparent breakdown in the patient's ability to function intellectually can also occur secondary to deficits in other related areas, such as attention, memory, and language.

Rehabilitation programs frequently involve attempts to address these deficits in a hierarchical manner, as originally proposed by Luria (1963). Ben-Yishay and Diller (1983) developed a two-tiered approach that defines five basic deficit areas—arousal and attention, memory, underlying skill structure, language and thought, and feeling tone—and two domains of higher-level problem solving. Deficits in the higher-level skills are often produced by core deficits, and the patient's behavior is likely to depend on an interaction between the two domains (Goldstein and Levin 1987). Stablum et al. (2000) reported the effects of a treatment of executive dysfunction by training and practice in a dual-task procedure. They found improvements in executive function for both patients with closed head injury and patients with anterior communicating artery aneurysms, with maintenance of the gains at 3 months for the former patients and at 12 months for the latter patients.

Speech and Language

Disorders of speech and language are common when the dominant (usually left) hemisphere is injured. Patients who receive speech therapy after a stroke have been shown to improve more than patients who do not (Basso et al. 1979).

An important consideration in designing treatment for speech and language impairment is the reason for the observed speech deficit; that is, it is not sufficient simply to identify the behavioral deficit and attempt to increase the rate of production (Franzen 1991). For example, Giles et al. (1988) increased appropriate verbalizations in a patient with head injury by providing cuing to keep verbalization short and to pause in planning his speech. The remediation attempted to affect the mediating behavior rather than to decrease unwanted behavior through extinction.

Molar Behaviors

The final test of rehabilitation efforts is frequently the change in ecologically relevant molar behaviors—that is, in behaviors that would be used in the open environment. Standardized testing may account for most of the variance reported for molar behaviors, such as driving skill (Galski et al. 1997). However, the improvement in these molar behaviors also may depend on treatment aimed directly at the production of the behaviors, even when the component cognitive skills have been optimized. Giles et al. (1997) used behavioral techniques to improve washing and dressing skills in a series of individuals with severe brain injury.

Use of Computers in Cognitive Rehabilitation

The microcomputer has great potential for use in rehabilitation settings (Gourlay et al. 2000; Grimm and Bleiberg 1986). Computers have a significant potential advantage in their capacity to present precise stimuli and conditions and to readily measure and record the effects of the treatments (Rizzo and Buckwalter 1997), and the use and quality of computer programs in cognitive rehabilitation are increasing (Gontkovsky et al. 2002). Reports have been published of the effectiveness of computerized rehabilitation programs for patients with Parkinson's disease (Sinforiani et al. 2004), closed head injury (Grealy et al. 1999), and schizophrenia (Bellucci et al. 2003; da Costa and de Carvalho 2004).

Disorders and Associated Treatments

Birnboim and Miller (2004) reported that patients with multiple sclerosis have specific deficits in working strategies and that interventions aimed at improving the capacity to develop and use these strategies may necessarily precede other cognitive rehabilitation interventions. Amato and Zipoli (2003) reviewed limited evidence in support of existing programs that attempt to moderate the cognitive impairment associated with multiple sclerosis, provided suggestions for future attempts, and reported optimism on the part of investigators involved in then-current research. Cuesta (2003) reviewed published studies involving the treatment of memory impairment following stroke and reported generally positive but moderate results. Particular interest has been focused on treatment of the dementias, especially Alzheimer's dementia (Clare et al. 2003). Some of these advances have involved novel pharmacological approaches, such as nicotinic substances, that can be combined with behavioral approaches (Newhouse et al. 1997).

Another study involved the combination of cognitive rehabilitation methods with the use of cholinesterase inhibitors (Loewenstein et al. 2004). In this study, gains were reported at the end of 12 weeks of treatment and were maintained at a 3-month follow-up. Certain disorders may have their own specific considerations. For example, greater awareness of deficit is associated with greater improvement from cognitive rehabilitation in patients with Alzheimer's disease (Clare et al. 2002, 2004).

Patients with schizophrenia demonstrate significant cognitive impairment. This cognitive impairment can interfere with other treatment efforts, and cognitive rehabilitation has been reported to improve general aspects of other symptoms and problems exhibited by patients with schizophrenia (Lewis et al. 2003). A review of attempts to rehabilitate the attention deficits associated with schizophrenia indicated generally positive results (Suslow et al. 2001). The evidence is mixed regarding the extent to which brain perfusion changes as a result of cognitive rehabilitation in patients with schizophrenia (Penades et al. 2000). However, a quantitative review of studies indicated that cognitive rehabilitation not only improves cognitive operations on experimental tasks but also generalizes to improvement on tasks outside the experimental setting (Krabbendam and Aleman 2003).

Behavioral Dysfunction After Brain Injury

Research studies (Levin et al. 1982; Lishman 1978; Weddell et al. 1980) have shown that behavioral dysfunction is often associated with reduced abilities to comply with rehabilitation programs, to return to work, to engage in recreational and leisure activities, and to sustain positive interpersonal relationships. Levin and Grossman (1978) reported behavior problems that were present 1 month after TBI and that occurred in areas such as emotional withdrawal, conceptual disorganization, motor slowing, unusual thought content, blunt affect, excitement, and disorientation. Six months after injury, those patients who had poor social and occupational recovery continued to manifest significant cognitive and behavioral disruption. Complaints of tangential thinking, fragmented speech, slowness of thought and action, depressed mood, increased anxiety, and marital and/or family conflict also were frequently noted (Levin et al. 1979).

Other behavioral changes reported to have the potential to cause psychosocial disruption include increased irritability (Rosenthal 1983), social inappropriateness (Lewis et al. 1988), aggression (Mungas 1988), and expansiveness, helplessness, suspiciousness, and anxiety (Grant and Alves 1987). Rapoport et al. (2005) have described the deleterious effect of depressive reactions on cognitive functions in individuals who experienced mild to moderate closed head injury.

Patients with lesions in specific brain regions secondary to other pathological conditions also can have characteristic patterns of dysfunctional behavior. For example, frontal lobe dysfunction secondary to stroke, tumor, or other disease processes is often associated with a cluster of symptoms, including social disinhibition, reduced attention, distractibility, impaired judgment, affective lability, and more pervasive mood disorder (Bond 1984; Stuss and Benson 1984). In contrast, Prigatano (1987) noted that individuals with temporal lobe dysfunction can show heightened interpersonal sensitivity, which can evolve into frank paranoid ideation. Perhaps not too surprisingly, individuals with mild head injuries are less prone to debilitating behavioral changes but still can experience physical, cognitive, and affective changes of sufficient magnitude to affect their ability to return to preaccident activities (Dikmen et al. 1986; Levin et al. 1987).

Adjustment after brain injury appears to be related to a multitude of neurological and non-neurological factors, each of which requires consideration in the choice of an appropriate intervention. In addition to the extent and severity of the neurological injury itself, some of the other factors that can contribute to the presence and type of behavioral dysfunction include the amount of time elapsed since the injury, premorbid psychiatric and psychosocial adjustment, financial resources, social supports, and personal awareness of (and reaction to) acquired deficits (Eames 1988; Goldstein and Ruthven 1983; Gross and Schutz 1986; Meier et al. 1987).

Given the large number of factors that influence recovery from brain injury, a multidimensional approach to the behavioral treatment of patients with brain injury is likely to result in an optimal recovery. Individuals with more severe cognitive impairments are more likely to profit from highly structured behavioral programs. Those whose neuropsychological functioning is more intact, in contrast, may profit from interventions with a more active cognitive component that requires them to use abstract thought as well as self-evaluative and self-corrective processes. Not surprisingly, therapeutic approaches that fall under the general heading of behavior therapy are gaining increasing interest as a component of the overall treatment plan for patients with neuropsychiatric impairment. Ackerman (2004) presented a case study of treatment for a patient with mild TBI and posttraumatic stress disorder in which the treatment required coordinated application of cognitive rehabilitation techniques, biofeedback, and psychotherapy.

Behavior Therapy for Patients With Brain Impairment

Behavioral assessment and treatment have been adapted for use with numerous special populations, most recently including persons with brain injuries (Bellack and Hersen 1985a; Haynes 1984; Hersen and Bellack 1985, 1988; Kazdin 1979). Despite a broadening scope that has included the treatment of patients with neurological impairment, behavioral approaches remain committed to the original principles derived from experimental and social psychology. They also emphasize the empirical and objective implementation and evaluation of treatment (Bellack and Hersen 1985b).

The following are the general assumptions about the nature of behavior disorders that form the basis of behavioral approaches (Haynes 1984):

- Disordered behavior can be expressed through overt actions, thoughts, verbalizations, and physiological reactions.
- These reactions do not necessarily vary in the same way for different individuals or for different behavior disorders.
- Changing one specific behavior may result in changes in other related behaviors.
- Environmental conditions play an important role in the initiation, maintenance, and alteration of behavior.

Intervention focuses on the active interaction between the individual and the environment. The goal of treatment is to alter those aspects of the environment that have become associated with the initiation or maintenance of maladaptive behaviors or to alter the patient's response to those aspects of the environment in some way. The application of a behavioral intervention with a neuropsychiatric patient requires careful consideration of both the neuropsychological and the environmental aspects of the presenting problem. Few clinicians have the training, time, or energy to become and remain equally competent in both neuropsychology and behavioral psychology.

At present, the accumulated body of evidence remains limited regarding the specific types of behavioral interventions that are most effective in treating the various dysfunctional behaviors. Despite this limitation, there is optimism, based on the current literature, that behavior therapy can be effective for patients with brain injuries (Horton and Miller 1985). Indeed, an increasing number of books, primarily on the rehabilitation of patients with brain injuries, describe the potential applications of behavioral approaches for persons with neurological impairment (Edelstein and Couture 1984; Goldstein and Ruthven 1983; Frank and Elliott 2000; Seron 1987; Stuss et al. 2008; Wood 1984) and reviews (Cattelani et al. 2010). Such sources provide an excellent introduction to the basic models, methods, and limitations of behavioral treatments for patients with brain injuries.

Behavioral approaches can be broadly classified into at least three general models (Calhoun and Turner 1981): a traditional behavioral approach, a social learning approach, and a cognitive-behavioral approach.

Traditional Behavioral Approach

The traditional behavioral approach emphasizes the effects of environmental events that occur after (consequences) as well as before (antecedents) a particular behavior of interest. We address these two aspects of environmental influence separately.

Interventions Aimed at the Consequences of Behavior

A consequence that increases the probability of a specific behavior occurring again under similar circumstances is termed a *reinforcer*. Consequences can either increase or decrease the likelihood of a particular behavior occurring again.

A behavior followed by an environmental consequence that increases the likelihood that the behavior will occur again is called a *positive reinforcer*. A behavior followed by the removal of a negative or aversive environmental condition is called a *negative reinforcer*. A behavior followed by an aversive environmental event is termed a *punishment*. The effect of punishment is to reduce the probability that the behavior will occur under similar conditions. There has often been confusion concerning the difference between negative reinforcers and punishments. It is useful to remember that reinforcers (positive or negative) always increase the likelihood of the behavior occurring again, whereas punishments decrease the likelihood of a behavior occurring again. When the reliable relation between a specific behavior and an environmental consequence is removed, the behavioral effect is to reduce the target behavior to a near-zero level of occurrence. This process is called *extinction*. Self-management skills (relaxation training, biofeedback) have been used in the treatment of ataxia (Guercio et al. 1997).

Interventions Aimed at the Antecedents of Behavior

Behavior is controlled or affected not only by the consequences that follow it but also by events that precede it. These events are called *antecedents*. For example, an aggressive patient may have outbursts only in the presence of the nursing staff and never in the presence of the physician. In this situation, treatment is structured to decrease the likelihood of an outburst by restructuring the events that lead to the violent behavior. Some patients are able to learn to anticipate these antecedents themselves, whereas for others, it becomes the task of the treatment staff to identify and modify the antecedents that lead to unwanted behavior. For example, if the stress of verbal communication leads to aggressive behavior in an aphasic patient, the patient may be initially trained to use an alternative form of communication, such as writing or sign language (Franzen and Lovell 1987).

Other Behavioral Approaches

Yet another class of approaches involves the use of differential reinforcement of other behaviors. In this approach, the problem behavior is not consequated. Instead, another behavior that is inconsistent with the problem target behavior is reinforced. As the other behavior increases in frequency, the problem behavior decreases. Hegel and Ferguson (2000) reported the successful use of this approach in reducing aggressive behavior in a subject with brain injury. Differential reinforcement of low rates of responding also may be used to reduce undesired behaviors (Alderman and Knight 1997). Finally, noncontingent reinforcement in the form of increased attention to a subject resulted in a decrease in aggression toward others and a decrease in self-injurious behaviors (Persel et al. 1997).

Social Learning Approach

With the social learning approach, cognitive processes that mediate between environmental conditions and behavioral responses are included in explanations of the learning process. Social learning approaches take advantage of learning through modeling. Socially skilled behavior is generally divided into three components: 1) social perception, 2) social problem solving, and 3) social expression. Training can occur at any one of these levels. For the patient who has lost the ability to interact appropriately using conversational skills, this behavior may be modeled by staff members. (For a comprehensive review, see Bandura 1977.)

Cognitive-Behavioral Approach

The term *cognitive-behavioral approach* refers to a heterogeneous group of procedures that emphasizes the individual's cognitive mediation (self-messages) in explaining behavioral responses within environmental contexts. Treatment focuses on changing maladaptive beliefs and increasing an individual's self-control within the current social environment by changing maladaptive thoughts or beliefs. This approach is particularly useful with patients who have relatively intact language and self-evaluative abilities. For example, Suzman et al. (1997) used cognitive-behavioral methods to improve the problem-solving skills of children with cognitive deficits following TBI.

Assessment of Treatment Effects

In addition to providing a set of methodologies to affect the disordered behavior produced by cognitive deficits, the literature on behavior therapy has provided a conceptual scheme for evaluating the effects of intervention. One of the most influential products of the tradition of behavior therapy has been the development of single-subject designs to evaluate the effect of interventions. Although originally conceived as a method for evaluating the effect of environmental interventions, the single-subject design has been successfully applied in the evaluation of pharmacological interventions as well. Because each patient is an individual and treatment of cognitive dysfunction is still a relatively nascent endeavor, interventions often need to be specifically tailored to the individual patient. Interventions often must be applied before the period of spontaneous recovery has ended, and a method to distinguish the effects of intervention from the effects of recovery from acute physiological disturbance is needed. The multiple-baseline design is a single-subject design that addresses these issues (Franzen and Iverson 1990).

The design of multiple baselines across behaviors involves the evaluation of more than one behavior taking place at the same time. However, only one of the behaviors is targeted for intervention at a time. In this way, the nontargeted behaviors are used as control comparisons for the targeted behaviors. For example, behavior A is targeted for intervention first, and monitors on behaviors B and C are used as control comparisons. After completion of the treatment phase for behavior A, an intervention is implemented for behavior B, and monitors on behaviors A and C are used as control comparisons.

In an application of the multiple-baseline design to the treatment of a patient with brain injury, Franzen and Harris (1993) reported a case in which a patient had deficits in attention-based memory and in abstraction and planning as the result of a closed head injury. This patient was first seen 23 days after the closed head injury occurred. He was seen for a series of weekly appointments. At these appointments, the emotional adjustment was discussed and support was provided. Additionally, the patient received psychotherapy in the form of anger control training and social reinforcement for increasing his daily level of activity and self-initiated social interactions, two areas identified as problems during the evaluation. Finally, cognitive retraining exercises were implemented and taught to the patient and his family so that home practice could take place on a daily basis. The family was instructed in the methods used to record the scores from the exercises, which were then entered into a daily log.

Conclusion

Neuropsychological and behavioral dysfunction associated with brain injury can be varied and complex. Effective intervention requires an integrated interdisciplinary approach that focuses on the individual patient and his or her specific needs. There may be an interactive effect in that improvement in cognitive operations may result in improvement in emotional and behavioral adaptation. Behaviorally based formulations can provide a valuable framework from which to understand the interaction between an individual with compromised physical, neuropsychological, and emotional functioning, and the psychosocial environment in which he or she is trying to adjust.

Much work remains to define the most effective cognitive and behaviorally based treatments for various neuropsychiatric disorders. Increasing evidence suggests that computerized approaches may be helpful. A combined behavioral and pharmacological approach may be more effective than either strategy alone. The evidence to date suggests that cognitive rehabilitation is indeed an area worthy of continued pursuit.

Recommended Readings

Halligan PW, Wade DT (eds): The Effectiveness of Rehabilitation for Cognitive Deficits. New York, Oxford University Press, 2005

High WM Jr, Sander AM, Struchen MA, et al (eds): Rehabilitation for Traumatic Brain Injury. New York, Oxford University Press, 2005

Klein R, McNamara P, Albert ML: Neuropharmacologic approaches to cognitive rehabilitation. Behav Neurol 17:1–3, 2006

León-Carrión J, von Wild KRH, Zitnay GA (eds): Brain Injury Treatment: Theories and Practices. New York, Taylor & Francis, 2006

Loewenstein D, Acevedo A: Training of cognitive and functionally relevant skills in mild Alzheimer's disease: an integrated approach, in Geriatric Neuropsychology: Assessment and Intervention. Edited by Attix DK, Welsh-Bohmer KA. New York, Guilford, 2006, pp 261–274

Murrey GJ: Alternate Therapies in the Treatment of Brain Injury and Neurobehavioral Disorders: A Practical Guide. New York, Haworth Press, 2006

References

Ackerman RJ: Applied psychophysiology, clinical biofeedback, and rehabilitation neuropsychology: a case study—mild traumatic brain injury and post-traumatic stress disorder. Phys Med Rehabil Clin N Am 15:919–931, 2004

Alderman N, Knight C: The effectiveness of DRL in the management of severe behaviour disorders following brain injury. Brain Inj 11:79–101, 1997

Amato MP, Zipoli V: Clinical management of cognitive impairment in multiple sclerosis: a review of current evidence. Int MS J 1072–1083, 2003

Anderson-Hanley C, Sherman ML, Riggs R, et al: Neuropsychological effects of treatments for adults with cancer: a meta-analysis and review of the literature. J Int Neuropsychol Soc 9:967–982, 2003

Azouvi P, Jokic C, Attal N, et al: Carbamazepine in agitation and aggressive behaviour following severe closed-head injury: results of an open trial. Brain Inj 13:797–804, 1999

Bandura A: Social Learning Theory. Englewood Cliffs, NJ, Prentice Hall, 1977

Basso A, Capotani E, Vignolo L: Influence of rehabilitation on language skills in aphasic patients. Arch Neurol 36:190–196, 1979

Bellack AS, Hersen M: Dictionary of Behavior Therapy Techniques. New York, Pergamon, 1985a

Bellack AS, Hersen M: General considerations, in Handbook of Clinical Behavior Therapy With Adults. Edited by Hersen M, Bellack AS. New York, Plenum, 1985b, pp 3–19

Bellack AS, Mueser KT: Psychosocial treatment for schizophrenia. Schizophr Bull 19:317–336, 1993

Bellucci DM, Glaberman K, Haslam N: Computer assisted cognitive rehabilitation reduces negative symptoms in the severely mentally ill. Schizophr Res 59:225–232, 2003

Benedict RH, Harris AE, Markow T, et al: Effects of attention training on information processing in schizophrenia. Schizophr Bull 20:537–546, 1994

Ben-Yishay Y, Diller L: Cognitive deficits, in in Rehabilitation of the Head Injured Adult. Edited by Rosenthal M, Griffith ER, Bond MR, et al. Philadelphia, PA, FA Davis, 1983, pp 167–183

Birnboim S, Miller A: Cognitive strategies application of multiple sclerosis patients. Mult Scler 10:67–73, 2004

Ble A, Volpato S, Zuliani G, et al: Executive function correlates with walking speed in older person: the InCHIANTI study. J Am Geriatr Soc 3:410–415, 2005

Bond M: The psychiatry of closed head injury, in Closed Head Injury: Psychosocial, Social and Family Consequences. Edited by Brooks PN. Oxford, UK, Oxford University Press, 1984, pp 148–178

Calhoun KS, Turner SM: Historical perspectives and current issues in behavior therapy, in Handbook of Clinical Behavior Therapy. Edited by Turner SM, Calhoun KS, Adams HE. New York, Wiley, 1981, pp 1–11

Cattelani R, Zettin M, Zoccolotti P: Rehabilitation treatments for adults with behavioral and psychosocial disorders following acquired brain injury: a systematic review. Neuropsychology Review 20(1):52–85, 2010

Chiaravalloti ND, Demaree H, Gaudino EA, et al: Can the repetition effect maximize learning in multiple sclerosis? Clin Rehabil 17:58–68, 2003

Cicerone KD, Dahlberg C, Kalmar K, et al: Evidence-based cognitive rehabilitation: recommendations for clinical practice. Arch Phys Med Rehabil 81:1596–1615, 2000

Clare L, Wilson BA, Carter G, et al: Relearning face-name associations in early Alzheimer's disease. Neuropsychology 16:538–547, 2002

Clare L, Carter G, Hodges JR: Cognitive rehabilitation as a component of early intervention in Alzheimer's disease: a single case study. Aging Ment Health 7:15–21, 2003

Clare L, Wilson BA, Carter G, et al: Awareness in early stage Alzheimer's disease: relation to outcome of cognitive rehabilitation. J Clin Exp Neuropsychol 26:215–226, 2004

Corrigan PW, Penn DL (eds): Social cognition and schizophrenia, in Cognitive Rehabilitation for Schizophrenia: Enhancing Social Cognition by Strengthening Neurocognitive Functioning. Washington, DC, American Psychological Association, 2001, pp 217–247

Crovitz H, Harvey M, Horn R: Problems in the acquisition of imagery mnemonics: three brain damaged cases. Cortex 15:225–234, 1979

Cuesta GM: Cognitive rehabilitation of memory following stroke. Adv Neurol 92:415–421, 2003

da Costa RM, de Carvalho LA: The acceptance of virtual realist devices for cognitive rehabilitation: a report of positive results with schizophrenia. Comput Methods Programs Biomed 73:173–182, 2004

Dikmen S, McLean A, Temkin N: Neuropsychological and psychosocial consequences of minor head injury. J Neurol Neurosurg Psychiatry 49:1227–1232, 1986

Diller L, Weinberg J: Hemi-inattention in rehabilitation: the evolution of a rational remediation program. Adv Neurol 18:63–82, 1977

Eames P: Behavior disorders after severe head injury: their nature, causes and strategies for management. J Head Trauma Rehabil 3:1–6, 1988

Edelstein BA, Couture ET: Behavioral Assessment and Rehabilitation of the Traumatically Brain-Damaged. New York, Plenum, 1984

Flesher S: Cognitive habilitation in schizophrenia: a theoretical review and model of treatment. Neuropsychol Rev 1:223–246, 1990

Frank RG, Elliott TR (eds): Traumatic brain injury, in Handbook of Rehabilitation Psychology. Washington, DC, American Psychological Association, 2000, pp 49–74

Franzen MD: Behavioral assessment and treatment of brain-impaired individuals, in Progress in Behavior Modification. Edited by Hersen M, Eisler RM. Newbury Park, CA, Sage, 1991, pp 56–85

Franzen MD, Harris CV: Neuropsychological rehabilitation: application of a modified multiple baseline design. Brain Inj 7:525–534, 1993

Franzen MD, Haut MW: The psychological treatment of memory impairment: a review of empirical studies. Neuropsychol Rev 2:29–63, 1991

Franzen MD, Iverson GL: Applications of single subject design to cognitive rehabilitation, in Neuropsychology Across the Lifespan. Edited by Horton AM. New York, Springer, 1990, pp 155–174

Franzen MD, Lovell MR: Behavioral treatments of aggressive sequelae of brain injury. Psychiatr Ann 17:389–396, 1987

Galski T, Ehle HT, Williams JB: Off-road driving evaluations for persons with cerebral injury: a factor analytic study of predriver and simulator testing. Am J Occup Ther 51:352–359, 1997

Gardner H: The Shattered Mind: The Person After Brain Damage. London, Routledge & Kegan Paul, 1977

Gianutsos R, Matheson P: The rehabilitation of visual perceptual disorders attributable to brain injury, in Neuropsychological Rehabilitation. Edited by Meier MJ, Benton AL, Diller L. New York, Guilford, 1987, pp 202–241

Gianutsos R, Glosser D, Elbaum J, et al: Visual imperception in brain injured adults: multifaceted measures. Arch Phys Med Rehabil 64:456–461, 1983

Giles GM, Pussey I, Burgess P: The behavioral treatment of verbal interaction skills following severe head injury: a single case study. Brain Inj 2:75–79, 1988

Giles GM, Ridley JE, Dill A, et al: A consecutive series of adults with brain injury treated with a washing and dressing retraining program. Am J Occup Ther 51:256–266, 1997

Glasgow RE, Zeiss RA, Barrera M, et al: Case studies on remediating memory deficits in brain damaged individuals. J Clin Psychol 33:1049–1054, 1977

Glen MB: Methylphenidate for cognitive and behavioral dysfunction after traumatic brain injury. J Head Trauma Rehabil 13:87–90, 1998

Glisky EL, Schacter DL: Remediation of organic memory disorders: current status and future prospects. J Head Trauma Rehabil 4:54–63, 1986

Goldstein FC, Levin HS: Disorders of reasoning and problem solving ability, in Neuropsychological Rehabilitation. Edited by Meier MJ, Benton AL, Diller L. New York, Guilford, 1987, pp 327–354

Goldstein G, Ruthven L: Rehabilitation of the Brain-Damaged Adult. New York, Plenum, 1983

Gontkovsky ST, McDonald NB, Clark PG, et al: Current directions in computer-assisted cognitive rehabilitation. NeuroRehabilitation 17:195–199, 2002

Gordon W, Hibbard M, Egelko S, et al: Perceptual remediation in patients with right brain damage: a comprehensive program. Arch Phys Med Rehabil 66:353–359, 1985

Gourlay D, Lun KC, Liya G: Telemedicinal virtual reality for cognitive rehabilitation. Stud Health Technol Inform 77:1181–1186, 2000

Gouvier WD, Webster JS, Blanton PD: Cognitive retraining with brain damaged patients, in The Neuropsychology Handbook: Behavioral and Clinical Perspectives. Edited by Wedding D, Horton AM, Webster J. New York, Springer, 1986, pp 278–324

Grant I, Alves W: Psychiatric and psychosocial disturbances in head injury, in Neurobehavioral Recovery From Head Injury. Edited by Levin HS, Grafman J, Eisenberg HM. New York, Oxford University Press, 1987, pp 222–246

Grealy MA, Johnson DA, Rushton SK: Improving cognitive function after brain injury: the use of exercise and virtual reality. Arch Phys Med Rehabil 80:661–667, 1999

Grimm BH, Bleiberg J: Psychological rehabilitation in traumatic brain injury, in Handbook of Clinical Neuropsychology, Vol 2. Edited by Filskov SB, Boll TJ. New York, Wiley, 1986, pp 495–560

Gross Y, Schutz LF: Intervention models in neuropsychology, in Clinical Neuropsychology of Intervention. Edited by Uzzell BP, Gross Y. Boston, MA, Martinus Highoff, 1986, pp 179–204

Gualtieri CT: Pharmacotherapy and the neurobehavioural sequelae of traumatic brain injury. Brain Inj 2:101–129, 1988

Guercio J, Chittum R, McMorrow M. Self-management in the treatment of ataxia: a case study in reducing ataxic tremor through relaxation and biofeedback. Brain Inj 11:353–362, 1997

Harris JE: Methods of improving memory, in Clinical Management of Memory Problems. Edited by Wilson BA, Moffat N. Rockville, MD, Aspen, 1984, pp 46–62

Haynes SN: Behavioral assessment of adults, in Handbook of Psychological Assessment. Edited by Goldstein G, Hersen M. New York, Pergamon, 1984, pp 369–401

Hegel MT, Ferguson RJ: Differential reinforcement of other behavior (DRO) to reduce aggressive behavior following traumatic brain injury. Behav Modif 24:94–101, 2000

Hersen M, Bellack AS: Handbook of Clinical Behavior Therapy With Adults. New York, Plenum, 1985

Hersen M, Bellack AS: Dictionary of Behavioral Assessment Techniques. New York, Pergamon, 1988

Ho MR, Bennett TL: Efficacy of neuropsychological rehabilitation of mild-moderate traumatic brain injury. Arch Clin Neuropsychol 12:1–11, 1997

Holzer JC: Buspirone and brain injury (letter). J Neuropsychiatry Clin Neurosci 10:113, 1998

Horton AM, Miller WA: Neuropsychology and behavior therapy, in Progress in Behavior Modifications. Edited by Hersen M, Eisler R, Miller PM. New York, Academic Press, 1985, pp 1–55

Kazdin AE: Fictions, factions, and functions of behavior therapy. Behav Ther 10:629–654, 1979

Khouzam HR, Donnelly NJ: Remission of traumatic brain injury–induced compulsions during venlafaxine treatment. Gen Hosp Psychiatry 20:62–63, 1998

Kolata G: Brain-grafting work shows promise (letter). Science 221:1277, 1983

Krabbendam L, Aleman A: Cognitive remediation in schizophrenia: a quantitative review of controlled studies. Psychopharmacology (Berl) 169:376–382, 2003

Kraus MF, Maki M: Effect of amantadine hydrochloride on symptoms of frontal lobe dysfunction in brain injury: case studies and review. J Neuropsychiatry Clin Neurosci 9:222–230, 1997

Levin HS, Grossman RG: Behavioral sequelae of closed head injury: a quantitative study. Arch Neurol 35:720–727, 1978

Levin HS, Grossman RG, Rose JE, et al: Long-term neuropsychological outcome of closed head injury. J Neurosurg 50:412–422, 1979

Levin HS, Benton AL, Grossman RG: Neurobehavioral Consequences of Closed Head Injury. New York, Oxford University Press, 1982

Levin HS, Mattis S, Ruff R, et al: Neurobehavioral outcome following minor head injury: a three center study. J Neurosurg 66:234–243, 1987

Lewis FD, Nelson J, Nelson C, et al: Effects of three feedback contingencies on the socially inappropriate talk of a brain-injured adult. Behav Ther 19:203–211, 1988

Lewis L, Unkefer EP, O'Neal SK, et al: Cognitive rehabilitation with patients having severe psychiatric disabilities. Psychiatr Rehabil J 26:325–331, 2003

Lezak MD: Neuropsychological Assessment, 3rd Edition. New York, Oxford University Press, 1995

Liepert J, Bauder H, Miltner WHR, et al: Treatment-induced cortical reorganization after stroke in humans. Stroke 31:1210–1216, 2000

Lishman WA: Organic Psychiatry. St Louis, MO, Blackwell Scientific, 1978

Loewenstein DA, Acevedo AS, Czaja SJ, et al: Cognitive rehabilitation of mildly impaired Alzheimer's disease patients on cholinesterase inhibitors. Am J Geriatr Psychiatry 12:395–402, 2004

Luria AR: Restoration of Function After Brain Injury. New York, Macmillan, 1963

Luria AR, Tsvetkova LS: The Neuropsychological Analysis of Problem Solving. Orlando, FL, Paul Deutsch, 1990

Marson D, Harrell L: Executive dysfunction and loss of capacity to consent to medical treatment in patients with Alzheimer's disease. Semin Clin Neuropsychiatry 4:41–49, 1999

McIntosh GC: Medical management of noncognitive sequelae of minor traumatic brain injury. Appl Neuropsychol 4:62–68, 1997

Medd J, Tate RL: Evaluation of an anger management therapy programme following acquired brain injury: a preliminary study. Neuropsychol Rehabil 10:185–201, 2000

Meier MJ, Strauman S, Thompson WG: Individual differences in neuropsychological recovery: an overview, in Neuropsychological Rehabilitation. Edited by Meier MJ, Benton AL, Diller L. New York, Guilford, 1987, pp 71–110

Mendez MF, Nakawatase TV, Brown CV: Involuntary laughter and inappropriate hilarity. J Neuropsychiatry Clin Neurosci 11:253–258, 1999

Muldoon MF, Waldstein SR, Ryan CM, et al: Effects of six anti-hypertensive medications on cognitive performance. J Hypertens 20:1643–1652, 2002

Mungas D: Psychometric correlates of episodic violent behaviour: a multidimensional neuropsychological approach. Br J Psychiatry 152:180–187, 1988

Newhouse PA, Potter A, Levin ED: Nicotinic system involvement in Alzheimer's and Parkinson's diseases: implications for therapeutics. Drugs Aging 11:206–228, 1997

NIH Consensus Statement: Rehabilitation of Persons With Traumatic Brain Injury, Vol 16, No 1, October 26–28, 1998. Available at: http://consensus.nih.gov/1998/1998TraumaticBrainInjury109html.htm. Accessed March 4, 2011.

O'Sullivan M, Morris RG, Huckstep B, et al: Diffusion tensor MRI correlates with executive dysfunction in patients with ischaemic leukoaraiosis. J Neurol Neurosurg Psychiatry 75:441–447, 2004

Penades R, Boget T, Lomena F, et al: Brain perfusion and neuropsychological changes in schizophrenic patients after cognitive rehabilitation. Psychiatry Res 98:127–132, 2000

Persel CS, Persel CH, Ashley MJ, et al: The use of noncontingent reinforcement and contingent restraint to reduce physical aggression and self-injurious behaviour in a traumatically brain injured adult. Brain Inj 11:751–760, 1997

Prigatano GP: Personality and psychosocial consequences after brain injury, in Neuropsychological Rehabilitation. Edited by Meier MJ, Benton AL, Diller L. New York, Guilford, 1987, pp 355–378

Rapoport MJ, McCullagh S, Shami P, et al: Cognitive impairment associated with major depression following mild and moderate traumatic brain injury. J Neuropsychiatry Clin Neurosci 17:61–65, 2005

Rizzo AA, Buckwalter JG: Virtual reality and cognitive assessment and rehabilitation: the state of the art. Stud Health Technol Inform 44:123–145, 1997

Rosenthal M: Behavioral sequelae, in Rehabilitation of the Head Injured Adult. Edited by Rosenthal M, Griffith ER, Bond MR, et al. Philadelphia, PA, FA Davis, 1983, pp 297–308

Schmitter-Edgecombe M, Fahy JF, Whelan JP, et al: Memory remediation after severe closed head injury: notebook training versus supportive therapy. J Consult Clin Psychol 63:484–489, 1995

Schneider WN, Drew-Cates J, Wong TM, et al: Cognitive and behavioural efficacy of amantadine in acute traumatic brain injury: an initial double-blind placebo-controlled study. Brain Inj 13:863–872, 1999

Seron X: Operant procedures and neuropsychological rehabilitation, in Neuropsychological Rehabilitation. Edited by Meier MJ, Benton AL, Diller L. New York, Guilford, 1987, pp 132–161

Sinforiani E, Banchieri L, Zuchella C, et al: Cognitive rehabilitation in Parkinson's disease. Arch Gerontol Geriatr Suppl 9:387–391, 2004

Sivak M, Hill C, Henson D, et al: Improved driving performance following perceptual training of persons with brain damage. Arch Phys Med Rehabil 65:163–167, 1985

Stablum F, Umilta C, Mogentale C, et al: Rehabilitation of executive deficits in closed head injury and anterior communicating artery aneurysm patients. Psychol Res 63:265–278, 2000

Stuss DT, Benson DF: Neuropsychological studies of the frontal lobes. Psychol Bull 95:3–28, 1984

Stuss DT, Winocur G, Robertson IH (eds): Cognitive Neurorehabilitation: Evidence and Application, 2nd Edition. Cambridge, UK, Cambridge University Press, 2008

Suslow T, Schonauer K, Arolt V: Attention training in the cognitive rehabilitation of schizophrenic patients: a review of efficacy studies. Acta Psychiatr Scand 103:15–23, 2001

Suzman KB, Morris RD, Morris MK, et al: Cognitive remediation of problem solving deficits in children with acquired brain injury. J Behav Ther Exp Psychiatry 28:203–212, 1997

Wade SL, Walz NC, Carey J, et al: A randomized trial of teen online problem solving for improving executive function deficits following pediatric traumatic brain injury. J Head Trauma Rehabil 25:409–415, 2010

Wall P, Egger M: Mechanisms of plasticity of connection following damage in adult mammalian nervous systems, in Recovery of Function: Theoretical Considerations for Brain Injury Rehabilitation. Edited by Bach-y-Rita P. Baltimore, MD, University Park Press, 1971, pp 117–129

Walsh JK, Randazzo AC, Stone KL, et al: Modafinil improves alertness, vigilance, and executive function during simulated night shifts. Sleep 27:434–439, 2004

Weddell R, Oddy M, Jenkins D: Social adjustment after rehabilitation: a two year follow up of patients with severe head injury. Psychol Med 10:257–263, 1980

Williams SE, Ris DM, Ayyangar R, et al: Recovery in pediatric brain injury: is psychostimulant medication beneficial? J Head Trauma Rehabil 13:73–81, 1998

Wilson B: Success and failure in memory training following a cerebral vascular accident. Cortex 18:581–594, 1982

Wilson B: Identification and remediation of everyday problems in memory-impaired patients, in Neuropsychology of Alcoholism: Implications for Diagnosis and Treatment. Edited by Parsons GA, Butters N, Nathan PE. New York, Guilford, 1987, pp 322–338

Wood RL: Behavior disorders following severe brain injury: their presentation and psychological management, in Closed Head Injury: Psychological, Social and Family Consequences. Edited by Brooks N. New York, Oxford University Press, 1984, pp 195–219

Wroblewski BA, Joseph AB, Kupfer J, et al: Effectiveness of valproic acid on destructive and aggressive behaviours in patients with acquired brain injury. Brain Inj 11:37–47, 1997

Index

*Page numbers printed in **boldface** type refer to tables or figures.*